ON CALL
OBSTETRICS
AND GYNECOLOGY

Be *on call* with confidence!

Successfully managing on-call situations requires a masterful combination of speed, skills, and knowledge. Rise to the occasion with **W.B. SAUNDERS COMPANY'S On Call Series!** These pocket-size resources provide you with immediate access to the vital, step-by-step information you need to succeed!

Other titles in the On Call series

Adams & Bresnick: *On Call Surgery*

Adams & Bresnick: *On Call Procedures*

Bernstein et al: *On Call Psychiatry*

Khan: *On Call Cardiology*

Lewis & Nocton: *On Call Pediatrics*

Marshall & Mayer: *On Call Neurology*

Marshall & Ruedy: *On Call: Principles and Protocols, 3rd Edition*

ON CALL

OBSTETRICS
AND GYNECOLOGY

HOMER G. CHIN,
MD, FACOG

Professor and Vice Chairman
Director, Division of Obstetrics and Gynecology
Department of Reproductive Medicine
University of California,
San Diego, School of Medicine
San Diego, California

W.B. SAUNDERS COMPANY
A Division of Harcourt Brace & Company
Philadelphia London Toronto Montreal Sydney Tokyo

W.B. SAUNDERS COMPANY
A Division of Harcourt Brace & Company

The Curtis Center
Independence Square West
Philadelphia, Pennsylvania 19106

Library of Congress Cataloging-in-Publication Data

Chin, Homer G.
On call obstetrics and gynecology / Homer G. Chin.—1st ed.

    p.   cm.

Includes index.

ISBN 0–7216–1316–0

1. Obstetrical emergencies.   2. Gynecologic emergencies.   I. ON
    CALL: OBSTETRICS AND GYNECOLOGY   [DNLM: 1. Pregnancy
    Complications.   2. Genital Diseases, Female.
    WQ 240 C539o 1977]

RG571.C46 1997   618'.0425—dc20

DNLM/DLC   96–16716

Cover illustration is OPUS 1971, enamel on steel, by Virgil Cantini, PhD, with permission from the artist, owned by Mr. and Mrs. Anthony Haradin, Pittsburgh, PA.

On Call Obstetrics and Gynecology   ISBN 0–7216–1316–0

Printed in the United States of America.

Last digit is the print number: 9   8   7   6   5   4   3   2   1

To my wife, Vicki,
for her support, encouragement, and enthusiasm.
To my daughters, Stephanie and Meredith,
who put up with my many hours on the computer.

PREFACE

On-call responsibility has been and remains an important aspect of the training of medical students and housestaff in every medical specialty. This is especially true of obstetrics and gynecology training programs because the practice of obstetrics takes place during all hours of the day and night. Individuals on call are responsible not only for caring for patients admitted to an obstetrics and gynecology service, but also for providing consultations requested by other medical services with female patients. Those on call are frequently called to assess and consult on female patients in the emergency department.

On Call Obstetrics and Gynecology covers the diagnosis and management of problems commonly encountered by medical students and housestaff on call for obstetrics and gynecology patients. The patient-related problems covered in this book will also be pertinent to physicians in emergency departments and urgent care facilities who do not have immediate access to obstetrical and gynecological consultants.

After a discussion of the book's format, *On Call Obstetrics and Gynecology* begins with a chapter on the female reproductive system from conception to menopause and another on the maternal physiological changes in pregnancy. It is important to fully understand what is normal for both pregnant and non-pregnant women before considering abnormal and disease states. Next, patient-related problems are divided into two sections: obstetrical problems and gynecological problems. Each patient-related problem is presented in a manner that allows those on call to quickly, logically, and efficiently make the diagnosis and formulate a management plan. The organization of each chapter emphasizes the presentation of key information in a clear and concise manner that will make this book valuable as a quick reference book for those on call.

At the end of the book are three appendices that can be used for quick reference as well as for a rapid review in preparations for rounds or examinations. Two appendices consist of key charts, tables, illustrations, and guidelines for obstetrics and gynecology, respectively. The third appendix is a formulary of drugs commonly prescribed to obstetric and gynecologic patients and includes all drugs referred to in this book.

On Call Obstetrics and Gynecology will be a valuable aid for all individuals who care for patients with acute obstetrical and gynecological problems regardless of their level of training and area of specialty.

Homer G. Chin

NOTICE

Obstetrics and gynecology is an ever-changing field. Standard safety precautions must be followed, but as new research and clinical experience broaden our knowledge, changes in treatment and drug therapy become necessary or appropriate. The editors of this work have carefully checked the generic and trade drug names and verified drug dosages to ensure that the dosage information in this work is accurate and in accord with the standards accepted at the time of publication. Readers are advised, however, to check the product information currently provided by the manufacturer of each drug to be administered to be certain that changes have not been made in the recommended dose or in the contraindications for administration. This is of particular importance in regard to new or infrequently used drugs. It is the responsibility of the treating physician, relying on experience and knowledge of the patient, to determine dosages and the best treatment for the patient. The editors cannot be responsible for misuse or misapplication of the material in this work.

THE PUBLISHER

COMMONLY USED ABBREVIATIONS

AB	abortus
ABG	arterial blood gas
AC	before meals
AFI	amniotic fluid index
AFP	alpha-fetoprotein
AIDS	acquired immunodeficiency syndrome
ARDS	adult respiratory distress syndrome
AROM	artificial rupture of membranes
ART	artificial reproductive technologies
BE	barium enema
BID	two times per day
BP	blood pressure
BPP	biophysical profile
BSO	bilateral salpingo-oophorectomy
BST	breast stimulation test
BTL	bilateral tubal ligation
CA-125	cancer antigen-125
CBC	complete blood count
CHF	congestive heart failure
CIN	cervical intraepithelial neoplasia
CLE	continuous lumbar epidural
CIS	carcinoma in situ
CMV	cytomegalovirus
CNS	central nervous system
CO	cardiac output
CrCL	creatinine clearance
C&S	culture and sensitivity
CSF	cerebrospinal fluid

CST	contraction stress test
CT	computed tomography
CVS	chorionic villus sampling
CXR	chest x-ray
D&C	dilatation and curettage
D5LR	5% dextrose in lactated Ringer's
D5NS	5% dextrose in normal saline
D5W	5% dextrose in water
DES	diethylstilbestrol
DIC	disseminated intravascular coagulation
DUB	dysfunctional uterine bleeding
DVT	deep vein thrombosis
E_1	estrone
E_2	estradiol
E_3	estriol
EBL	estimated blood loss
EDC	estimated date of confinement
ECG	electrocardiogram
EMB	endometrial biopsy
ESR	erythrocyte sedimentation rate
FCA	fetal cardiac activity
FFP	fresh frozen plasma
FHR	fetal heart rate
FSE	fetal scalp electrode
FSH	follicle-stimulating hormone
FSP	fibrin split products
FTA-ABS	fluorescent treponemal antibody absorption
G	gravida
GC	gonorrhea
GI	gastrointestinal
GIFT	gamete intrafallopian tube transfer
GnRH	gonadotropin-releasing hormone

GTN	gestational trophoblastic neoplasia
GTT	glucose tolerance test
hCG	human chorionic gonadotropin
HDL	high-density lipoprotein
HIV	human immunodeficiency virus
HPV	human papillomavirus
HSG	hysterosalpingogram
HSV	herpes simplex virus
IM	intramuscular
ITP	idiopathic thrombocytopenic purpura
IUD	intrauterine device
IUFD	intrauterine fetal demise
IUP	intrauterine pregnancy
IUPC	intrauterine pressure catheter
IV	intravenous
IVF	in vitro fertilization
IVH	intraventricular hemorrhage
IVP	intravenous pyelogram
LAVH	laparoscopically assisted vaginal hysterectomy
LC	living children
L&D	labor and delivery
LDL	low-density lipoprotein
LEEP	loop electrosurgical excision procedure
LGV	lymphogranuloma venereum
LH	luteinizing hormone
LLETZ	large loop excision of the transformation zone
LMP	last menstrual period
L/S	lecithin/sphingomyelin
LT C/S	low transverse cesarean section
MHA	microhemagglutination assay
MLE	midline episiotomy
MMK	Marshall-Marchetti-Kranz retropubic urethropexy

MRI	magnetic resonance imaging
MVP	mitral valve prolapse
NG	nasogastric
NPO	nothing by mouth
NS	normal saline
NSAID	nonsteroidal anti-inflammatory drug
NST	nonstress test
NSVD	normal spontaneous vaginal delivery
OA	occiput anterior
OP	occiput posterior
OT	occiput transverse
P	parity or para
PC	after meals
Pco_2	partial pressure of carbon dioxide
PDA	patent ductus arteriosus
PG	phosphatidylglycerol
PI	phosphatidylinositol
PID	pelvic inflammatory disease
PIH	pregnancy-induced hypertension
PMN	polymorphonuclear cell
PMS	premenstrual syndrome
PO	per os
Po_2	partial pressure of oxygen
PR	per rectum
PRL	prolactin
PRN	as necessary
PROM	premature rupture of membranes
PT	prothrombin time
PTL	preterm labor
PTT	partial thromboplastin time
PVC	premature ventricular contraction
QHS	each bedtime

QID	four times per day
RBC	red blood cell
RDS	respiratory distress syndrome
RPR	rapid plasma reagin
RR	respiratory rate
SAB	spontaneous abortion
SC	subcutaneous
SIL	squamous intraepithelial lesion
SL	sublingual
SLE	systemic lupus erythematosus
SO	salpingo-oophorectomy
S/P	status post
SROM	spontaneous rupture of membranes
STD	sexually transmitted disease
T	testosterone
T_3	triiodothyronine
T_4	thyroxine
TAB	therapeutic abortion
TAH	total abdominal hysterectomy
TB	tuberculosis
TID	three times per day
TPI	*Treponema pallidum* immobilization (test)
TOA	tubo-ovarian abscess
TPN	total parenteral nutrition
TSH	thyroid-stimulating hormone
TSS	toxic shock syndrome
TVH	total vaginal hysterectomy
UTI	urinary tract infection
VDRL	Venereal Disease Research Laboratory
VTX	vertex
WBC	white blood cell

CONTENTS

PATIENT-RELATED GYNECOLOGICAL PROBLEMS: THE COMMON CALLS

APPENDICES

INTRODUCTION

APPROACH TO ON-CALL OBSTETRICAL AND GYNECOLOGICAL PROBLEMS

There exists a vast array of clinical problems that are unique to women, both pregnant and nonpregnant. A comprehensive understanding of the female reproductive system is critical in order to make the correct diagnosis and properly manage these problems. Knowledge of the profound physiological, anatomical, and endocrinological maternal adaptations to pregnancy is crucial for the management of obstetrical disorders. Furthermore, because obstetrical disorders impact two patients concurrently, the mother and the fetus, the welfare of both must be considered. The optimum management of an obstetrical problem might favor one but be detrimental to the other. Many obstetrical and gynecological problems present acutely in a labor and delivery suite, emergency room, or urgent care clinic. In this book, acute and urgent obstetrical and gynecological problems are presented in a concise format that will aid those who are on call. Each chapter is divided into sections as described below.

■ BACKGROUND AND DEFINITIONS

Although this book is not intended to be a comprehensive reference book, the knowledge of key background information and the understanding of terminologies and definitions are essential to the understanding and management of these disease processes.

■ CLINICAL PRESENTATION

Because most of the clinical problems are presented as diagnoses rather than as symptoms, this section describes the presenting signs and symptoms of each clinical problem.

■ PHONE CALL

The on-call physician will most likely be contacted initially by telephone. This section is intended to aid in quickly obtaining important information about the patient and also in initiating care for the patient before she is able to be examined. This section is divided into three parts.

Questions

Questions that should be asked initially over the telephone are listed.

Orders

Orders that can be given to initiate patient care and laboratory studies are enumerated.

Degree of Urgency

This part addresses how quickly the patient should be seen.

■ ELEVATOR THOUGHTS

This section consists of information that should be reviewed while on the way to see the patient. This includes the differential diagnosis as well as other key information that might help in confirming the diagnosis and in treating the patient. This section is presented as lists to allow for a quick review.

■ MAJOR THREAT TO LIFE

This section lists the means by which a patient's life is threatened by a clinical problem. With obstetrical problems, the lives of the mother and fetus are addressed separately.

■ BEDSIDE

Assessment of the patient and medical chart should be performed in a careful and yet timely and efficient manner. This section deals with the key elements in assessing a patient in an urgent and acute situation. There are four parts to this assessment.

Quick Look Test

This is the initial part of the patient assessment in which a quick evaluation is performed to determine the severity of the patient's condition. The severity will often dictate how the patient is managed.

Vital Signs

Many of the clinical problems presented in this book are associated with abnormal vital signs, especially those consistent with shock from hemorrhage.

Selective History and Chart Review

This section lists the key information that should be obtained when taking the patient's history and when reviewing her medical record and hospital chart. This information will assist in confirming the diagnosis and will impact the management of the patient.

Selective Physical Examination

This section lists the findings on physical examination that are consistent with and sometimes pathognomonic of the diagnosis.

■ DIAGNOSTIC TESTING

Because there are many diagnostic tests that are unique to obstetrics and gynecology, a separate section listing all the pertinent diagnostic tests and the information they provide is included. These tests might help in confirming the diagnosis or determining the appropriate management for a patient. These tests include laboratory tests, radiographic studies, and diagnostic procedures. Inclusion of a test or procedure in this section should not imply that the test must always be ordered. The decision on which test is ordered or which procedure is performed is dependent on the individual patient's condition.

■ MANAGEMENT

This section covers the management of the patient once the diagnosis has been confirmed. In many conditions, there are several management strategies that can be used. In such cases, all management plans are listed and discussed. Which management plan is chosen will depend on the individual patient's condition and needs and also the physician's personal experience and training.

At the end of the book, the following three appendices are included:

■ APPENDIX A: GUIDELINES, ILLUSTRATIONS, AND TABLES FOR OBSTETRICS

■ APPENDIX B: GUIDELINES, ILLUSTRATIONS, AND TABLES FOR GYNECOLOGY

These appendices contain guidelines, illustrations, and tables that are pertinent to both normal and abnormal patients. These appendices can be used for quick reference as well as for a rapid review in preparation for rounds or examinations.

■ APPENDIX C: FORMULARY FOR OBSTETRICS AND GYNECOLOGY

This formulary contains drugs commonly prescribed to obstetrical and gynecological patients, including drugs recommended in this book for the treatment of clinical problems.

2

THE FEMALE REPRODUCTIVE SYSTEM: CONCEPTION TO MENOPAUSE

■ SEXUAL DIFFERENTIATION AND ENDOCRINOLOGY IN THE FETUS

Even though genetic gender is determined at the time of conception, the fetal gonads remain undifferentiated until 4 to 5 weeks of gestation. At this time, testicular development is initiated in males, under the influence of the Y chromosome. A plasma membrane histocompatibility antigen known as the H-Y antigen appears to be the testes-determining factor. In the absence of the Y chromosome and H-Y antigen, the ovaries and müllerian duct system develop in females. Ovarian differentiation begins at 6 to 8 weeks of gestation with the multiplication of germ cells. The number of oocytes reaches a peak of 6 to 7 million at approximately 20 weeks of gestation. This represents the maximum egg content of the ovaries. At the same time, there is an elevation in the gonadotropins, luteinizing hormone (LH), and follicle-stimulating hormone (FSH) (Fig. 2–1). This elevation in gonadotropins results in varying degrees of oocyte maturation. Furthermore, there is ovarian estrogen production, although the amount is minor when compared with placental estrogen. Over the next 50 years, eggs are gradually depleted and the nadir is reached at menopause. The process of egg atresia and depletion begins as early as 15 weeks of gestation. The major mechanism for egg

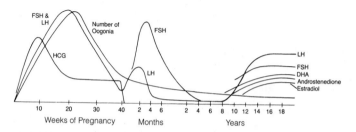

Figure 2–1 □ Changes in gonadotropins and oocytes from fetal life to puberty. (Adapted from Speroff L, Glass RH, Kase NG: Neuroendocrinology. In: Clinical Gynecologic Endocrinology and Infertility. Baltimore, Williams & Wilkins, 1989, © 1989, the Williams & Wilkins Co, Baltimore.)

depletion in the fetus is loss through the ovarian capsule into the peritoneal cavity.

■ NEONATAL AND CHILDHOOD PERIODS

At birth, the number of oocytes has fallen to approximately 2 million. The ovary is close to 1 cm in diameter, and varying degrees of oocyte maturation are present. After birth, the loss of exposure to placental and maternal estrogens results in a rise in gonadotropins, which peak at 3 months of age and then gradually fall to a plateau at 2 to 4 years of age. LH and FSH remain suppressed between the ages of 4 and 10 years.

■ PUBERTY

At the beginning of puberty, the number of oocytes remaining is approximately 300,000. Puberty represents a transition between the immature reproductive system of childhood and the mature reproductive system of adulthood. It is characterized by a reactivation of the hypothalamic-pituitary axis, which had been active in the fetal period and suppressed in the childhood period. As a result, puberty is associated with the appearance of pulsatile gonadotropin-releasing hormone (GnRH) and episodic LH secretion during sleep. In puberty, secondary sexual characteristics develop and fertility is achieved.

The stages of pubertal development require an average of 4.5 years with a range of 1.5 to 6 years and consist of the following events (Table 2–1):

1. **Thelarche (breast budding)**—occurs at a mean age of 9.8 years with a range of 8 to 13 years and is usually the first physical sign of puberty. The stages of breast development can be defined by Tanner stages (Fig. 2–2).
2. **Adrenarche or pubarche (pubic or axillary hair)**—occurs at

Table 2–1 □ **STAGES OF PUBERTAL DEVELOPMENT**

Stage	Mean Age (yr)	Age Range (yr)
Thelarche (breast budding)	9.8	8–13
Adrenarche (pubic or axillary hair)	11	8–14
Peak height velocity (maximal growth)	11.5	10–14
Menarche	13	9–16
Mature pubic hair	14	12–18
Mature breasts	14.5	12–18

Figure 2–2 □ Tanner stages of breast development. Stage 1: Pre-adolescent—elevation of the papilla only. Stage 2: Breast bud stage—elevation of the breast and papilla with enlargement of the areolar region. Stage 3: Further enlargement of the breast and areola without separation of their contours. Stage 4: Projection of the areola and papilla to form a secondary mound above the level of the breast. Stage 5: Mature stage—projection of the papilla only, resulting from recession of the areola to the general contour of the breast. (From Hacker NF, Moore JG: Essentials of Obstetrics and Gynecology, 2nd ed. Philadelphia, WB Saunders Co, 1992, p 515.)

a mean age of 11 years with a range of 8 to 14 years. In approximately 20% of girls, the appearance of pubic hair is the first sign of puberty. Pubic hair usually appears first, with axillary hair appearing about 2 years later. The stages of female pubic hair development can be defined by Tanner stages (Fig. 2–3).

3. **Peak height velocity or maximal growth**—occurs at a mean age of 11.5 years with a range of 10 to 14 years; it usually occurs 2 years after thelarche and 1 year before menarche. It occurs in females approximately 2 years earlier than in males. The average patient can increase her height between 2 and 4 inches in 1 year. This accelerated growth is mediated by growth hormone, estradiol, and insulin-like growth factor-I (IGF-I) or somatomedin-C. Very low levels of estrogen are required to stimulate long-bone cortical growth.

4. **Menarche (beginning of menses)**—occurs at a mean age of 13 years with a range of 9 to 16 years; first menses is typically anovulatory and therefore irregular and often heavy and prolonged (see Chapter 23). Adolescents can have anovulatory cycles for as long as 12 months.

5. **Mature pubic hair**—usually achieved by 14 years of age with a range of 12 to 18 years.

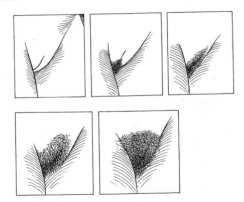

Figure 2–3 □ Tanner stages of female pubic hair development. Stage 1: Preadolescent—absence of pubic hair. Stage 2: Sparse hair along the labia. Stage 3: Hair sparsely over the junction of the pubes. Hair is darker and coarser. Stage 4: Adult-type hair without spread to the medial surface of the thighs. Stage 5: Adult-type hair with spread to the medial thighs. (From Hacker NF, Moore JG: Essentials of Obstetrics and Gynecology, 2nd ed. Philadelphia, WB Saunders Co, 1992, p 516.)

6. **Mature breasts**—usually achieved by age 14.5 years of age with a range of 12 to 18 years.

Precocious puberty is defined as the appearance of pubertal changes before 8 years of age, which represents 2.5 standard deviations below the expected age of pubertal development. Maximal growth is often the first sign of precocious puberty.

The final milestone in puberty is development of positive feedback by estrogen on the hypothalamus and pituitary. This results in estrogen stimulation of the LH surge, which in turn stimulates ovulation and the regular menses that are associated with ovulatory cycles.

■ ADULTHOOD: REPRODUCTIVE MATURITY

Adulthood and reproductive maturity in women is characterized by regular menstrual cycles of follicular maturation, ovulation, and corpus luteum formation during the next 30 to 40 years. The normal menstrual cycle is characterized by an intricate coordination of gonadotropin release, ovarian steroidogenesis, follicular maturation and ovulation, and histophysiological changes in the uterine endometrium (Fig. 2–4).

The Normal Menstrual Cycle

The normal ovulatory menstrual cycle begins with the first day of menstrual bleeding, which by convention is referred to as "day

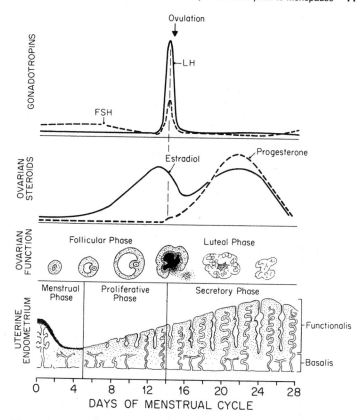

Figure 2–4 □ Events of the normal menstrual cycle. (From Hacker NF, Moore JG: Essentials of Obstetrics and Gynecology, 2nd ed. Philadelphia, WB Saunders Co, 1992, p 39.)

1." The average length of the menstrual cycle is 28 days with a normal range of 21 to 35 days. The normal duration of bleeding is 4 to 5 days with a normal range of 3 to 7 days. The average blood loss during menses is 35 ml with a normal range of 20 to 80 ml. The normal menstrual cycle can be divided into the follicular phase and the luteal phase. The luteal phase is the more constant phase with a mean duration of 14 days and range of 12 to 16 days, and the follicular phase has a range of 7 days to more than 21 days.

1. Follicular phase

This phase begins with the onset of menses and concludes with the preovulatory LH surge. Folliculogenesis and an increase in FSH actually begin in the last few days of the luteal phase of the previous cycle. The initial rise in FSH is the result of escape of FSH secretion from the negative feedback provided by estrogen and progesterone when levels of these steroids decrease secondary to the regression of the corpus luteum from the preceding cycle. Rising FSH initiates recruitment and growth of a cohort of 3 to 30 follicles from which a single dominant follicle is chosen for ovulation. After the selection of the dominant follicle, the remaining follicles of the cohort undergo atresia or degeneration. LH begins to rise several days after the rise in FSH. LH continues to increase slowly in the follicular phase secondary to positive feedback from rising estradiol produced in the granulosa cells of the enlarging follicle. In contrast, FSH begins to decrease in the late follicular phase due to negative feedback from rising estradiol. Rising estrogen levels result in proliferation of the endometrium and increased cervical vascularity and edema. Furthermore, the amount of cervical mucus is increased, as is the elasticity of the mucus, referred to as "spinnbarkeit." The LH surge immediately precedes ovulation and marks the end of the follicular phase.

2. Ovulation (midcycle)

Ovulation, the release of the ovum from the mature dominant follicle, occurs 32 to 34 hours after the onset of the LH surge or the peak of estradiol. The site of ovulation is random and does not necessarily alternate between the two ovaries. If one ovary is removed, every ovulation will occur in the remaining ovary, and the number of ovulatory cycles in a woman's reproductive life is not decreased.

3. Luteal phase

The luteal phase begins after ovulation and is characterized by suppression of both LH and FSH secondary to negative feedback from rising levels of estrogen and progesterone. In the luteal phase, the corpus luteum develops from the luteinized granulosa and theca cells of the ovary. The corpus luteum secretes progesterone, which supports the ovum and induces histological changes of the endometrium that prepare it for implantation of the fertilized ovum. In response to progesterone, endometrial glands become coiled and secretory with increased vascularity. Progesterone peaks at a level greater than 10 ng/ml approximately 7 days after the LH surge. Progesterone increases the morning basal body temperature, and a rise of 0.3°C or greater over the nadir is presumptive evidence of ovulation. If fertilization does not occur, progesterone decreases and the corpus luteum regresses through a process referred to as luteolysis. This results in a fall in estrogen and progesterone, which causes endometrial edema, necrosis, and finally, bleeding that represents menses. Furthermore, this fall in estrogen and progesterone releases FSH from negative feedback. FSH begins to rise, and this rise continues into the follicular phase of the next menstrual cycle.

Fertilization and Implantation

After ovulation, the ovum can be fertilized for 12 to 24 hours. After ejaculation, sperm can fertilize an egg for up to 48 hours. Even though several hundred million sperm are ejaculated into the vagina, less than 200 actually reach the egg, and usually only one will fertilize the egg. The zona pellucida that surrounds the egg contains species-specific sperm receptors and undergoes zona reaction, which makes the zona impervious to other sperm once fertilization has occurred. Fertilization occurs in the ampullary portion of the fallopian tube. The fertilized ovum reaches the uterine cavity approximately 2 to 3 days after fertilization. Implantation begins 2 to 3 days after the fertilized ovum enters the uterine cavity. At the time of implantation, the zona pellucida is shed and the conceptus is at the blastocyst stage. Human chorionic gonadotropin (hCG) is produced by the conceptus at about the time of implantation. The blastocyst has an outer mass of cells that become trophoblasts and an inner cell mass that becomes the embryo. The trophoblasts proliferate and invade the decidua. Maternal blood vessels are trapped to form lacunae, which are filled with maternal blood. At approximately 12 days after fertilization, primitive villi are present traversing the lacunae. The primitive villi eventually develop into the placenta.

The endometrium undergoes changes referred to as decidual changes under the influence of progesterone. Endometrial stroma cells develop into enlarged, round decidual cells, and during pregnancy, the decidua reaches a thickness of 5 to 10 mm. Decidual basalis refers to the decidua at the implantation site, and decidua capsularis refers to the decidua overlying the conceptus (Fig. 2–5). Decidual parietalis or vera lines the remaining uterine cavity. The decidua capsularis and decidua parietalis fuse at 14 to 16 weeks of gestation, and the uterine cavity becomes obliterated.

■ CLIMACTERIC AND MENOPAUSE

Climacteric refers to the period of decreasing ovarian function beginning as early as the age of 40. It is characterized by decreased fertility and progressive tissue atrophy and aging from decreasing estrogen production. Climacteric culminates in menopause, which is defined as the cessation of menstruation. The median age of menopause in the United States is 51 years with a range of 45 to 55. Menopause before the age of 40 is defined as premature ovarian failure. The diagnosis of menopause should

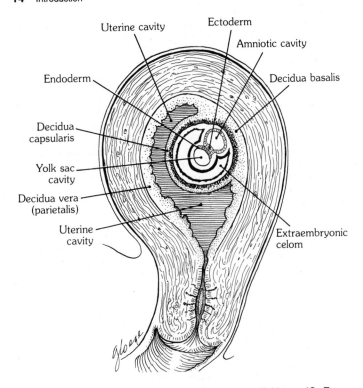

Uterine cavity

Ectoderm

Amniotic cavity

Endoderm

Decidua basalis

Decidua capsularis

Yolk sac cavity

Decidua vera (parietalis)

Uterine cavity

Extraembryonic celom

Figure 2–5 □ The early conceptus. (From Hacker NF, Moore JG: Essentials of Obstetrics and Gynecology, 2nd ed. Philadelphia, WB Saunders Co, 1992, p 46.)

be suspected in any patient in this age group who has had 6 to 12 months of amenorrhea. The basic feature of menopause is the depletion of ovarian follicles. This leads to the inability of the ovaries to respond to gonadotropins and a decrease in ovarian production of estrogen, progesterone, and androstenedione. Even in the perimenopausal years preceding menopause, women have lower estradiol levels and higher FSH levels. Women in this age group will commonly have anovulation or oligo-ovulation. Even when ovulation occurs, the quality of the ovum decreases as a woman ages. This results in a decrease in fertilization and an increase in the incidence of chromosomal abnormalities in the embryo when fertilization does occur. Furthermore, decreased progesterone production by the ovum results in shorter menstrual cycles and irregular bleeding.

Postmenopausal women have elevated gonadotropins and decreased estrogens, progesterone, and androgens (Table 2–2). FSH is increased by 10- to 20-fold, and a level of greater than 40 mIU/ml is diagnostic of menopause. LH is increased only threefold because it is cleared much faster than FSH. The half-life of LH is approximately 30 minutes, whereas the half-life of FSH is close to 4 hours. Serum estradiol is decreased to 5 to 25 pg/ml, and serum estone falls to 30 to 70 pg/ml. Serum progesterone falls to less than 1 ng/ml. Serum testosterone decreases from 20 to 80 ng/dl to 10 to 40 ng/dl. Ovarian production of testosterone remains unchanged when a woman enters menopause, and the decrease in serum testosterone is the result of diminished production from the adrenal glands. Plasma androstenedione decreases from approximately 150 ng/dl to close to 90 ng/ml. This decrease is a result of decreased production from both the adrenal glands and the ovaries. The clinical manifestations of menopause include the following:

1. **Vasomotor symptoms**

   Also referred to as hot flashes or flushes, vasomotor symptoms are experienced by close to 75% of postmenopausal women. Approximately 10% of women experience vasomotor symptoms before menopause. Vasomotor symptoms are caused by a relative decrease in estrogen levels, rather than a specific level of estrogen. Patients with gonadal dystrophy and who produce no endogenous estrogen do not experience vasomotor symptoms unless they are given exogenous estrogen and then it is withdrawn. The cause of vasomotor symptoms is an alteration of the central thermoregulatory mechanism.

2. **Atrophic genital and urological changes**

   Vaginal dryness and irritation, dysuria, and atrophic vaginitis are caused by decreased circulating estrogen. Atrophy of the vaginal epithelium can also result in dyspareunia and vaginal bleeding. Furthermore, the support for the uterus

Table 2–2 □ GONADOTROPIN AND STEROID LEVELS

	Follicular Phase	Midcycle	Luteal Phase	Postmenopausal
Serum FSH (mIU/ml)	5–20	10–40	5–20	>40
Serum LH (mIU/ml)	5–20	15–60	5–20	>40
Serum estradiol (pg/ml)	25–75	200–600	100–300	5–25
Serum progesterone (ng/ml)	<1	<1	5–20	<1
Serum testosterone (ng/dl)	20–80	20–80	20–80	10–40

and urethra can be weakened, resulting in uterine descensus and stress urinary incontinence.

3. Osteoporosis

Osteoporosis is a reduction in the quantity of bone mass and develops when osteoclastic activity exceeds osteoblastic activity. Estrogen deficiency is the major cause for osteoporosis in postmenopausal women. It has been estimated that at least 75% of the bone mass loss in women in the first 20 years of menopause is caused by the loss of estrogen rather than by aging. As a result, women who have been postmenopausal for more than 10 years have a fracture rate that is three to five times greater than men of comparable ages. High-risk factors for the development of osteoporosis include white or Asian ethnicity, smoking, slender and small body frame, sedentary lifestyle, steroid use, and a diet that is low in calcium and vitamin D and high in alcohol, caffeine, and protein. In women with high-risk factors, approximately 1 to 1.5% of bone mass is lost each year after menopause. Most calcium is lost from trabecular bone, where there may be a loss in bone mass of up to 50%. In contrast, osteoporosis in cortical bone occurs later, and there is a loss in bone mass of only 5%. Therefore, the spinal column and femoral neck are the most vulnerable to fracture. The incidence of hip or femur fractures rises from 0.3/1000 to 20/1000 between the ages of 45 and 85. Spinal compression fractures result in loss of height, pain, and postural deformities. Close to one-third of women over the age of 65 have spinal compression fractures, and the average postmenopausal woman who is not on estrogen replacement shrinks 2.5 inches in height. Colles' fractures of the distal forearm increase 10-fold in the postmenopausal years in women who do not take estrogen replacement.

Estrogen replacement protects against osteoporosis probably by decreasing bone resorption. In postmenopausal women who take estrogen, there is a slight increase in the levels of serum calcium and phosphorus and a decrease in the levels of parathyroid hormone and 1,25-dihydroxyvitamin D, the active form of vitamin D. The amount of estrogen necessary to prevent osteoporosis is 0.625 mg of equine estrogen or 1.25 mg of piperazine estrone sulfate. Calcium supplementation is also helpful in preventing osteoporosis, although it is not as critical as estrogen. Estrogen users should take 1000 mg of calcium supplementation per day, whereas nonusers should take 1500 mg per day. The average daily diet contains approximately 800 mg of calcium. The protective effects of estrogen are present only while the patient is taking estrogen. If estrogen is taken initially and

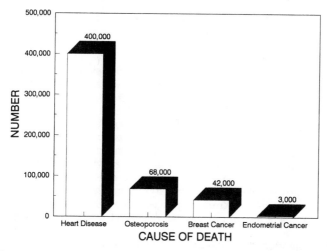

Figure 2–6 □ Causes of death among women in the United States. (From Copeland LJ: *Textbook of Gynecology*. Philadelphia, WB Saunders Co, 1993, p 622.)

then discontinued, there is an accelerated rate of osteoporosis.

4. Increased cardiovascular disease

In women, cardiovascular disease is by far the leading cause of death (Fig. 2–6). Premenopausal women have a significantly lower incidence of cardiovascular disease than men of the same age. However, in postmenopausal women, the incidence of heart disease rises such that 6 to 10 years after the onset of menopause, this incidence is the same as it is for men. Furthermore, the relative risk of cardiovascular disease increases with earlier age at menopause. In women who undergo bilateral oophorectomy before the age of 35, the relative risk of myocardial infarction is 7.2, almost three times higher than in women between the ages of 35 and 39 years who do not undergo bilateral oophorectomy.

Cholesterol, low-density lipoprotein (LDL), and high-density lipoprotein (HDL) are important in the development of coronary heart disease. High levels of cholesterol and LDL are positively correlated with the risk of coronary heart disease. In contrast, HDL is protective against atherosclerosis, and the level of HDL is inversely related to the risk of heart disease. It has been estimated that there is a 3 to 5% decrease in the risk of coronary heart disease for every 1-mg/dl increase in HDL level. There is a 2% decrease in the risk of coronary heart disease for every 1% decrease in total cholesterol level. In menopausal women who do not take estrogen replacement, lipid changes are atherogenic. Serum cholesterol, LDL, and triglycerides increase, whereas HDL decreases.

Estrogen replacement decreases the risk of cardiovascular disease by 50 to 65% in postmenopausal women. Estrogen ingestion is associated with a slight increase in serum cholesterol, but more important, there is an increase in HDL and a decrease in LDL. In addition to its effects on lipid levels, estrogen may have a local effect on arteries and protect against intimal plaque formation. Unfortunately, progestins, which are given along with estrogen to postmenopausal patients who have not had prior hysterectomies, result in a decrease in HDL and therefore blunt the protective effects of estrogen. Micronized progesterone (200 mg/day) appears to have less of this unfavorable effect than medroxyprogesterone.

5. **Emotional and psychological changes**

Menopause is associated with the following emotional and/or psychological changes:

- Insomnia
- Poor memory
- Mental confusion
- Lethargy
- Irritability
- Nervousness
- Fatigue
- Dizziness
- Inability to cope
- Loss of libido

These symptoms may be caused by a decrease in estrogen and androgens or may be caused at least partially by the presence of significant vasomotor symptoms.

3

MATERNAL PHYSIOLOGICAL CHANGES IN PREGNANCY

Profound anatomical, endocrinological, and physiological maternal changes occur during pregnancy. These changes adapt the mother to the needs of the fetus. Many of these adaptations begin early in pregnancy. To understand the many pathological conditions encountered in pregnancy, it is necessary first to understand these maternal adaptations that occur in normal pregnancy.

■ HEMATOLOGICAL SYSTEM

Blood Volume—Increased

Maternal blood volume increases by approximately 45% near term because of an increase in plasma volume and a slightly smaller increase in red blood cell mass. This increase begins in the first trimester, reaches the greatest rate of increase in the second trimester, and reaches a plateau near term. Plasma volume begins to increase as early as 6 weeks of gestational age and peaks at a volume of close to 5 L at term, an increase of 45%. Red blood cell mass increases by 300 to 400 ml by term, an increase of 20 to 30%.

Hematocrit and Hemoglobin—Decreased

Because the increase in plasma volume is usually greater than the increase in red blood cell volume, both hematocrit and hemoglobin decrease despite accelerated erythropoiesis. This dilutional effect can result in a decrease in hemoglobin concentration to 11.0 g/dl.

White Blood Cell Count—Increased

The normal white blood cell count in pregnancy is 5000 to 12,000/mm^3. However, during labor, the white blood cell count increases to approximately 15,000/mm^3 and can be as high as 25,000/mm^3.

Coagulation Factors

Serum fibrinogen increases to 300 to 600 mg/dl, a 50% rise over normal nonpregnant levels. This increase in fibrinogen results in an increase in erythrocyte sedimentation rate (ESR) in normal pregnancy. Levels of factors II, VII, VIII, IX, and X are also increased in normal pregnancy. Levels of factors XI and XIII are slightly decreased. Platelet count is slightly decreased, to between 150,000 and 400,000/mm^3.

Iron Requirements—Increased

The total iron requirement for a normal singleton pregnancy is approximately 1 g. This 1 g consists of 300 mg for the fetus, 500 mg for the increased red blood cell volume, and 200 mg that is lost through normal excretion. The total iron requirement translates to a daily requirement of 6 to 7 mg/day in the second half of pregnancy. The normally low absorption rate of iron through the gastrointestinal tract is only modestly increased in pregnancy. Therefore, the iron absorbed from diet and available from iron stores is not sufficient to meet the requirements imposed by pregnancy, and iron supplementation must be provided.

■ CARDIOVASCULAR SYSTEM

Anatomical Changes

The cardiac apex is displaced upward and to the left by the elevating diaphragm. There is also an increase in the size of the cardiac silhouette.

Heart Rate—Increased

The resting heart rate increases by 10 to 18 beats/min during pregnancy. The heart rate begins to increase late in the first trimester and reaches a plateau in the mid-second trimester (Fig. 3–1).

Stroke Volume—Increased

Cardiac stroke volume increases by 10 to 30%. Stroke volume starts to increase as early as 10 weeks of gestational age, peaks at approximately 20 weeks, and decreases slightly near term (see Fig. 3–1).

Cardiac Output—Increased

Cardiac output, a product of heart rate and stroke volume, increases by 33 to 50%. This increase in cardiac output peaks in the early second trimester.

Figure 3–1 □ Changes in heart rate and stroke volume in pregnancy. (Adapted from Robson SC, Hunter S, Boys RJ, et al: Serial study of factors influencing changes in cardiac output during human pregnancy. Am J Physiol 256:H1060, 1989.)

Heart Sound Changes (Fig. 3–2)

1. Exaggerated splitting of S_1 in 88% of patients
2. Systolic murmur in 96% of patients
3. Diastolic murmur in 18% of patients
4. Prominent S_3 in 84% of patients

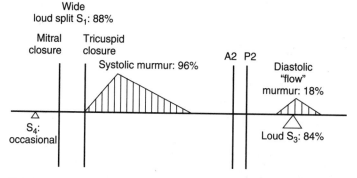

Figure 3–2 □ Changes in heart sounds in pregnancy. (Redrawn from Cutforth R, MacDonald CB: Heart sounds and murmurs in pregnancy. Am Heart J 71:741, 1966.)

Blood Pressure

Arterial blood pressure decreases in pregnancy as early as the first trimester. This decrease is caused primarily by a fall in systemic vascular resistance. Systolic blood pressure decreases by 4 to 6 mm Hg, and diastolic blood pressure decreases by 8 to 15 mm Hg. The nadir is reached between 24 and 32 weeks of gestation.

Systemic Vascular Resistance—Decreased

Systemic vascular resistance (SVR) is decreased in pregnancy due to the low-resistance uteroplacental circulation and the vasodilatatory effect of progesterone. SVR is calculated by using the following equation:

$$\text{SVR (dynes} \times \text{sec} \times \text{cm}^{-5}) = \frac{(\text{mean arterial pressure} - \text{central venous pressure}) \times 80}{\text{cardiac output}}$$

The decrease in SVR reaches a nadir between 14 and 24 weeks.

■ RESPIRATORY SYSTEM

Changes in lung volumes during pregnancy are summarized in Table 3–1.

Tidal Volume—Increased

Tidal volume is increased by close to 40%.

Functional Residual Capacity—Decreased

Functional residual capacity is decreased due to elevation of the diaphragm.

Residual Volume—Decreased

Residual volume is decreased by approximately 20% due to elevation of the diaphragm.

Total Body Oxygen Consumption—Increased

Oxygen consumption is increased by 15 to 20%. Close to 50% of this increase is due to the uterus, placenta, and fetus. The increased work by the maternal heart, lungs, and kidneys accounts for most of the remaining increase in oxygen consumption.

Table 3–1 □ CHANGES IN PULMONARY VOLUMES AND CAPACITIES IN PREGNANCY

Test	Definition	Change in Pregnancy
Respiratory rate	—	No significant change
Tidal volume	The volume of air inspired and expired at each breath	Progressive rise throughout pregnancy of 0.1–0.2 L
Expiratory reserve volume	The maximum volume of air that can be additionally expired after a normal expiration	Lowered by about 15% (0.55 L in late pregnancy compared with 0.65 L postpartum)
Residual volume	The volume of air remaining in the lungs after a maximum expiration	Falls considerably (0.77 L in late pregnancy compared with 0.96 L postpartum)
Vital capacity	The maximum volume of air that can be forcibly inspired after a maximum expiration	Unchanged, except for possibly a small terminal diminution
Inspiratory capacity	The maximum volume of air that can be inspired from resting expiratory level	Increased by about 5%
Functional residual capacity	The volume of air in lungs at resting expiratory level	Lowered by about 18%
Minute ventilation	The volume of air inspired or expired in 1 minute	Increased by about 40% as a result of the increased tidal volume and unchanged respiratory rate

Adapted from Main DM, Main EK: Obstetrics and Gynecology. A Pocket Reference. Chicago, Year Book, 1984, p 14.

Because PaO_2 is unchanged and arteriovenous oxygen difference actually decreases, this increased oxygen consumption is accompanied by increased cardiac output and increased ventilation through an increase in tidal volume.

Arterial Pco_2—Decreased

$PaCO_2$ is decreased because of hyperventilation, which is due to an increased tidal volume and not to an increased respiratory rate. $PaCO_2$ decreases from a nonpregnant level of 35 to 40 mm Hg to a pregnant level of approximately 30 mm Hg.

■ RENAL SYSTEM

Anatomical Changes

Renal dilatation and hydronephrosis is found in 90% of pregnant patients and is most prominent on the right side. The kidneys of a pregnant patient are approximately 1.5 cm longer than those of a nonpregnant patient. These changes are the result of both the relaxation of smooth muscle of the ureters due to progesterone and the obstruction of the ureters at the pelvic brim by the enlarging uterus.

Renal Plasma Flow—Increased

Renal plasma flow (RPF) increases by 60 to 80% by the mid-second trimester and then falls slightly to 50% over the nonpregnant level in the third trimester (Fig. 3–3).

Glomerular Filtration Rate—Increased

Glomerular filtration rate (GFR) increases beginning as early as 6 weeks of gestational age. It peaks at 50% over the nonpregnant level at 16 to 20 weeks of gestational age (see Fig. 3–3). Creatinine clearance peaks at close to 150 ml/min.

Serum Creatinine and Blood Urea Nitrogen—Decreased

Both serum creatinine and blood urea nitrogen (BUN) are decreased from nonpregnant levels becaused of increased glomerular filtration rate.

Urinalysis

Glucosuria in pregnancy is not necessarily abnormal. The increased glomerular filtration rate and impaired tubular reabsorp-

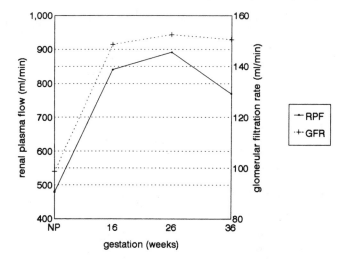

Figure 3–3 □ Changes in renal plasma flow and glomerular filtration rate in pregnancy. (Adapted from Dunlop W: Serial changes in renal hemodynamics during normal human pregnancy. Br J Obstet Gynecol 88:1, 1981.)

tion of glucose result in glucosuria in 15% of normal pregnant women.

■ ENDOCRINE SYSTEM

Pancreas—Insulin and Carbohydrate Metabolism

Fetal growth, development, and maturation require profound changes in maternal metabolic regulation. Pregnancy can be diabetogenic; pre-existing diabetes mellitus may be aggravated or new-onset diabetes may appear. Approximately 2 to 3% of pregnancies are complicated by diabetes, and 90% of these cases are caused by gestational diabetes. The following are usually found in normal pregnancy:

- Hyperinsulinemia and pancreatic beta cell hypertrophy
- Progressive insulin resistance
- Mild fasting hypoglycemia
- Postprandial hyperglycemia

Rising estrogen and progesterone levels result in pancreatic beta cell hypertrophy and hyperinsulinemia as early as 10 weeks of gestational age. This results in a mean decrease in fasting serum glucose of close to 10 mg/dl in pregnancy when compared with the nonpregnant state. In the second half of pregnancy, progressive insulin resistance develops as a result of rising levels of human chorionic somatomammotropin (hCS) and prolactin from the placenta and maternal cortisol and glucagon (Table 3–2).

Thyroid Gland

The thyroid gland is moderately enlarged during normal pregnancy. Rising levels of estrogen result in higher levels of thyroxine-binding globulin (TBG). Increased TBG results in a decrease in the level of triiodothyronine resin uptake (T_3RU) and increases in the levels of both thyroxine (T_4) and triiodothyronine (T_3). Levels of total T_4 begin to increase in the first trimester and eventually reach levels of 9 to 16 $\mu g/dl$ compared with 5 to 12 $\mu g/dl$ in the nonpregnant women. Although total T_3 and T_4 are elevated, free T_3 and T_4 as well as TSH are in the normal nonpregnant range, and pregnant patients are normally euthryoid.

Pituitary Gland

The pituitary gland is enlarged close to 135% during pregnancy. The anterior lobe may increase in size to two to three times the size in nonpregnant women. This is due primarily to hyperplasia and hypertrophy of prolactin-secreting cells. Serum prolactin increases in pregnancy to a mean level of 150 ng/ml, or close to 10 times greater than in the normal nonpregnant woman.

Adrenal Glands

Levels of corticosteroid-binding globulin or transcortin are increased threefold in pregnancy secondary to rising estrogen levels. Both adrenocorticotropic hormone (ACTH) and cortisol are elevated beginning in the late first trimester. Free cortisol, aldosterone, and deoxycorticosterone are also elevated in pregnancy.

■ GASTROINTESTINAL SYSTEM

Anatomical Changes

The stomach and intestines are displaced upward by the enlarging uterus. The appendix is displaced upward and laterally, sometimes reaching the right flank (Fig. 3–4). This results in a change in the clinical presentation of appendicitis in pregnant patients. The change in the position of the stomach also contributes to the higher incidence of esophageal reflux and pyrosis or heartburn. Intragastric pressures are increased and intraesophageal pressures are decreased in pregnancy.

Table 3–2 □ CARBOHYDRATE METABOLISM IN LATE PREGNANCY

Hormonal Change	Effect	Metabolic Changes
↑ hCS	"Diabetogenic" ↓ glucose tolerance	Facilitated anabolism during feeding and ↓ Accelerated starvation during fasting
↑ Prolactin	Insulin resistance	
↑ Bound and free cortisol	↓ Hepatic glycogen stores ↑ Hepatic glucose production	Ensures glucose and amino acids to fetus

From Creasy RK, Resnik R: Maternal-Fetal Medicine: Principles and Practice. Philadelphia, WB Saunders Co, 1994, p 938.

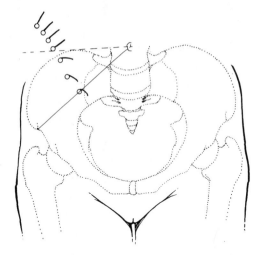

Figure 3–4 □ Location of the appendix in pregnancy. (From Plauche WC, Morrison JC, O'Sullivan M: Surgical Obstetrics, Philadelphia, WB Saunders Co, 1992, p 236.)

Table 3–3 □ **LIVER FUNCTION TESTS IN NORMAL PREGNANCY**

Serum Tests	Levels in Pregnancy
Prothrombin time	
Total bilirubin	
AST/SGOT	No change
ALT/SGPT	
Alkaline phosphatase (liver)	
Gamma GT	
5-Nucleotidase	
	Increase
Total alkaline phosphatase	Accelerated 3rd trimester*
Globulins alpha and beta	Progressive to term
Lipids	Progressive to term
Fibrinogen	Progressive to term
Ceruloplasmin	
Transferrin	
	Decrease
Albumin	20% first trimester
Globulins: gamma	Minor or unchanged

AST = aspartate aminotransferase; ALT = alanine aminotransferase; GT = glutamyl transpeptidase.
*Placental and skeletal isoenzymes only.
Modified from Creasy RK, Resnik R: Maternal-Fetal Medicine: Principles and Practice. Philadelphia, WB Saunders Co, 1994, p 1040.

Gastric Emptying

Gastric emptying and intestinal transit time are delayed in pregnancy. This delay may be caused by the effects of progesterone on the relaxation of smooth muscle or by mechanical effects of the enlarging pregnant uterus on the gastrointestinal tract.

Liver

No morphological changes in the liver are associated with normal pregnancy. Furthermore, liver size and hepatic blood flow do not change significantly in pregnancy. However, the levels of some liver function tests are altered in normal pregnancy (Table 3–3). Total serum alkaline phosphatase is normally elevated almost twofold due to placental production of alkaline phosphatase. Albumin is normally decreased by approximately 20%.

Gallbladder

Gallbladder contractility is decreased and there is an increase in residual volume. This effect is probably due to increased levels of progesterone and its effect on increased smooth muscle relaxation. The end result is increased stasis, which in turn increases the frequency of gallstones.

PATIENT-RELATED OBSTETRICAL PROBLEMS: THE COMMON CALLS

□ **4** □

ABNORMAL FETAL HEART RATE
PATTERNS

■ BACKGROUND AND DEFINITIONS

Intrapartum fetal heart rate monitoring is used to detect abnormal fetal heart rate patterns that may be associated with hypoxia, acidosis, and fetal asphyxia. Fetal heart rate patterns can be described as "reassuring" or "nonreassuring."

Fetal asphyxia: Hypoxia with metabolic acidosis

Baseline fetal heart activity: Baseline characteristics of the fetal heart rate

Periodic fetal heart rate activity: Characteristics of the fetal heart rate that are associated with uterine contractions

Abnormalities of baseline fetal heart activity include the following:

1. **Rate.** The normal baseline fetal heart rate in the third trimester is 120 to 160 beats/min. Occasional accelerations are associated with a normal fetal heart rate pattern (Fig. 4–1).

   Mild bradycardia: Baseline rate of 100 to 119 beats/min
   Moderate bradycardia: Baseline rate of 80 to 99 beats/min for at least 3 minutes (Fig. 4–2)

Figure 4–1 □ Normal fetal heart rate with accelerations. (From Creasy RK, Resnik R: Maternal-Fetal Medicine: Principles and Practice, 3rd ed. Philadelphia, WB Saunders Co, 1994, p 306.)

Figure 4–2 ◻ Prolonged fetal bradycardia. (From Creasy RK, Resnik R: Maternal-Fetal Medicine: Principles and Practice, 3rd ed. Philadelphia, WB Saunders Co, 1994, p 307.)

        Severe bradycardia: Baseline rate of <80 beats/min for at least 3 minutes
        Mild tachycardia: Baseline rate of 161 to 180 beats/min
        Severe tachycardia: Baseline rate of >180 beats/min
  2. **Beat-to-beat variability.** Variability is the oscillatory appearance of the fetal heart rate when recorded on graph paper. It is regulated by the fetal autonomic nervous system and is an index of fetal cardiovascular function.

        Short-term variability: Instantaneous change in fetal heart rate from one beat to the next. Short-term variability can be detected only by internal electronic fetal monitoring. Normal short-term variability is a beat-to-beat change of 3 to 7 beats/min, and increased short-term variability is a beat-to-beat change of >7 beats/min. Both are reassuring of fetal well-being. Decreased or absent short-term variability can be an indication of fetal compromise, especially if it is persistent (Fig. 4–3).
        Long-term variability: Oscillatory changes in fetal heart

Figure 4–3 ◻ Absence of variability. (From Creasy RK, Resnik R: Maternal-Fetal Medicine: Principles and Practice, 3rd ed. Philadelphia, WB Saunders Co, 1994, p 308.)

rate over 1 minute, resulting in a wavy baseline. The normal frequency of the "waves" or cycle changes is 3 to 5/min. Decreased long-term variability is defined as <2 cycle changes/min. Decreased or absent long-term variability, if persistent, can indicate fetal distress.

3. **Cardiac arrhythmia.** Fetal cardiac arrhythmias are found in approximately 1% of patients monitored and can be detected only by electronic monitoring. Most arrhythmias are supraventricular and resolve spontaneously in the neonatal period. Ventricular arrhythmias are infrequent in fetuses. Most fetal cardiac arrhythmias are of little clinical significance if fetal cardiac failure, manifested by the presence of hydrops, is absent. However, the presence of cardiac arrhythmias can make interpretation of fetal heart rate patterns difficult.

4. **Sinusoidal heart rate pattern.** A distinct pattern consisting of regular oscillations resembling a sine wave with a frequency of 3 to 5 cycles/min, amplitude of 5 to 15 beats/min, absence of short-term variability, and duration of at least 10 minutes (Fig. 4–4). When this pattern is persistent, it is usually associated with fetal acidosis and hypoxia. However, a sinusoidal heart rate pattern can also be associated with fetal anemia and the administration of alphaprodine.

Abnormalities of periodic fetal heart rate activity include the following:

1. **Early deceleration.** A smooth and symmetrical fall in fetal heart rate, beginning and ending with the uterine contraction and resembling a mirror image of the contraction (Fig. 4–5). Rarely does the absolute heart rate fall to <100 beats/

Figure 4–4 □ Sinusoidal pattern. (From Creasy RK, Resnik R: Maternal-Fetal Medicine: Principles and Practice, 3rd ed. Philadelphia, WB Saunders Co, 1994, p 318.)

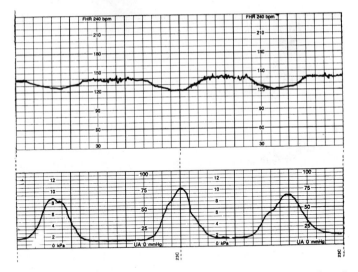

Figure 4–5 □ Early decelerations. (From Newton M, Newton ER: Complications of Gynecologic and Obstetric Management. Philadelphia, WB Saunders Co, 1988, p 272.)

min or >30 beats below the baseline. Early decelerations are caused by fetal head compression and do not indicate fetal distress.

2. **Late deceleration.** A uniform, smooth fall in the fetal heart rate, beginning at or after the peak of the uterine contraction and returning to baseline after the end of the contraction (Figs. 4–6 and 4–7). Late decelerations can be subtle, with a fall of only 10 to 20 beats below the baseline. The heart rate

Figure 4–6 □ Late decelerations. (From Creasy RK, Resnik R: Maternal-Fetal Medicine: Principles and Practice, 3rd ed. Philadelphia, WB Saunders Co, 1994, p 309.)

Figure 4–7 □ Late decelerations with loss of variability. (From Newton M, Newton ER: Complications of Gynecologic and Obstetric Management. Philadelphia, WB Saunders Co, 1988, p 273.)

rarely falls more than 30 to 40 beats below the baseline. Occasional late decelerations are of no clinical significance. However, repetitive late decelerations can be an indication of fetal asphyxia.

3. **Variable deceleration.** A rapid fall in fetal heart rate, with a steep downslope and a rapid return to baseline. A variable deceleration resembles the shape of the letter U or the letter V and is variable in duration, depth, and shape from one contraction to the next (Fig. 4–8). This type of deceleration is the most common type detected in labor. It is caused by cord compression and is present frequently in the second stage of labor. Variable decelerations are rarely indicative of fetal asphyxia unless they are severe. Severe variable decelerations are defined by the "rule of 60s," as follows: (1) the rate falls to <60 beats/min, or (2) the rate falls ≥60 beats below the baseline, or (3) the duration of the deceleration is >60 seconds.

■ CLINICAL PRESENTATION

Abnormal fetal heart rate patterns are not necessarily associated with any specific symptoms. Patients in whom fetal distress is

Figure 4–8 □ Variable decelerations. (From Creasy RK, Resnik R: Maternal-Fetal Medicine: Principles and Practice, 3rd ed. Philadelphia, WB Saunders Co, 1994, p 312.)

caused by placental abruption might have vaginal bleeding, uterine pain, or uterine tenderness. Likewise, patients with uterine hypertonus, excessive uterine contractions, or uterine rupture might have increased uterine pain. In many situations, conduction analgesia can mask these symptoms of uterine pain.

■ **PHONE CALL**

Questions

1. **What are the patient's vital signs?**
   Maternal hypotension can result in abnormal fetal heart rate patterns.
2. **Does the patient appear to be in hypovolemic shock?**
   Hypovolemic shock caused by placental abruption or uterine rupture can cause abnormal fetal heart rate patterns.
3. **Does the patient appear to be in an excessive amount of pain?**
   Excessive pain can result from hyperstimulation of the uterus, caused by oxytocin administration, placental abruption, or uterine rupture. These are all potential causes of abnormal fetal heart rate patterns.

Orders

1. Start an intravenous (IV) fluid infusion if the patient does not already have one
2. Turn the patient on her side to increase blood return through the inferior vena cava

3. Administer supplemental oxygen to the mother, with a face mask and at an oxygen flow rate of 8 to 10 L/min
4. Have available a fetal scalp electrode for internal fetal heart rate monitoring

Degree of Urgency

A patient whose fetus has abnormal heart rate patterns should be seen immediately.

■ ELEVATOR THOUGHTS

What are the causes of abnormal fetal heart rate patterns?
1. Maternal hypoperfusion
   - Hypotension from the use of conduction analgesia
   - Decreased blood return due to uterine compression of the vena cava in the supine position
2. Excessive uterine activity, usually from oxytocin administration
   - Hypertonus with elevated resting uterine tone
   - Excessively frequent uterine contractions with inadequate rest periods (lasting <1 minute) between contractions
   - Prolonged uterine contractions (lasting >90 seconds)
3. Uterine rupture
4. Decreased umbilical cord blood flow
   - Umbilical cord compression
   - Umbilical cord knot
   - Umbilical cord prolapse
5. Placental dysfunction
   - Maternal hypertension
   - Maternal diabetes mellitus
   - Maternal autoimmune disorders
   - Placental abruption

■ MAJOR THREAT TO FETAL LIFE

- Fetal asphyxia
  Abnormal fetal heart rate patterns can indicate fetal asphyxia with possible neonatal morbidity and mortality.

■ BEDSIDE

Quick Look Test

What types of abnormal fetal heart rate patterns are present?
Certain fetal heart rate patterns, such as early decelerations and mild, variable decelerations, can be detected in normal pregnancies and are not worrisome. Other patterns, such as

recurrent late decelerations and sinusoidal patterns, are suggestive of fetal distress.

How long have the abnormal fetal heart rate patterns been present?

Occasional isolated abnormal heart rate patterns are usually of no significance, whereas recurrent abnormal patterns are more ominous.

Is the patient in labor, and if so, what is the quality and frequency of her contractions?

Hyperstimulation of the uterus by oxytocin administration can cause abnormal heart rate patterns. Excessively frequent contractions (occurring more frequently than every 3 minutes), prolonged contractions (lasting >90 seconds), and an elevated uterine resting tone are indicative of hyperstimulation.

How much is the patient's cervix dilated and how close is the patient to delivery?

If the patient has a nonreassuring heart rate pattern and is also close to delivery, facilitation of delivery by forceps or by vacuum should be considered.

Vital Signs

Hypotension caused by poor blood return in a supine position, placental abruption, and uterine rupture can result in abnormal heart rate patterns.

Selective History and Chart Review

1. Does the patient have any medical conditions such as hypertension, diabetes mellitus, or collagen-vascular disorders that cause chronic placental dysfunction?
2. Has there been evidence of intrauterine growth restriction?
   Intrauterine growth restriction can result from chronic placental dysfunction, which may in turn result in fetal distress during labor.

Selective Physical Examination

Abdominal	Tender in placental abruption
Pelvic	
External genitalia and vagina	Normal unless there is excessive vaginal bleeding or meconium passage
Cervix	Usually normal
Uterus and adnexae	Normal unless there is uterine tenderness, irritability, or hypertonus caused by placental abruption, hyperstimulation, or uterine rupture

■ DIAGNOSTIC TESTING

1. Electronic fetal heart rate monitoring

Fetal heart rate can be monitored either with continuous electronic monitoring or with intermittent auscultation. In low-risk patients, the fetal heart rate tracing should be evaluated every 30 minutes in the first stage of labor and every 15 minutes in the second stage of labor. If intermittent auscultation is used, the fetal heart rate should be auscultated and recorded every 30 minutes in the first stage of labor and every 15 minutes in the second stage of labor. In high-risk patients, the fetal heart rate should be evaluated every 15 minutes in the first stage of labor and every 5 minutes in the second stage of labor. When auscultation of the heart rate is nonreassuring and abnormalities are suspected, fetal heart rate should be monitored electronically.

■ MANAGEMENT

If abnormal fetal heart rate patterns suggestive of fetal distress are present, the following conservative steps should first be taken:

1. Place the patient in the lateral position

Placement of the patient in the lateral position displaces the uterus from the midline and relieves compression of the vena cava, resulting in increased blood return to the heart.

2. Administer supplemental oxygen

Oxygen should be administered at a flow rate of 8 to 10 L/min via a face mask. Although arterial PO_2 in the fetus is approximately one-fourth of the arterial PO_2 in the mother, fetal blood can deliver a large amount of oxygen from the placenta because of the high concentration of fetal hemoglobin and its high oxygen affinity. Supplemental oxygen will increase total blood oxygen content in the fetus by at least 30 to 40%.

3. Decrease uterine contractions

a. Discontinue oxytocin

Every uterine contraction is associated with a transient decrease in blood flow to the placenta, and subsequently the fetus. Therefore, if the patient is receiving oxytocin, discontinuation of the infusion will decrease both the intensity and the frequency of uterine contractions and increase uterine blood flow. Discontinuation of oxytocin is also the best treatment for uterine hyperstimulation and uterine hypertonus.

b. Administer a tocolytic agent

Tocolytic drugs such as terbutaline sulfate or magnesium sulfate can be administered to decrease both the intensity and the frequency of uterine contractions, regardless of whether the patient is receiving oxytocin.

(1) Terbutaline sulfate 0.25 mg subcutaneously once.

   If a decrease in uterine activity is not achieved in 15 to 30 minutes, a second dose can be administered.

(2) Magnesium sulfate 2.0 g IV over 10 minutes.

4. Correct maternal hypotension

Maternal hypotension can decrease uterine blood flow, which in turn can cause abnormal fetal heart rate patterns. Hypotension is often the result of conduction analgesia used during labor.

a. **Increase IV infusion rate.**

b. **Administer ephedrine sulfate 25 to 50 mg intramuscularly or IV.**

If the above steps do not resolve the abnormal fetal heart rate patterns, then the fetal status should be ascertained, as follows:

1. **Fetal scalp blood sampling**

Measurement of capillary blood pH can be used to identify a fetus with acidosis (Table 4–1). The cervix must be dilated at least 2 to 3 cm, and the membranes must be ruptured, to perform fetal scalp blood sampling. An endoscope with a light source is inserted into the vagina and is placed against the fetal scalp. The scalp is then wiped clean and coated with a silicone gel, which causes the fetal blood to form into globules. A punch incision is made, with a special blade, into the fetal scalp to a depth of approximately 2 mm, and the blood is collected with a heparinized glass capillary tube. If fetal capillary blood pH is >7.25, it is reassuring, and labor is allowed to proceed with continuous electronic monitoring of the fetal heart rate (Table 4–2). If the pH range is 7.20 to 7.25, the fetal scalp blood sampling should be repeated within approximately 30 minutes, depending on the subsequent fetal heart rate tracing. If the fetal heart rate pattern becomes more ominous, then fetal scalp sampling should be repeated sooner. If the fetal heart rate pattern becomes normal, then fetal scalp sampling can be delayed. If the pH is <7.20, the fetus should be delivered either immediately or after a repeated fetal scalp sampling performed immediately shows that acidemia is still present.

2. **Fetal scalp stimulation test**

If fetal scalp sampling is not possible, fetal scalp stimulation

Table 4–1 □ INDICATIONS FOR FETAL SCALP BLOOD SAMPLING

Absent or decreased short-term variability
Late decelerations persistent for more than 10 minutes
Persistent, severe variable decelerations
Sinusoidal heart rate pattern
Heart rate patterns nonreassuring due to difficulties in interpretation

Table 4–2 □ FETAL SCALP BLOOD VALUES IN LABOR*

	Early First Stage	Late First Stage	Second Stage
pH	7.33 ± 0.03	7.32 = 0.02	7.29 ± 0.04
P_{CO_2} (mm Hg)	44 ± 4.05	42 = 5.1	46.3 ± 4.2
P_{O_2} (mm Hg)	21.8 ± 2.6	21.3 = 2.1	16.5 ± 1.4
Bicarbonate (mmol/L)	20.1 ± 1.2	19.1 = 2.1	17 ± 2
Base excess (mmol/L)	3.9 ± 1.9	4.1 = 2.5	6.4 ± 1.8

*Mean ± standard deviation.
From Creasy RK, Resnik R: Maternal Fetal Medicine: Principles and Practice, 3rd ed. Philadelphia, WB Saunders Co, 1994, p 352. Abstracted from Huch R, Huch A: In: Beard RW, Nathanielsz PW, eds: Fetal Physiology and Medicine. New York, Marcel Dekker Inc, 1984.

can be performed instead. Acceleration of the fetal heart rate, in response to pinching of the fetal scalp with a surgical instrument such as an Allis clamp, is almost always associated with a normal scalp blood pH. However, the converse is not always true. Absence of an acceleration is not always associated with fetal acidemia.

If there is evidence of fetal acidemia, the fetus should be delivered immediately. This can be done by either cesarean delivery or, when possible, vaginal delivery assisted by forceps or vacuum extraction if the patient is in the second stage of labor. **When nonreassuring fetal heart rate patterns are present without fetal acidemia in the second stage of labor, vaginal delivery should be performed if it can be accomplished safely.**

5

ABNORMAL LABOR

■ BACKGROUND AND DEFINITIONS

Basic Labor

Labor: Uterine contractions that result in progressive effacement and dilatation of the cervix

Dystocia: Abnormally slow labor or difficult delivery

Latent phase of labor: From onset of regular uterine contractions to the beginning of the active phase of labor

Active phase of labor: From the onset of rapid cervical dilatation, usually 3 to 4 cm, to full dilatation

First stage of labor: From the onset of labor to full cervical dilatation; also referred to as 10 cm of cervical dilatation

Second stage of labor: From full cervical dilatation to delivery of the infant

Third stage of labor: From delivery of the infant to delivery of the placenta

The latent phase of labor begins when the patient notices the onset of regular uterine contractions. During this phase of labor, a small amount of cervical dilatation may occur, but the predominant changes are cervical softening and effacement. The latent phase of labor ends when criteria for the active phase of labor are fulfilled, based on extent of cervical dilatation and rate of dilatation. This usually occurs after the cervix has dilated to 3 to 4 cm. In the active phase of labor, nulliparous patients should dilate at the rate of ≥ 1.2 cm/hr, and multiparous patients should dilate at the rate of ≥ 1.5 cm/hr (Table 5–1). The duration of the second stage of labor varies from 2 hours in nulliparous patients

Table 5–1 □ NORMAL DURATION OF THE STAGES OF LABOR

Stages of Labor	Nullipara	Multipara
First stage		
Latent phase	≤ 20 hr	≤ 14 hr
Active phase	5–8 hr	2–5 hr
Rate of dilatation	≥ 1.2 cm/hr	≥ 1.5 cm/hr
Second stage	≤ 2 hr	≤ 1 hr
Third stage	≤ 30 min	≤ 30 min

to 1 hour in multiparous patients. The third stage of labor can last 30 minutes in both nulliparous and multiparous patients.

Abnormal Labor

Prolonged latent phase of labor: Latent phase lasts >20 hours in a nulliparous patient or >14 hours in a parous patient

Protracted active phase dilatation: Rate of cervical dilatation is <1.2 cm/hr in a nulliparous patient or <1.5 cm/hr in a parous patient

Arrest of dilatation: No cervical dilatation in 2 hours in the active phase of labor

Protracted descent: Rate of descent of the fetus is <1 cm/hr in a nulliparous patient or <2 cm/hr in a parous patient

Arrest of descent: No descent of the fetus in 1 hour

Prolonged latent phase of labor is encountered in approximately 3 to 4% of patients and is not usually associated with an increase in maternal or fetal morbidity or mortality. Abnormalities in the active phase of labor are the most common types of labor abnormalities. Approximately 25% of nulliparous labors and 15% of multiparous labors are complicated by an abnormality in the active phase of labor.

■ CLINICAL PRESENTATION

Patients with abnormal labor cannot be distinguished from patients with normal labor based on clinical findings. They can be distinguished only by differences in their labor curves. A labor curve can be drawn by simply plotting cervical dilatation and descent of the fetal presenting part against time. Figure 5–1 shows a normal labor curve.

■ PHONE CALL

Questions

1. **What type(s) of labor abnormality does the patient exhibit on her labor curve?**
2. **Is conduction analgesia being administered?**
   The use of conduction analgesia such as a lumbar epidural can prolong the latent phase of labor. It can also cause protracted descent because both the sensory and the motor blocks of conduction analgesia may interfere with the patient's ability to push in the second stage of labor.

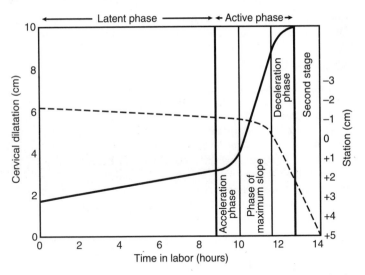

Figure 5–1 □ Normal labor curves. Solid line, cervical dilatation; dashed line, station. (Redrawn from Cohen WR, Friedman EA: Management of Labor. Gaithersburg, MD, Aspen Publishers, Inc, 1983, p 13.)

Orders

1. Start intravenous (IV) oxytocin infusion if the uterine contractions are clearly inadequate
2. Prepare the patient for placement of an intrauterine pressure monitor if suboptimal uterine contractions are suspected
3. Type and crossmatch for 2 units of blood if cesarean section is anticipated

Degree of Urgency

The patient and her labor curve should be evaluated as soon as possible, but the patient does not need to be seen immediately if there is no evidence of fetal distress.

■ ELEVATOR THOUGHTS

What factors are associated with the prolonged latent phase of labor?
- Excessive sedation
- Excessive or early administration of conduction anesthesia
- Unfavorable cervical status: cervix is undilated, uneffaced, and firm

What are the causes of abnormal labor?
- Abnormalities of the fetus
    Macrosomia
    Malpresentation
    Congenital anomalies
- Abnormalities of the maternal pelvis
    An abnormally small or contracted pelvis can result in cephalopelvic disproportion (CPD), which in turn causes abnormal labor. The same is true with a normal pelvis when the fetus is macrosomic.
- Abnormalities of the expulsive forces
    Inadequate uterine contractions
        Contractions of inadequate strength
        Contractions of inadequate frequency
    Inadequate pushing effort in the second stage of labor
- Abnormalities of the uterus, cervix, vagina, or vulva
    Uterine leiomyomata (fibroids)
    Cervical stenosis
    Vaginal septum
    Extensive vulvar condylomata acuminata

■ MAJOR THREAT TO FETAL LIFE

- Fetal asphyxia
    In rare cases, prolonged or arrested labor is associated with fetal distress.

■ MAJOR THREAT TO MATERNAL LIFE

- Hemorrhage and hypovolemic shock
    If abnormal labor is ignored, uterine rupture can occur, resulting in hemorrhage and in significant maternal and fetal morbidity. Prolonged labor is associated with an increased risk of postpartum uterine atony, resulting in postpartum hemorrhage and, possibly, in hypovolemic shock.

■ BEDSIDE

Quick Look Test

Does the patient appear to be having adequate uterine contractions?
    If the patient has not already received analgesia, her level of discomfort is often a good indicator of the quality of her uterine contractions. Although it is not as helpful as internal uterine

pressure monitoring, external uterine monitor tracing can also be used to evaluate quickly the quality and the frequency of a patient's uterine contractions.

What is the estimated fetal weight?

Patients with large fetuses are at greater risk for CPD, which is manifested by abnormal labor.

If the patient is pushing in the second stage of labor, is she pushing with adequate effort?

A patient who is exhausted or has excessive sensory and motor nerve block from conduction anesthesia will often not push adequately.

Are there any abnormal fetal heart rate patterns that suggest fetal distress?

Management of some types of abnormal labor is expectant as long as fetal distress is not suspected.

Vital Signs

Vital signs are usually normal.

Selective History and Chart Review

1. Has the patient given birth previously, and if so, what was that infant's birth weight and method of delivery?

   The birth weights of previous infants delivered vaginally can provide information concerning the adequacy of the patient's pelvis. Previous abnormal labor resulting in cesarean delivery of an infant with a normal birth weight suggests a small maternal pelvis.

2. Was the patient's prior pregnancy complicated by abnormal labor?

   Certain causes of abnormal labor, such as small pelvis and poor expulsive forces due to either inadequate uterine contractions or poor pushing in the second stage of labor, may exist in subsequent pregnancies.

3. Does the patient have diabetes mellitus?

   Diabetes mellitus and gestational diabetes can cause fetal macrosomia.

4. Does the patient have an abnormality of the birth canal that predisposes to abnormal labor, such as cervical stenosis, uterine leiomyomata, or a vaginal septum?

Selective Physical Examination

Abdominal   The fetus should be palpated for estimated birth weight.

Pelvic

External genitalia and vagina — Vaginal and vulvar lesions, such as vaginal septum and extensive condylomata acuminata, can cause abnormal labor by obstructing descent of the fetus.

Cervix — **Cervical dilatation** (cm), **effacement** (%), and the **station** of the presenting fetal part, in relation to the ischial spine of the maternal pelvis ($"-x"$ or $"+x"$), should be determined by digital examination. A station of $-x$ means that the presenting fetal part is x cm above the level of the ischial spine, and $+x$ means that the presenting fetal part is x cm below the level of the ischial spine. **Fetal position**, which refers to the relationship between a point on the fetal presenting part and the maternal pelvis, should also be determined. This point is the fetal occiput, chin, and sacrum, for vertex, face, and breech presentations, respectively. Figure 5–2 illustrates fetal positions for vertex, face, and breech presentations.

Uterus and adnexae — Palpation of the uterus should be performed to determine the strength and the frequency of uterine contractions. Examination will also reveal uterine leiomyomata and ovarian masses, which might cause abnormal labor by obstructing descent of the fetus.

■ DIAGNOSTIC TESTING

The diagnosis of abnormal labor is based on an abnormal labor curve. Diagnostic tests may help in determining the cause(s) of abnormal labor.

1. Ultrasound examination

Ultrasound examination can be used to diagnose some of the fetal causes of dystocia. Fetal measurements can provide an estimated fetal weight and can thereby help in diagnosis of macrosomia. Abnormal fetal presentation and congenital anomalies can also be diagnosed by ultrasound, as can some uterine and ovarian causes of abnormal labor, such as leiomyomata and ovarian masses.

2. Internal uterine pressure monitor

Manual palpation of the uterus and external uterine monitoring can help determine the adequacy of uterine contractions.

Left Occipito-Anterior	Left Occipito-Transverse	Left Occipito-Posterior

Right Occipito-Anterior	Right Occipito-Transverse	Right Occipito-Posterior

Left Sacro-Anterior	Right Sacro-Anterior	Right Sacro-Posterior

Figure 5–2 □ Fetal positions. *A*, Left positions in occiput presentations, with the fetal head viewed from below. *B*, Right positions in occiput presentations. *C*, Left and right positions in breech presentations. (From Pritchard JA, MacDonald PC: Williams' Obstetrics, 16th ed. East Norwalk, CT, Appleton-Century-Crofts, 1980.)

However, internal uterine pressure monitoring is superior, because it provides quantitative measurements of both the strength and the frequency of uterine contractions (Fig. 5–3). Adequate uterine contractions reach an amplitude at least 25 mm Hg above the resting or baseline pressure and occur at a frequency of not less than every 4 to 5 minutes.

An alternative means of measuring uterine contractions is by Montevideo units. Montevideo units are calculated by subtracting the baseline uterine pressure from the peak uterine pressure, for each contraction in a 10-minute period as measured by an internal uterine pressure catheter, and by adding these pressure differences (Fig. 5–4). Adequate labor usually generates 95 to 395 Montevideo units.

The following two criteria must be met before arrest of dilatation can be diagnosed: (1) The patient must have com-

Figure 5–3 □ Intrauterine pressure monitoring. (From Hacker NF, Moore JG: Essentials of Obstetrics and Gynecology, 2nd ed. Philadelphia, WB Saunders Co, 1992, p 252.)

pleted the latent phase of labor and have cervical dilatation ≥4 cm, and (2) a uterine contraction pattern attaining ≥200 Montevideo units must be present for ≥2 hours without change in cervical dilatation.

3. Pelvimetry

Radiographic pelvimetry can be performed by either conventional x-ray or computed tomography (CT) scan to determine adequacy of the bony pelvis. The anteroposterior and transverse diameters of the pelvic inlet and of the midpelvis are measured (Fig. 5–5). The minimum diameters are listed in Table 5–2. Pelvimetry is currently used in patients with breech presentations of the fetus, but it is rarely used in patients with vertex presentations of the fetus. For vertex presentations, adequacy of the patient's pelvis is determined by allowing labor to proceed and by ruling out other causes of abnormal labor if such labor is encountered.

■ MANAGEMENT

1. Prolonged latent phase of labor
   a. Rest and sedation
      (1) **Morphine sulfate 10 to 15 mg intramuscularly (IM) every 4 hours** or
      (2) **Meperidine hydrochloride (Demerol) 50 to 100 mg IM every 4 hours** or
      (3) **Pentobarbital sodium (Nembutal) 100 mg capsule by mouth**

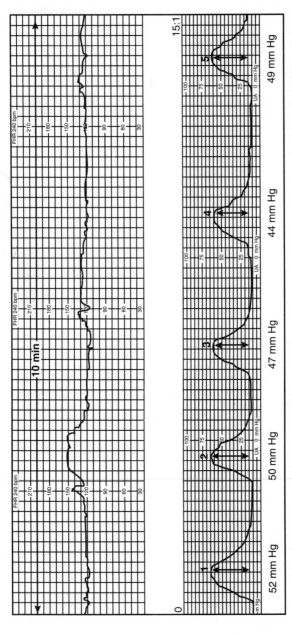

Figure 5–4 □ Calculation of Montevideo units. Montevideo units are calculated by subtracting the baseline uterine pressure from the peak contraction pressure for each contraction in a 10-minute window and adding the pressures generated by each contraction. In the example shown, five contractions occurred, producing pressure changes of 52, 50, 47, 44, and 49 mm Hg, respectively. The sum of these five contractions is 242 Montevideo units. (Redrawn from American College of Obstetricians and Gynecologists: Dystocia. Technical Bulletin No. 137. Washington, DC, ACOG, © 1989.)

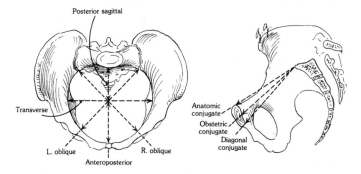

Figure 5–5 □ Pelvic inlet diameters. (From Hacker NF, Moore JG: Essentials of Obstetrics and Gynecology, 2nd ed. Philadelphia, WB Saunders Co, 1992, p 113.)

Because most patients with prolonged latent phases are exhausted and frustrated, rest and sedation can be therapeutic. Most patients will wake up refreshed and in active labor. This conservative management is appropriate only if the fetal heart rate pattern is reassuring.

b. Oxytocin IV infusion

An alternative to rest and sedation is infusion of oxytocin by IV to induce labor. This management has been called "active management of labor" and can be used in any patient, but it is absolutely indicated for a patient with a nonreassuring fetal heart rate pattern.

2. Protracted active phase dilatation or **protracted descent**

Protracted labor abnormalities can be managed expectantly if the patient is stable and there is no evidence of fetal distress. Uterine contractions should be optimized.

a. Oxytocin IV infusion

Oxytocin should be infused if uterine contractions have an amplitude of less than 25 mm Hg above the resting pressure or occur at a frequency of less than every 4 to 5 minutes. A solution of **10 IU oxytocin in 1000 ml of 5% dextrose and lactated Ringer's solution,** or in 1000 ml of

Table 5–2 □ **NORMAL PELVIMETRY MEASUREMENTS**

	Anteroposterior Diameter (cm)	Transverse Diameter (cm)
Pelvic inlet	≥10.5	≥11.5
Midpelvis	≥11.5	≥10.0

5% dextrose and 0.5 normal saline, is used. This solution has an oxytocin concentration of 10 mIU/ml and is infused starting at a rate of 0.1 ml/min or 1 mIU/min and is increased until regular uterine contractions are achieved. The infusion rate is increased by 1 mIU/min every 20 to 30 minutes, to a dose of 8 mIU/min. After this dose, the rate can be increased in increments of 2 mIU/min every 20 to 30 minutes, to a dose of 20 mIU/min. If higher doses are required, it should be remembered that oxytocin has an antidiuretic effect, and high doses given over a prolonged period of time can cause water intoxication. These patients should, therefore, have fluids restricted, and oxytocin should be administered in a more concentrated solution to restrict fluids further.

3. Arrest of dilatation or arrest of descent

When protracted labor abnormalities are encountered, uterine contractions should be optimized in amplitude and frequency if they are inadequate.

a. Oxytocin IV infusion

The oxytocin infusion described above should be administered if uterine contractions are inadequate.

b. Cesarean section

If a patient has arrest of dilatation or arrest of descent, despite the presence of adequate uterine contractions, a cesarean section should be performed. Operative vaginal delivery can be attempted in patients with complete cervical dilatation.

c. Operative vaginal delivery

If the patient has reached complete cervical dilatation but has arrest of descent, despite the presence of adequate uterine contractions, operative vaginal delivery with forceps or with vacuum assistance should be considered if it can be performed safely. The safety of operative vaginal delivery depends on estimated fetal size, station of the vertex, position, skill of the operator, and fetal status. If operative vaginal delivery cannot be done safely, then a cesarean section should be performed.

6

AMNIOTIC FLUID EMBOLISM

■ BACKGROUND AND DEFINITION

Amniotic fluid embolism: Entrance of amniotic fluid into the maternal circulation, resulting in hypoxemia, cardiovascular collapse, and disseminated intravascular coagulation (DIC)

Although it is a rare complication with an incidence rate of 1 in 7000 to 1 in 30,000 deliveries, amniotic fluid embolism comprises 4 to 10% of all maternal deaths. Amniotic fluid embolism usually occurs in the third trimester of pregnancy either during delivery or during the immediate postpartum period. However, it has also been encountered as early as in the first trimester, during suction curettage for pregnancy termination, and as late as several days postpartum. For amniotic fluid embolism to develop, there must first exist open endocervical or uterine veins, a tear through the fetal membranes, and enough of a pressure gradient to force amniotic fluid into the maternal circulation. The severity of this complication is directly related to the amount of debris and other particulate matter in the fluid, such as meconium, fetal lanugo, and fetal squamous cells. Amniotic fluid embolism results in a biphasic pattern of hemodynamic abnormalities. The first phase consists of **vasospasm of the pulmonary vasculature**, resulting in pulmonary hypertension, hypoxia, and right-side heart failure. In this initial phase, pulmonary hypertension develops from the shower of occlusive emboli that causes increased pulmonary vascular resistance. Pulmonary hypertension may also result from pulmonary vasoconstriction caused by a vasoactive substance in the amniotic fluid. This initial phase comprises 50% of maternal deaths in the first hour. The second phase consists of **left-side heart failure** with secondary elevation of pulmonary arterial pressure. Coagulopathy occurs in up to 40% of patients and is caused by the thromboplastin effects of trophoblasts.

■ CLINICAL PRESENTATION

Sudden onset of dyspnea
Cyanosis
Hypotension out of proportion to blood loss
Seizures
Hemorrhage
Patient often states that she feels she is going to die

■ PHONE CALL

Questions

1. How ill does the patient appear?

Although severe cases are often lethal, milder and sublethal cases have been reported. In these cases, the patient's symptoms are self-limiting, and with supportive care, survival is the rule.

Orders

1. Order complete blood count (CBC)
2. Order platelet count
3. Order serum fibrinogen level
4. Order fibrin split products
5. Prepare for placement of a pulmonary artery catheter (Swan-Ganz catheter)
6. Place the patient on oxygen supplementation at a flow rate of 8 to 10 L/min via a face mask
7. Insert Foley catheter
8. Type and crossmatch for whole blood or packed red blood cells
9. Order fresh frozen plasma

Degree of Urgency

Amniotic fluid embolism is one of the most catastrophic conditions encountered in obstetrics. Patients should be seen immediately.

■ ELEVATOR THOUGHTS

What factors predispose for amniotic fluid embolism?
- Tumultuous labor
- Use of oxytocin
- Advanced maternal age
- Multiparity

What other obstetrical complications can mimic amniotic fluid embolism?
- Placental abruption
- Preeclampsia

  Placental abruption can also result in hypovolemic shock out of proportion to the amount of visible bleeding. Preeclampsia can lead to eclampsia or seizures. Both placental abruption and severe preeclampsia can cause disseminated intravascular coagulation.

■ MAJOR THREAT TO FETAL LIFE

- Fetal asphyxia

  If amniotic fluid embolism occurs before delivery, maternal

hypoxia and cardiovascular collapse can result in fetal asphyxia and fetal death.

■ MAJOR THREAT TO MATERNAL LIFE

- Hypoxia
- Hypovolemic shock
- Cardiac failure
- DIC

Overall, amniotic fluid embolism has a maternal mortality rate
of approximately 85%.

■ BEDSIDE

Quick Look Test

Has the patient suffered cardiorespiratory arrest?
  Cardiopulmonary resuscitation should be initiated immediately in patients who have had cardiorespiratory arrest.

Vital Signs

Hypotension out of proportion to bleeding may occur.
Cardiorespiratory arrest may be encountered.

Selective History and Chart Review

1. Does the patient have any other obstetrical complications,
   such as placental abruption and severe preeclampsia, that
   might mimic amniotic fluid embolism?
2. Has the patient's labor been complicated by meconium passage?
     Amniotic fluid embolism is much more catastrophic in the
   presence of thick meconium.

Selective Physical Examination

General	Cyanotic, often unconscious and unresponsive. Patients will almost always suffer cardio-respiratory arrest.
	Bleeding from IV and venipuncture sites if DIC has developed
Abdominal	Normal
Pelvic	
External genitalia and vagina	Bleeding may be present if the patient has developed DIC
Cervix	Normal for the intrapartum or postpartum pe-

| | riod. Heavy bleeding from the cervix may be present if the patient has developed DIC. |
| Uterus and adnexae | Normal for the intrapartum or postpartum period |

■ DIAGNOSTIC TESTING

The diagnosis of amniotic fluid embolism is made by the patient's clinical presentation. The diagnosis can often be confirmed retrospectively in two ways.

1. **Smear of buffy coat suspension of central blood**

   Blood should be obtained from the pulmonary artery via the Swan-Ganz catheter, and a smear of the buffy coat of the aspirated blood should be made. Special stains can be used to help identify fetal squamous cells and fat cells. Standard staining with hematoxylin and eosin may not reveal these diagnostic findings. Instead, special stains, such as Alcian blue stain and others that stain for acid mucopolysaccharide, keratin, and fat, must be used.

2. **Autopsy**

   In women who die from amniotic fluid embolism, fetal squamous cells and fat cells can be found on autopsy not only in the lungs, but also in the vascular systems of the uterus, heart, brain, kidneys, and ovaries. As is true with blood smears, hematoxylin and eosin stains may be insufficient for diagnosis.

■ MANAGEMENT

Treatment of a patient with amniotic fluid embolism has the following three general goals: oxygenation of the patient, maintenance of cardiac output and blood pressure, and treatment of coagulopathy.

1. **Perform cardiopulmonary resuscitation.**

   Cardiopulmonary resuscitation (CPR) should be initiated immediately if the patient has suffered cardiorespiratory arrest.

2. **Intubate and oxygenate the patient.**

   The patient should be intubated and given 100% oxygen if she has had respiratory arrest.

3. **Place pulmonary artery catheter (Swan-Ganz catheter).**

   A pulmonary artery catheter provides the intensive hemodynamic monitoring necessary for maintenance of cardiac output and blood pressure. Normal hemodynamic measurements obtained by pulmonary artery catheter are listed in Table 6–1.

Table 6–1 □ **NORMAL CENTRAL HEMODYNAMIC MEASUREMENTS IN NONPREGNANT AND PREGNANT PATIENTS**

	Nonpregnant	Pregnant
Cardiac output (L/min)	4.3 ± 0.9	6.2 ± 1.0
Heart rate (beats/min)	71 ± 10.0	83 ± 10.0
Systemic vascular resistance (dyne $\times$ cm $\times$ sec^{-5})	1530 ± 520	1210 ± 266
Pulmonary vascular resistance (dyne $\times$ cm $\times$ sec^{-5})	119 ± 47.0	78 ± 22
Colloid oncotic pressure (mm Hg)	20.8 ± 1.0	18.0 ± 1.5
Colloid oncotic pressure–pulmonary capillary wedge pressure (mm Hg)	14.5 ± 2.5	10.5 ± 2.7
Mean arterial pressure (mm Hg)	86.4 ± 7.5	90.3 ± 5.8
Pulmonary capillary wedge pressure (mm Hg)	6.3 ± 2.1	7.5 ± 1.8
Central venous pressure (mm Hg)	3.7 ± 2.6	3.6 ± 2.5
Left ventricular stroke work index (g $\times$ m $\times$ m^{-2})	41 ± 8	48 ± 6

From Clark SL, Cotton DB, Lee W, et al: Central hemodynamic assessment of normal term pregnancy. Am J Obstet Gynecol 1989;161:1439.

4. **Treat cardiogenic shock.**
   a. **Infusion of IV fluids**
      Fluid resuscitation will improve cardiac output by increasing preload.
   b. **Dopamine 5 μg/kg/min by IV infusion, with dose increases of 5 μg/kg/min to a maximum of 50 μg/mg/min**
      Dopamine, a vasoactive amine, has a positive inotropic effect and increases both myocardial contractility and heart rate. Dopamine also increases organ perfusion by vasodilation of renal, mesenteric, coronary, and cerebral vasculatures. The dose is monitored by Swan-Ganz catheter measurements of pulmonary artery and wedge pressure.
5. **Treat coagulopathy and blood loss.**
   a. **Red blood cells**
      Red blood cells (RBCs) are transfused to increase oxygen-carrying capacity in anemic patients. Each unit of packed red blood cells and of whole blood has a volume of 250 and 450 ml, respectively. Each unit of RBCs should increase the hematocrit by 3% and the hemoglobin by 1 g/dl. Coagulation studies should be obtained after every 5 to 10 units of RBCs transfused.
   b. **Platelets**
      Platelets are transfused for a patient with a platelet count of $<20,000/mm^3$ or for a patient with a platelet count of $<50,000/mm^3$ in whom a cesarean section is planned. Each

unit of platelets should increase the platelet count by 5000 to 10,000/mm³.

c. **Fresh frozen plasma**

Fresh frozen plasma is transfused for coagulopathy due to a deficiency of clotting factors, usually manifested by a prothrombin time (PT) or partial thromboplastin time (PTT) that is >1.5 times normal. Each unit of fresh frozen plasma will increase any clotting factor by 2 to 3%. The usual initial dose is 2 units, and each unit has a volume of 200 to 250 ml.

d. **Cryoprecipitate**

Cryoprecipitate is transfused for coagulopathy due to deficiency of factor VIII, von Willebrand factor, factor XIII, fibrinogen, and/or fibronectin. Cryoprecipitate is concentrated from fresh frozen plasma, and each bag has a volume of 10 to 15 ml. Each bag contains at least 150 mg of fibrinogen.

6. **Perform electronic fetal monitoring.**

Amniotic fluid embolism is often accompanied by fetal asphyxia, and therefore, continuous electronic fetal monitoring should be used to follow the fetal status. If the patient has attained complete cervical dilatation, operative vaginal delivery should be performed if it can be accomplished quickly and safely. Delivery will benefit the fetus and will furthermore facilitate efforts to resuscitate the mother. If the cervix is not completely dilated and delivery can be accomplished only by cesarean section, the gestational age and the status of the fetus, the condition of the mother, and the effects of the cesarean section on the mother must all be considered in making the decision to perform surgery.

7

FETAL DEATH

■ BACKGROUND AND DEFINITIONS

Fetal death, intrauterine fetal demise (IUFD), or **stillbirth:** No signs of life present at or after birth in fetuses beyond 20 weeks of gestational age

Neonatal death: The death of a live-born infant before 29 days of life

Perinatal mortality rate: The sum of fetal and neonatal deaths per 1000 total births

The fetal death rate in the United States in 1992 was 7.4 per 1000 total births, representing over one-half the perinatal mortality rate, which was 12.8 per 1000 total births. Most states require the reporting of fetal death after 20 weeks of gestation, and many states require the recording of birth weight. The major risk of fetal demise for the mother is consumptive coagulopathy, presumably caused by the release of thromboplastin from the dead fetus and the placenta. This complication occurs rarely before 1 month after fetal death, and even then, the incidence of coagulopathy is only approximately 25%.

■ CLINICAL PRESENTATION

Absence of fetal movement detected by the patient
Absence of fetal cardiac activity as recorded by auscultation with a fetoscope or by Doppler monitoring

■ PHONE CALL

Questions

1. **What attempts have been made to document fetal cardiac activity?**
   Fetal cardiac activity is not usually detected by auscultation with a fetoscope until after 20 weeks of gestational age. Furthermore, fetal movement is not usually felt by the mother until after 20 weeks.
2. **Was the patient being monitored while in active labor when fetal heart tones were lost?**
   The loss of fetal heart tones during labor is usually caused

by movement of the patient that displaces the monitoring device, rather than by fetal death, especially in the absence of abnormal fetal heart rate patterns.

3. Does the patient have any bleeding suggesting the presence of coagulopathy?

Orders

1. Obtain a complete blood count (CBC) with differential
2. Obtain coagulation studies: prothrombin time (PT), partial thromboplastin time (PTT), platelet count, fibrinogen, fibrin split products
3. Obtain serum glucose
4. Obtain a Kleihauer–Betke stain of maternal blood
5. Obtain a Venereal Disease Research Laboratory (VDRL) test
6. Obtain blood type and Rh
7. Obtain antibody screen

Degree of Urgency

Fetal death is not life threatening to the patient unless she has disseminated intravascular coagulation (DIC). Nevertheless, patients are extremely anxious when confronted with the possibility of fetal demise, and therefore, the patient should be seen as soon as possible.

■ ELEVATOR THOUGHTS

What characteristics of the patient and the pregnancy are associated with an increased risk of fetal death?
- Multiple gestation
- Young maternal age
- Advanced maternal age
- Unmarried status
- Male fetal gender

What are the most common causes of fetal death?
1. Maternal conditions
   - Diabetes mellitus
   - Chronic hypertension
   - Pregnancy-induced hypertension
   - Viral and bacterial infections
     Cytomegalovirus
     Listeria monocytogenes
     Syphilis
   - Rh isoimmunization
   - Phospholipid antibodies or lupus anticoagulant

Also referred to as anticardiolipin antibodies, these phospholipid antibodies cause increased coagulation and are associated with an increased risk for both spontaneous abortion and fetal death.
  - Thyroid disease
2. Fetal disease
  - Congenital abnormalities
    As many as 35% of fetal deaths are associated with congenital abnormalities.
3. Placental, umbilical cord, and uterine complications
  - Placenta previa
  - Placental abruption
  - Prolapsed umbilical cord
  - Umbilical cord knot
  - Uterine rupture
4. Fetal–maternal hemorrhage
  Fetal–maternal hemorrhage is found in 3 to 5% of all fetal deaths. Fetal–maternal hemorrhage is detected by Kleihauer–Betke staining of a blood smear of peripheral maternal blood.

■ MAJOR THREAT TO MATERNAL LIFE

  - Hemorrhage secondary to DIC

■ BEDSIDE

Quick Look Test

Does the patient appear to be bleeding?
  Bleeding may be a result of placental abruption, placenta previa, uterine rupture, or DIC.

Is the patient having pelvic pain consistent with placental abruption or uterine rupture?

Does the patient appear to be ill from a systemic infection?

Vital Signs

Vital signs are usually normal unless the patient has developed hypovolemic shock with hypotension and tachycardia from blood loss secondary to coagulopathy, placental abruption, or placenta previa.

Selective History and Chart Review

1. What is the gestational age?
   The gestational age will determine the method of delivery.

2. Does the patient have any of the medical conditions that are associated with an increased risk of fetal death, i.e., diabetes mellitus, chronic hypertension, pregnancy-induced hypertension, systemic bacterial or viral infection, or Rh isoimmunization?
3. Does the patient have a history of fetal losses?
    Patients with multiple pregnancy losses are more likely to have a recurrent cause. Causes of recurrent pregnancy loss include chromosomal abnormalities in the mother or the father or both, chronic medical conditions such as diabetes and hypertension, and the presence of circulating phospholipid antibodies.

Selective Physical Examination

Fetal death is often asymptomatic.

Abdominal	Usually negative
	Tenderness with placental abruption or uterine rupture
Pelvic	Usually negative
External genitalia, vagina, and cervix	Bleeding from placental abruption, placenta previa, or uterine rupture
Uterus and adnexae	Usually normal
	Uterine tenderness with placental abruption or uterine rupture

■ DIAGNOSTIC TESTING

1. Ultrasound examination
    Real-time ultrasound examination is used to detect fetal cardiac activity. The absence of cardiac activity is diagnostic of fetal death.

■ MANAGEMENT

Management of a patient with fetal death has three goals. First is safe and timely delivery of the fetus. Timely delivery is especially important because of the emotional trauma associated with fetal death. Second is appropriate support throughout the grieving process for the patient and her partner. And third is an investigation to determine the cause of fetal death.

1. Delivery of the fetus
    Approximately 80 to 90% of patients who have suffered a fetal death will begin spontaneous labor within 2 weeks. The

time between fetal death and onset of labor, however, increases proportionately with the degree of prematurity of the fetus.

a. Vaginal prostaglandin E_2 (PGE$_2$) suppositories

In pregnancies of <28 weeks' duration, delivery can be facilitated by PGE$_2$ 20-mg suppositories inserted into the vagina every 4 hours until the patient begins to labor. Side effects of PGE$_2$ include diarrhea, fever, and vomiting, and therefore, administration of prophylactic medications should be considered.

b. Oxytocin IV infusion

Intravenous infusion of dilute oxytocin is a well-established and safe method for inducing labor, although it is less successful the more premature the fetus. A solution of **10 IU of oxytocin in 1000 ml of 5% dextrose and lactated Ringer's solution or in 1000 ml of 5% dextrose and 0.5 normal saline** is used. This solution has an oxytocin concentration of 10 mIU/ml and is infused, starting at a rate of 0.1 ml/min or 1 mIU/min, and is increased until regular uterine contractions are achieved. The infusion rate is increased by 1 mIU/min every 20 to 30 minutes, to a dose of 8 mIU/min. After this dose, the rate can be increased, in increments of 2 mIU/min every 20 to 30 minutes, to a dose of 20 mIU/min. If higher doses are required, patients should have their fluid intake restricted, and the oxytocin solution should be concentrated. These precautions should be taken because high doses of oxytocin can result in water intoxication due to the antidiuretic effect of oxytocin.

If cervical dilatation and delivery are not accomplished despite the prolonged use of either PGE$_2$ suppositories or IV oxytocin, ectopic pregnancy and especially abdominal pregnancy should be considered.

2. Grief and emotional support

The classic grief reaction to a fetal death includes shock, guilt, anger, disorientation, and reorganization. All health care providers must recognize and meet the emotional needs of the parents and the family members going through the grieving process. It should be emphasized to patients that neither they nor their health care providers are to blame for most cases of fetal death. After the delivery of the fetus, the parents and the family members should be given the opportunity to hold the infant, to name the infant, and to take something as a keepsake such as a lock of hair or the blanket with which the infant is wrapped. The parents should be given the opportunity to arrange for a funeral service. At the time of discharge from the hospital, patients should be given the telephone numbers of support groups that provide ongoing help.

3. **Investigation of the cause(s) of the fetal death**

All patients who have suffered a fetal death should have the following tests performed:

a. **Blood antibody screen**—The presence of a maternal blood group antibody can cause hemolytic disease of the fetus.

b. **Kleihauer-Betke stain of maternal blood**—Significant fetal–maternal hemorrhage is a cause of fetal death even in the absence of trauma.

c. **VDRL**—Congenital syphilis can result in fetal death.

d. **Serum glucose**—Poorly controlled diabetes mellitus can be complicated by fetal death.

e. **Urine toxicology screen**—Illicit drug use can cause fetal death.

Depending on the patient's history and the findings of the physical examination, some of the following tests might reveal the cause of fetal death:

f. **Cytomegalovirus acute and convalescent titers (immunoglobulins M and G)**

g. **Karyotype of fetal tissue**—A normal karyotype rules out a chromosomal abnormality and makes karyotyping of the parents unnecessary.

h. **Lupus anticoagulant or anticardiolipin antibody**

i. **Thyroid function tests**—Both hypothyroidism and hyperthyroidism have been associated with fetal death.

j. **Cultures for *Listeria monocytogenes***—Maternal blood and placental cultures are the best tests for ruling out listeriosis.

8

HYPERTENSIVE DISORDERS

■ BACKGROUND AND DEFINITIONS

Hypertensive disorders in pregnancy are responsible for approximately 12% of all maternal mortality. The classifications of hypertensive disorders associated with pregnancy are as follows:

Preeclampsia and eclampsia
Chronic or pre-existent hypertension
Preeclampsia superimposed on chronic hypertension
Transient hypertension
Unclassified hypertension

Pregnancy-induced hypertension: A more general term that refers to all of the above disorders except chronic or pre-existent hypertension.

Toxemia of pregnancy: An old term for hypertensive disorders of pregnancy and other obstetrical disorders including liver disease and hyperemesis gravidarum.

Preeclampsia: A disorder unique to pregnancy and characterized by vasospasm that results in poor perfusion of vital organs including the placenta. The classic triad of clinical findings associated with preeclampsia consists of edema, hypertension, and proteinuria. This triad represents common signs of preeclampsia, not the causes of preeclampsia. Because impaired perfusion secondary to vasospasm is the underlying disease process, many organ systems including the kidneys, liver, and brain are affected by preeclampsia. Preeclampsia typically occurs after 20 weeks of gestation and has an incidence of approximately 5 to 7%. It usually occurs before labor but can also occur in the intrapartum or postpartum period. Preeclampsia can be present in either a mild form or a severe form. The cause of this disease is unknown.

Eclampsia: The occurrence of seizures in a patient with preeclampsia and no other condition that causes seizures. As is the case with preeclampsia, eclampsia can occur in the prepartum, intrapartum, or postpartum period.

Chronic or pre-existent hypertension: Hypertension that is diagnosed either before 20 weeks of gestation or after 42 days postpartum. This term is also used to refer to hypertension that existed before pregnancy.

Preeclampsia superimposed on chronic hypertension: Preeclampsia that develops in a patient with chronic or pre-existent hypertension. The prognosis for patients with preeclampsia superimposed on chronic hypertension is often worse than the prognosis for patients with preeclampsia or chronic hypertension alone.

Transient hypertension: Hypertension that develops for the first time during pregnancy or in the first 24 hours postpartum without any other signs or symptoms of preeclampsia.

Unclassified hypertension: A term used for patients in whom there is insufficient information for another classification. This term should be used for only a small minority of patients.

■ CLINICAL PRESENTATION

1. Preeclampsia
   a. Hypertension
      (1) Increase in systolic blood pressure of ≥30 mm Hg, or in diastolic blood pressure of ≥15 mm Hg, over a baseline blood pressure taken before 20 weeks of gestation, or
      (2) Blood pressure of ≥140/90 if prior blood pressures are not known, or
      (3) Increase in mean arterial pressure of 20 mm Hg over a baseline pressure taken before 20 weeks, or
      (4) Mean arterial pressure of ≥105 if prior blood pressure is unknown

      Any of the above elevations in blood pressure must be recorded on at least two measurements taken at least 6 hours apart. Mean arterial pressure can be calculated by the following formula:

      Mean arterial pressure = diastolic blood pressure + (1/3 × pulse pressure)

      where

      pulse pressure = systolic blood pressure − diastolic blood pressure

   b. Edema
      Edema of the face and hands is more commonly associated with sodium retention and is therefore a more reliable indicator of preeclampsia than edema of the lower extremities, which is more commonly influenced by gravity. A weight gain of ≥5 lb in 1 week may also be a sign of impending preeclampsia. The presence of edema cannot be used alone as a diagnostic indicator of preeclampsia because 10 to 15% of normal pregnant women have edema of the face and hands.

   c. Proteinuria
      (1) Urine protein of ≥0.1 g/L in a random specimen, or
      (2) Urine protein of ≥0.3 g/L in a 24-hour urine collection

d. Central nervous system (CNS) symptoms
   (1) Headache, usually frontal and not relieved by analgesics
   (2) Mental confusion
   (3) Dizziness
   (4) Drowsiness
e. Visual symtoms
   (1) Blurred vision
   (2) Scotomata
   (3) Diplopia
   (4) Flashes of light in the visual field
   (5) Blindness
f. Gastrointestinal (GI) symptoms
   (1) Epigastric pain from distention of the hepatic capsule
   (2) Nausea
   (3) Vomiting
   (4) Hematemesis
g. Renal symptoms
   (1) Anuria
   (2) Oliguria
   (3) Hematuria

2. Severe preeclampsia
   a. Hypertension
      (1) Systolic blood pressure of $\geq$160 or diastolic blood pressure of $\geq$110 recorded on at least two occasions at least 6 hours apart
   b. Proteinuria
      (1) Urine protein of $\geq$5 g in a 24-hour collection
          This usually correlates with $3+$ or $4+$ on qualitative dipstick test.
   c. Oliguria
      (1) $\leq$500 ml in 24 hours
   d. CNS symptoms
   e. Visual symptoms
   f. Epigastric pain
   g. Pulmonary edema
   h. Thrombocytopenia
      (1) Platelet count <100,000/mm^3
   i. Intrauterine growth restriction
      (1) Manifested by low estimated fetal weight, abnormally low interval growth, or decreased amniotic fluid or oligohydramnios

3. Eclampsia
   a. Signs and symptoms of either mild or severe eclampsia
   b. Seizures
   c. Convulsions
   d. Common symptoms that precede eclampsia are listed in Table 8–1.

Table 8–1 □ **FREQUENCY OF SYMPTOMS THAT PRECEDE ECLAMPSIA**

Symptom	Percentage of Patients with Symptom (%)
Headache	83
Hyperreflexia	80
Proteinuria	80
Edema	60
Clonus	46
Visual signs	45
Epigastric pain	20

Adapted from Sibai BM, Lipshitz J, Anderson GD, Dilts PV Jr: Reassessment of intravenous MgSO₄ therapy in preclampsia-eclampsia. Obstet Gynecol 1981;57:199.

4. Chronic or pre-existing hypertension
  #### a. Hypertension
  (1) Blood pressure of ≥140/90 recorded before 20 weeks of gestation or after 42 days postpartum or documented before pregnancy.
5. Transient hypertension
  #### a. Hypertension
  (1) Blood pressure of ≥140/90 recorded transiently during pregnancy or in the first 24 hours postpartum without any signs or symptoms of preeclampsia.

■ PHONE CALL

Questions

1. **What is the patient's blood pressure?**
2. **What is the result of her urine dipstick test for qualitative protein?**
3. **Does the patient complain of epigastric or right upper quadrant pain?**

    These complaints are ominous because they may be caused by distention of the liver capsule.

4. **Does the patient complain of any neurological or visual symptoms?**

    Severe neurological or visual symptoms are indicative of poor perfusion of the central nervous system and possibly impending seizures.

5. **Does the patient have any signs of bleeding from any site?**

    Bleeding may be indicative of coagulopathy, which is associated with severe preeclampsia.

Orders

1. Obtain a complete blood count (CBC)
2. Perform urinalysis
3. Perform renal functions tests: serum creatinine, serum uric acid, and blood urea nitrogen (BUN)
4. Perform twenty-four-hour urine collection for protein and creatinine clearance
5. Perform liver function tests: serum glutamic-oxaloacetic transaminase (SGOT) and serum glutamic-pyruvic transaminase (SGPT)
6. Perform coagulation studies: platelet count, prothrombin time (PT), partial thromboplastin time (PTT), fibrinogen, fibrin split products
7. Check the patient's deep tendon reflexes

Degree of Urgency

Patients with chronic hypertension, transient hypertension, or mild preeclampsia should be seen as soon as possible. Mild preeclampsia can progress to severe preeclampsia quickly and without warning. Patients with severe preeclampsia must be seen immediately.

■ ELEVATOR THOUGHTS

What factors are associated with an increased risk of pre-eclampsia and eclampsia?
- Nulliparity
- Young maternal age
- Advanced maternal age
- Family history of preeclampsia or eclampsia
- Lower socioeconomic status

    Lower socioeconomic status has not been shown in all studies to be associated with a higher risk of preeclampsia, but it has been clearly shown to be associated with an increased risk of eclampsia.
- Diabetes mellitus
- Chronic or pre-existent hypertension
- Multiple pregnancy
- Hydatidiform mole

What complications can result from preeclampsia?
- Coagulopathy

    The cause of coagulopathy in patients with preeclampsia is unclear. Vascular damage caused by vasospasm may in turn cause DIC. Approximately 10% of patients with either preeclampsia or eclampsia develop DIC.

- Abnormal renal function
    The cause of renal dysfunction in patients with preeclampsia is probably the abnormal renal perfusion that is caused by vasospasm. Abnormal renal function can progress to renal failure.
- Placental abruption
- Eclampsia
- Hepatic rupture
    Distention of the liver capsule, hepatomegaly, liver tenderness, and abnormal liver function tests may be signs of impending hepatic rupture. The maternal mortality rate from hepatic rupture is close to 65%.
- HELLP syndrome
    Hemolysis, elevated liver enzymes, and low platelet count (HELLP) syndrome is a rare but morbid variant of preeclampsia and of eclampsia. It is usually found in multiparous patients in whom the gestational age of the fetus is less than 36 weeks. HELLP syndrome can be found in as many as 15% of all patients with preeclampsia or eclampsia. Conversely, approximately 50% of the patients with HELLP syndrome have severe preeclampsia, 30% have mild preeclampsia, and 20% are normotensive.

■ MAJOR THREAT TO FETAL LIFE

- Asphyxia from placental insufficiency secondary to vasospasm or placental abruption
- Prematurity
    Delivery of the infant is the only true cure for preeclampsia and eclampsia. The severity of preeclampsia and the development of eclampsia are often indications for delivery even at a premature gestational age.

■ MAJOR THREAT TO MATERNAL LIFE

- Hypovolemic shock from hemorrhage due to placental abruption, rupture of the liver, or DIC
- Eclampsia
- Stroke

■ BEDSIDE

Quick Look Test

How ill does the patient appear?

Does the patient have an altered mental status with confusion and drowsiness?

The patient who appears ill or toxemic and who has an altered mental status is at risk for the development of eclampsia.

Does the patient appear to be having abdominal or epigastric pain?

Both placental abruption and distention of the liver capsule can cause abdominal pain.

Vital Signs

The patient is hypertensive but otherwise has normal vital signs, unless rupture of the liver or placental abruption has occurred. These complications usually lead to hypovolemic shock with hypotension and tachycardia.

Selective History and Chart Review

1. Does the patient have a history of chronic hypertension?
2. If the patient has been pregnant before, did she develop preeclampsia or eclampsia during a previous pregnancy?
3. Has the patient had an ultrasound examination during the pregnancy to document gestational age and to rule out multiple gestations or hydatidiform mole?
4. Does the patient have a history of neurological problems including seizures?

Selective Physical Examination

General	Generalized edema including facial and hand edema
	Altered mental status with drowsiness or confusion
	Bleeding from IV and venipuncture sites if DIC develops
Fundoscopic	Narrowing and segmental spasms of the retinal arterioles
Abdominal	Tender if hepatic rupture or placental abruption develops
	Hepatomegaly or liver tenderness may be a sign of hepatic capsular distention and impending hepatic rupture
Pelvic	
External genitalia and vagina	Normal
	Vaginal bleeding if placental abruption or DIC develops
Cervix	Normal
Uterus and adnexae	Irritable, tender, and hard if placental abruption develops

Neurological	Hyperactive reflexes
	Clonus
	Seizures if eclampsia develops

■ DIAGNOSTIC TESTING FOR PREECLAMPSIA

1. **Ultrasound examination**

   Ultrasound examination should be performed to confirm the gestational age, to determine fetal presentation, and to rule out multiple gestation. Knowing the gestational age of the fetus is important for proper management of the patient with preeclampsia.

2. **Renal function tests**

   Serum creatinine: Elevated (normal, 0.5–1.0 mg/dl)

   BUN: Elevated (normal, 5–10 mg/dl)

   Serum uric acid: Elevated (normal, 3.0–5.5 mg/dl)

   24-hour urine collection for creatinine clearance: Decreased, <100 ml/min (normal, 130–150 ml/min; borderline, 100–129 ml/min)

   24-hour urine collection for total protein: Elevated (≥0.3 g/24 hr is found in mild preeclampsia; >5 g/24 hr is found in severe preeclampsia)

   Urinalysis: Proteinuria (3+ or 4+ proteinuria on a qualitative dipstick test is one criterion of severe preeclampsia)

3. **Liver function tests**

   SGOT or serum aspartate aminotransaminase (AST): Elevated (normal, 8–20 mU/ml)

   SGPT or serum alanine aminotransferase (ALT): Elevated (normal, 8–20 mU/ml)

4. **Hematology tests**

   Hematocrit: Elevated secondary to hemoconcentration

   Hemolysis may be noted on blood smear

5. **Coagulation studies**

   Platelet count: Decreased (normal, 140,000–440,000/mm^3)

   Serum fibrinogen: Decreased (normal, 300–600 mg/dl)

   PT: Increased (normal, 11–12 seconds)

   PTT: Increased (normal, 24–36 seconds)

   Fibrin D-dimer: Elevated (normal, <0.05 μg/ml)

■ MANAGEMENT OF PREECLAMPSIA

The optimal management for the mother is always delivery, because preeclampsia is reversible and begins to resolve after delivery. The goal of management for the mother is the prevention of eclampsia. When the fetus is considered, however, the risk of fetal prematurity must be weighed against the maternal and the fetal risks of continuing a preeclamptic pregnancy.

1. Decision to deliver

The decision to deliver the infant or to manage the patient expectantly is based on the degree of severity of the patient's preeclampsia and the gestational age of the fetus. The route of delivery is determined by the usual obstetrical factors and should not usually be influenced by preeclampsia. If the fetus is stable, a vaginal delivery is preferable to a cesarean birth, because it does not impose surgical stress on a patient who is already ill.

a. Severe preeclampsia—Deliver

Because severe preeclampsia is associated with a high risk of eclampsia, hepatic rupture, and significant morbidity and mortality, infants of patients with severe preeclampsia should be delivered regardless of gestational age.

b. Mild preeclampsia

(1) Term gestational age—Deliver

In term patients with mild preeclampsia, there is little to be gained by delaying delivery. If the gestational age of the fetus is 33 to 35 weeks, amniocentesis and phospholipid analysis for fetal lung maturity should be considered. If phospholipid analysis shows that lung maturity has been attained, the infant should be delivered.

(2) Premature gestational age—Expectant management

In the absence of fetal distress or severe intrauterine growth retardation, a preterm patient with mild preeclampsia can be managed expectantly. Because worsening of the disease is likely, both the mother and the infant should be monitored closely. Bedrest is commonly recommended but is only palliative and will only slow the progression of preeclampsia, rather than cure the disease. If both maternal and fetal conditions are stable, the patient should be seen at least once a week. If there is evidence that the preeclampsia is progressing, the patient should be seen more often, as frequently as every 2 days. Hospitalization of these patients should be considered for closer monitoring. In these patients, the following maternal parameters should be monitored:

(a) Blood pressure

(b) Urine output

(c) Daily weights

(d) Repeat renal functions tests: Urinalysis, serum creatinine, BUN, uric acid, 24-hour creatinine clearance, and 24-hour urine protein

(e) Repeat liver function tests: SGOT or AST, SGPT or ALT

(f) Repeat coagulation studies: Platelet count, PT, PTT, serum fibrinogen, fibrin split products

(g) Onset of epigastric pain

(h) Onset of neurological symptoms such as headaches or confusion; visual symptoms

The fetus should be monitored with the following tests:

(a) Nonstress testing or

(b) Contractions stress testing with either oxytocin-stimulated or breast-stimulation contractions

(c) Ultrasound examination

Ultrasound examination is used to follow interval fetal growth and the amount of amniotic fluid present, because intrauterine growth restriction associated with preeclampsia is often accompanied by oligohydramnios. The amount of amniotic fluid can be followed quantitatively by measuring the amniotic fluid (amniotic fluid index [AFI]). AFI is determined by adding the lengths of the largest vertical fluid pockets not containing umbilical cord, in each of the four quadrants of the uterus. Normal AFI measurements for different gestational ages are shown in Figure 8–1.

Because preeclampsia usually worsens gradually, the use of corticosteroids should be considered in order to accelerate fetal lung maturity if the fetus is very premature. Antepartum corticosteroid therapy should be considered when the gestational age of the fetus is 24 to 34 weeks. Corticosteroid therapy reduces the incidence of respiratory distress syndrome and intraventricular hemorrhage in the neonate. Although the maximum benefits occur 24 hours after the start of treatment, some benefits can be gained sooner. Therefore, corticosteroid therapy should be begun unless delivery is imminent. **Administer 2 ml of Celestone Soluspan solution intramuscularly (IM); then repeat the dose in 24 hours** (1 ml of Celestone contains 3 mg of betamethasone sodium and 3 mg of betamethasone acetate). The effects of treatment last for 7 days, and therefore, a repeat dose should be administered if the infant is not delivered. If the severity of disease increases significantly, the infant should be delivered immediately, regardless of gestational age.

2. Intrapartum management

The key issues that must be addressed are as follows:

(1) management of fluids and intravascular volume, (2) prophylactic anticonvulsant therapy, and (3) treatment of hyper-

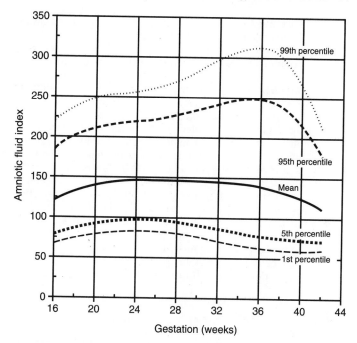

Figure 8–1 □ Mean and percentiles for amniotic fluid index. (Redrawn from Moore TR, Cayle JE: Amniotic fluid index in normal human pregnancy. Am J Obstet Gynecol 1990;162:1168.)

tension. In patients with severe preeclampsia, oliguria and coagulopathy must also be treated in a timely fashion.

a. Management of fluids and intravascular volume

In preeclamptic patients, vasospasm results in generalized vasoconstriction, contraction of the intravascular space, and increased vascular permeability. The end result is decreased intravascular fluid and increased extravascular fluid, making the preeclamptic patient extremely sensitive to fluid adminstration. Fluids must be given carefully to keep the contracted intravascular space expanded, without causing excessive spillage into the extravascular space resulting in pulmonary edema. Intrapartum management of fluids and intravascular volume should include the following:

(1) Placement of a Foley catheter
(2) Recording of input and output

(3) Intensive cardiovascular monitoring with either a Swan-Ganz catheter or central venous pressure (CVP) catheter (recommended in patients with eclampsia or severe preeclampsia.) Normal central hemodynamic measurements for the pregnancy are shown in Table 8–2.

b. **Prophylactic anticonvulsant therapy**

Most eclamptic seizures occur in the intrapartum and the postpartum periods. Therefore, prophylactic anticonvulsant therapy should be initiated in the intrapartum period and continued into the postpartum period. Prophylaxis should be given to all preeclamptic patients because there are no signs or symptoms that can be used with absolute reliability to predict the onset of seizures. Headaches are absent in 17% of patients who develop eclampsia, and hyperactive reflexes are absent in 20% (see Table 8–1). Magnesium sulfate is the most commonly used anticonvulsant agent. The effects of magnesium sulfate are threefold, as follows:

(1) Inhibition of neuromuscular transmission and the cardiac conducting system

(2) Reduction of smooth muscle contractility

Table 8–2 □ NORMAL CENTRAL HEMODYNAMIC MEASUREMENTS IN NONPREGNANT AND PREGNANT PATIENTS

	Nonpregnant	Pregnant
Cardiac output (L/min)	4.3 ± 0.9	6.2 ± 1.0
Heart rate (beats/min)	71 ± 10.0	83 ± 10.0
Systemic vascular resistance (dyne $\times$ cm $\times$ sec^{-5})	1530 ± 520	1210 ± 266
Pulmonary vascular resistance (dyne $\times$ cm $\times$ sec^{-5})	119 ± 47.0	78 ± 22
Colloid oncotic pressure (mm Hg)	20.8 ± 1.0	18.0 ± 1.5
Colloid oncotic pressure–pulmonary capillary wedge pressure (mm Hg)	14.5 ± 2.5	10.5 ± 2.7
Mean arterial pressure (mm Hg)	86.4 ± 75	90.3 ± 5.8
Pulmonary capillary wedge pressure (mm Hg)	6.3 ± 2.1	7.5 ± 1.8
Central venous pressure (mm Hg)	3.7 ± 2.6	3.6 ± 2.5
Left ventricular stroke work index (g $\times$ m $\times$ m^{-2})	41 ± 8	48 ± 6

From Clark SL, Cotton DB, Lee W, et al: Central hemodynamic assessment of normal term pregnancy. Am J Obstet Gynecol 1989; 161:1439.

(3) Depression of central nervous system irritability.

The following are the two regimens for the administration of magnesium sulfate:

(1) **Magnesium sulfate 2 to 4 g IV over 5 minutes, as a loading dose, followed by 1.0 g/hr IV, as the maintenance dose,** or

(2) **Magnesium sulfate 2 to 4 g IV over 2 to 4 minutes, concurrently with 10 g IM as the loading dose, followed by 5 g IM every 4 hours.**

Magnesium sulfate therapy should be continued after delivery for at least 24 hours. Undesired side effects of magnesium sulfate include flushing, nausea, and decreased uterine contractility. More serious complications resulting from magnesium toxicity include respiratory depression and cardiac arrest. Therefore, serum magnesium levels should be monitored. The desired serum level for anticonvulsant therapy is 4 to 7 mEq/L. Toxic effects of serum magnesium levels are listed in Table 8–3. If respiratory arrest or cardiac arrest develops, the magnesium sulfate infusion should be discontinued and calcium gluconate should be administered as follows:

Calcium gluconate (10% solution) 10 ml (1 g) IV over 3 minutes

c. **Treatment of hypertension**

Antihypertensive therapy is recommended only for patients in whom diastolic blood pressure is persistently >105 mm Hg. Treatment is recommended in these patients to prevent hemorrhagic strokes. There is no evidence that antihypertensive therapy prevents eclampsia. The goal of treatment is not to attain normal blood pressures but to lower the blood pressure to a safer level. Because patients with preeclampsia have a decreased intravascular volume, overly aggressive treatment of hypertension decreases cardiac output and uterine blood flow further and may result in fetal distress. Because they further reduce intravascular volume, diuretics are not appropriate antihypertensive agents for

Table 8–3 □ SERUM MAGNESIUM LEVELS AND CLINICAL EFFECTS

Clinical Effect	Serum Level (mEq/L)
Loss of patellar reflexes	10
Respiratory depression	10
Respiratory arrest	12
General anesthesia	15
Cardiac arrest	25

women with preeclampsia. Antihypertensive agents that can be used for acute hypertension in patients with pre-eclampsia are listed in Table 8–4. Hydralazine (Apresoline), an antihypertensive commonly used in preeclamptic patients, is a vasodilator. It increases cardiac output and uterine blood flow, and it should be administered as follows:

(1) **Hydralazine 1 mg IV over 1 minute, as a test dose to detect idiosyncratic hypotension; then 5 to 25 mg IV over 2 to 4 minutes.**

(2) After 20 minutes, if a diastolic blood pressure of between 90 and 100 mm Hg is not attained, a repeat dose or lower dose can be given.

In rare cases in which hydralazine is not effective, the following antihypertensive agents can be used:

(1) **Nifedipine 10 mg by mouth, and repeat in 4 to 8 hours**

(2) **Labetalol 20 mg IV bolus dose, followed by 10 to 50 mg IV every 10 minutes**

d. **Management of oliguria**

Oliguria in pregnancy is defined as a urine output of less than 20 to 30 ml/hr. Oliguria in preeclamptic patients may be of prerenal or renal origin. Furthermore, oliguria in pregnancy may be secondary to elevated antidiuretic hormone (ADH) due to stress or due to high-dose oxytocin administration, which also has an antidiuretic effect. If pulmonary edema is not present and there is no history of congestive heart failure, management of oliguria in the preeclamptic patient is as follows:

(1) Intensive cardiovascular monitoring with either a Swan-Ganz catheter or a central venous pressure (CVP) catheter, and

(2) **IV infusion of 500 to 1000 ml of isotonic crystalloid solution over 1 hour**

e. **Management of disseminated intravascular coagulation**

Laboratory evidence of DIC is found in 20% of patients with severe preeclampsia or eclampsia. Management of DIC and blood loss in preeclamptic or eclamptic patients consists of the following:

(1) Red blood cells

Units of packed red blood cells (RBCs) and whole blood have volumes of 250 ml and 450 ml, respectively. Each unit of RBCs should increase the hematocrit by 3% and hemoglobin by 1 g/dl. Coagulation studies should be obtained after every 5 to 10 units of RBCs transfused.

(2) Platelets

Platelets should be transfused for a platelet count of <20,000/mm^3, or for a platelet count of <50,000/mm^3 in patients for whom a cesarean section is planned. Each

Table 8-4 □ ANTIHYPERTENSIVE AGENTS USED IN PREECLAMPSIA

Drug	Time Course of Action			IM	Dosage IV	Interval Between Doses	Mechanism of Action
	Onset	Maximum	Duration				
Hydralazine	10–20 min	20–40 min	3–8 hr	10–50 mg	5–25 mg	3–6 hr	Direct dilatation of arterioles
Trimethaphan camsylate	1–2 min	2–5 min	10 min	—	IV solution, 2 g/L IV infusion rate, 1–5 mg/min		Ganglionic blockade
Sodium nitroprusside	$\frac{1}{2}$–2 min	1–2 min	3–5 min	—	IV solution, 0.01 g/L IV infusion rate, 0.2–0.8 mg/min		Direct dilatation of arterioles and veins
Labetalol	1–2 min	10 min	6–16 hr	—	20–50 mg	3–6 hr	Alpha- and beta-adrenergic blocker
Nifedipine	5–10 min	10–20 min	4–8 hr	—	10 mg orally	4–8 hr	Calcium channel blocker

From Creasy RK, Resnik R: Maternal-Fetal Medicine: Principles and Practice, 3rd ed. Philadelphia, WB Saunders Co, 1994, p 832.

unit of platelets should increase the platelet count by 5000 to 10,000/mm^3.

(3) Fresh frozen plasma

Fresh frozen plasma (FFP) should be given to patients with coagulopathy due to deficiency of clotting factors, usually if PT or PTT is >1.5 times normal. Each unit of FFP will increase any clotting factor by 2 to 3%. The usual initial dose is 2 units and each unit has a volume of 200 to 250 ml.

(4) Cryoprecipitate

Cryoprecipitate should be administered to patients with coagulopathy due to deficiency of factor VIII, von Willebrand factor, factor XIII, fibrinogen, and/or fibronectin. Cryoprecipitate is concentrated from FFP, and each bag has a volume of 10 to 15 ml. Each bag contains at least 150 mg of fibrinogen.

As is the case with fluid administration, the transfusion of blood products must be performed carefully in preeclamptic and eclamptic women to prevent fluid overload and pulmonary edema.

3. Treatment of eclampsia

Eclamptic seizures usually resolve spontaneously in 1 to 2 minutes, and therefore, protection of the patient from injury, prevention of aspiration, and establishment of an airway are the initial goals in addition to drug therapy. If seizures develop before the administration of prophylactic magnesium, the following should be given:

a. Magnesium sulfate 4 g IV or IM

A maintenance dose of either 1.0 g/hr IV or 5 g IM every 4 hours can then be given. If seizures develop while the patient is already receiving magnesium sulfate, treatment with one of the following anticonvulsant drugs should be initiated:

(1) Diazepam (Valium) 5 g IV, or

(2) Pentobarbital (Nembutal) 125 mg IV

9

INCOMPETENT CERVIX

■ BACKGROUND AND DEFINITION

Incompetent cervix: Painless cervical dilatation and/or efface-ment that occurs in the second or early-third trimester of preg-nancy in the absence of uterine contractions. The natural history includes the ballooning of the fetal membranes into the vagina with subsequent rupture of membranes and delivery of an imma-ture fetus. Incompetent cervix is a common cause of pregnancy loss in the second trimester (Table 9–1).

■ CLINICAL PRESENTATION

Painless cervical dilatation
Painless cervical effacement
Vaginal discharge
Vaginal bleeding or spotting
Premature rupture of membranes

■ PHONE CALL

Questions

1. **What is the gestational age of the fetus?**
2. **Has the patient had rupture of membranes?**
3. **Does the patient appear to be having uterine contrac-tions?**

Table 9–1 □ COMMON CAUSES OF PREGNANCY LOSS IN THE SECOND TRIMESTER

Incompetent cervix
Fetal chromosomal abnormality
Uterine anomaly
Uterine leiomyomata
Premature rupture of membranes
Premature labor
Systemic infection (pyelonephritis, appendicitis)

Orders

1. Place the patient at bedrest in Trendelenburg position
2. Start IV
3. Place the patient on electronic fetal heart rate monitoring and uterine monitoring

Degree of Urgency

Incompetent cervix can progress quickly from cervical dilatation to prolapse of the amniotic sac into the vagina to rupture of membranes, and, finally, to the delivery of an often nonviable fetus. The success of treatment of this condition is dependent on early diagnosis and intervention. Therefore, patients suspected of having incompetent cervix should be seen immediately.

■ ELEVATOR THOUGHTS

What are the causes of incompetent cervix?
- Previous cervical trauma
  1. Cervical conization or amputation
  2. Extensive cervical dilatation as done in second-trimester pregnancy terminations
  3. Cervical laceration at the time of a prior vaginal delivery
- In utero exposure to diethylstilbestrol (DES)

  DES exposure in utero has been associated with an increased risk of cervical incompetence, spontaneous abortion, and preterm labor and delivery. The absence of structural abnormalities commonly seen in DES-exposed patients, such as cervical collars, hoods, and cock's combs, does not necessarily preclude cervical incompetence.

■ MAJOR THREAT TO FETAL LIFE

- Prematurity

  Cervical incompetence is not life threatening to the mother but can result in delivery of a previable or premature infant.

■ BEDSIDE

Quick Look Test

Does the patient appear to be having uterine contractions?

Is there evidence of gross rupture of membranes?

Both rupture of membranes and uterine contractions are poor prognostic signs that make surgical intervention with cervical cerclage placement contraindicated.

Vital Signs

Vital signs are usually normal. The presence of a fever may be due to chorioamnionitis secondary to premature rupture of membranes.

Selective History and Chart Review

1. What is the gestational age of the fetus?
   The gestational age of the fetus will impact the management of the patient.
2. Has the patient had a prior ultrasound examination?
   A prior ultrasound examination can be used to confirm gestational age; more important, it can also be used to rule out fetal anomalies before placement of a cervical cerclage is performed.

Selective Physical Examination

Abdominal	Normal
Pelvic	
External genitalia and vagina	Normal or prolapsing of membranes into the vagina
Cervix	Dilated, effaced, and shortened
Uterus and adnexae	Normal unless patient is in labor or has chorioamnionitis, which results in uterine tenderness

■ DIAGNOSTIC TESTING

There are no specific diagnostic tests for incompetent cervix; the diagnosis is based on clinical findings.

1. Ultrasound examination
   Not only is an ultrasound examination useful for confirming gestational age of the fetus and for evaluating the fetus for fetal anomalies, but it can also be used to measure cervical length and dilatation. Serial ultrasound examinations can be used to detect change in cervical dilatation and change in cervical shortening. The length of the normal cervix remains constant at 5.2 ± 1.2 cm until 34 weeks of gestation, when gradual shortening of the cervix begins.

■ MANAGEMENT

1. Cervical cerclage

Cervical cerclage is best performed at a fetal gestational age of more than 14 weeks, so that the patient is beyond the first trimester, when spontaneous abortion of an abnormal fetus frequently occurs. The success of cervical cerclage is inversely related to the amount of cervical dilatation, and it is best performed before the cervix has dilated more than 2 cm. Cervical cultures for gonorrhea, for group B streptococcus, and for chlamydia should be performed, and positive cultures should be treated before cerclage placement. The two most common types of cervical cerclage are the McDonald cerclage and the Shirodkar cerclage. There is usually less cervical trauma and blood loss with the McDonald cerclage. The success rate for both procedures is 75 to 90%. After placement of the cerclage, tocolytics such as **terbutaline 2.5 mg PO every 4 hours** or **indomethacin 25 mg PO every 6 hours** can be administered for 24 hours, although the benefits of tocolytics have not been clearly established. Sexual intercourse should be prohibited for at least 1 week after the procedure. The patient should have cervical examinations every 1 to 2 weeks to detect any cervical dilatation in the presence of the cerclage.

Cervical cerclage is contraindicated if the patient has ruptured membranes, uterine contractions, vaginal bleeding of unknown cause, intrauterine infection, cervical infection, or fetal anomalies. Complications of cervical cerclage include rupture of membranes, chorioamnionitis, vesicovaginal and urethrovaginal fistulas, and displacement of the suture. Rupture of membranes usually occurs in the perioperative period but can also occur intraoperatively, especially if advanced cervical dilatation has occurred. The suture should be cut when the fetus has reached term, and preferably before onset of labor. If this is not performed before labor begins, the patient can incur uterine rupture or cervical laceration. Even after the removal of

Table 9–2 □ INCIDENCE RATES OF COMPLICATIONS OF CERVICAL CERCLAGE

Complication	Incidence (%)
Rupture of membranes	1–9
Chorioamnionitis	1–8
Cervical laceration	1–13
Displacement of the suture	3–13
Vesicovaginal or urethrovaginal fistulas	Rare
Uterine rupture	Rare
Abnormal cervical dilatation	Rare

the suture, the patient in labor can develop a cervical laceration because of the prior cerclage placement. Furthermore, there may be abnormal cervical dilatation secondary to scarring from the cerclage. The incidence rates of complications resulting from cervical cerclage are listed in Table 9–2.

2. Bedrest without cervical cerclage

If there are contraindications to the placement of a cervical cerclage, the patient should be managed expectantly with bedrest. This management can also be used for patients with advanced cervical dilatation. The tocolytic drugs described above can also be administered to these patients.

10

MALPRESENTATION

■ BACKGROUND AND DEFINITIONS

Malpresentation: Any fetal presentation other than vertex. The most common malpresentation is the breech presentation. Other abnormal presentations that are encountered less frequently are brow presentation, face presentation, transverse lie, oblique lie, and compound presentations.

Breech presentation: The presenting fetal part is the buttock, the sacrum, or the lower extremities (Fig. 10–1)

Frank breech: Both lower extremities are flexed at the hips but extended at the knees, resulting in a U-shaped fetus with the feet close to the head.

Complete breech: Both lower extremities are flexed at the hips and one or both of the knees are also flexed.

Incomplete breech: One or both of the lower extremities are extended at the hips and one or both knees are extended so that the knees or the feet are presenting.

Single footling breech: Incomplete breech presentation with one foot presenting

Double footling breech: Incomplete breech presentation with both feet presenting

Transverse lie: The axis of the fetus is perpendicular to that of the mother so that the shoulder is often the presenting part (Fig.

Complete   Frank   Footling

Figure 10–1 □ Complete, frank, and footling breech presentations. (From Hacker NF, Moore JG: Essentials of Obstetrics and Gynecology, 2nd ed. Philadelphia, WB Saunders Co, 1992, p 231.)

10–2). When a patient with a transverse lie is encountered before 39 weeks of gestational age, there is an 80 to 85% incidence of spontaneous conversion to a longitudinal lie, either vertex or breech.

Oblique lie: The axis of the fetus forms an acute angle with the axis of the mother. This malpresentation is usually transitory and converts to either a longitudinal lie, either vertex or breech, or a transverse lie. Therefore, it is also referred to as an **unstable lie.**

Face presentation: The presenting part is the fetal chin or the mentum (Fig. 10–3). This malpresentation is the result of full extension of the fetal head so that the occiput comes into contact with the fetal back.

Brow presentation: The presenting part is the fetal brow, that portion of the head between the anterior fontanel and the orbital ridge (Fig. 10–4). Brow presentation is caused by partial extension of the head.

Compound presentations: A fetal extremity, usually an arm or a hand and less often a lower extremity, prolapses down and presents simultaneously with the presenting part.

The most commonly encountered malpresentation is the breech presentation. Approximately 3 to 4% of singleton term pregnancies are complicated by this malpresentation. Other malpresen-

Figure 10–2 □ Transverse lie. (From Hacker NF, Moore JG: Essentials of Obstetrics and Gynecology, 2nd ed. Philadelphia, WB Saunders Co, 1992, p 239.)

Figure 10–3 □ Face presentation. (From Hacker NF, Moore JG: Essentials of Obstetrics and Gynecology, 2nd ed. Philadelphia, WB Saunders Co, 1992, p 238.)

tations occur much less frequently than breech presentation. Transverse lie has a frequency of 0.24 to 0.3%. The incidence of face presentation is between 0.17 and 0.2%; and brow presentation is encountered even less frequently, with an incidence of 0.02%. Compound presentations are found in 0.05 to 0.14% of pregnan-

Figure 10–4 □ Brow presentation. (From Hacker NF, Moore JG: Essentials of Obstetrics and Gynecology, 2nd ed. Philadelphia, WB Saunders Co, 1992, p 238.)

cies. The incidence of all malpresentations is increased in pregnancies of earlier gestational ages.

At every gestational age, the fetal morbidity and mortality rates are higher for breech fetuses, compared with vertex fetuses. The overall mortality rate for breech fetuses ranges from 8 to 25%, compared with 2.5% for vertex fetuses. This increase is a result not only of complications encountered during labor and delivery, but also of the increased incidence of preterm delivery, intrauterine growth restriction, and congenital anomalies in breech fetuses. Furthermore, it is possible that fetuses that do not spontaneously change their presentation to vertex may be abnormal and compromised in some way.

■ CLINICAL PRESENTATION

When the patient is not in labor or is in early labor, there are no specific symptoms that are associated with malpresentation.

- Prolapsed umbilical cord

  Malpresentation is associated with a higher incidence of umbilical cord prolapse once membranes are ruptured.

- Abnormal labor

  Malpresentation is associated with a greater frequency of abnormal labor.

■ PHONE CALL

Questions

1. **What is the fetus' gestational age?**

   If the fetus is not near term, breech presentation is a common and normal finding. If the patient is not in labor and membranes have not ruptured, the fetus may spontaneously turn to a vertex presentation. Therefore, these patients may be managed expectantly. As the gestational age approaches term, the likelihood of spontaneous version diminishes.

2. **Is the patient in active labor?**

   In the patient in active labor with a malpresentation, the decision on the route of delivery must be made. Active labor is a contraindication to external cephalic version of the fetus in the breech presentation.

3. **Is there evidence or a history of rupture of membranes?**

   Rupture of membranes makes external cephalic version technically more difficult. In patients with a breech presentation other than frank breech, rupture of membranes places the fetus at risk for prolapse of the umbilical cord.

4. **Is there evidence of fetal distress found on fetal heart rate monitoring?**

The presence of abnormal fetal heart rate patterns that suggest fetal distress is a contraindication to external cephalic version of a breech fetus. The management of patients with malpresentations and abnormal heart rate patterns should be the same as the management of patients with vertex presentations. The only exception is that internal fetal monitoring is not recommended in the patient with a face presentation because of potential scarring of the fetus' face.

Orders

1. Start an IV
2. Obtain a complete blood count (CBC)
3. Place the patient on continuous electronic fetal monitoring
4. Type and crossmatch blood
5. Notify the pediatrician and anesthesiologist of the possible need for an emergency cesarean section

Degree of Urgency

If the patient is in labor or has ruptured membranes, she should be evaluated immediately so that a plan for management in labor and the route of delivery can be made.

■ ELEVATOR THOUGHTS

What factors increase the incidence of breech presentation?
- Early gestational age
- Multiple gestation
- Fetal anencephaly
- Fetal hydrocephalus
- Polyhydramnios
- Oligohydramnios
- Uterine anomaly
- Uterine or pelvic mass
- Multiparity resulting in uterine relaxation
- Placenta previa
- Fundal or cornual implantation of the placenta
- Previous pregnancy with breech presentation

What complications are associated with abnormal presentations?
- Increased perinatal morbidity and mortality from difficult delivery

    Vaginal delivery of the breech infant is complicated because the diameter of the fetal head is normally larger than that of the buttocks. This discrepancy in size between the head and the buttocks is even greater when the fetus is premature. Furthermore, in the breech presentation, the fetal head does not undergo molding as it does in the vertex presentation. Therefore, the fetal buttocks and torso can be delivered through a cervix that is not dilated enough to allow delivery of the head. Once entrapment of the head occurs, if delivery is not accomplished soon, fetal hypoxia develops because of compression of the umbilical cord, which has been brought down into the vagina. If an excessive amount of traction is applied to the fetus in an attempt to facilitate delivery, fetal trauma can occur. The most commonly injured organs are the brain, spinal cord, liver, spleen, adrenal glands, and brachial plexus. Although cesarean delivery of the breech fetus is often less traumatic than vaginal delivery, it does not preclude birth injury, because the fetus still must be delivered as a breech through the uterine incision.

- Preterm delivery
- Congenital anomalies
  The incidence of congenital anomalies in pregnancies complicated by breech presentation is 6 to 7%, compared with 2 to 2.5% for pregnancies with normal presentations.
- Abnormal labor
  Labor usually progresses normally with a fetus in the frank breech presentation. However, with certain malpresentations, such as transverse lie and face presentation with the fetal chin posterior, referred to as the mentum posterior position, labor progresses abnormally and vaginal delivery is impossible.
- Increased risk of cesarean section
- Intrauterine growth restriction
- Umbilical cord prolapse
  Transverse lie, complete breech, and incomplete breech presentations are all associated with an increased risk of umbilical cord prolapse after rupture of membranes, because in these presentations, there is no fetal part that is applied to the dilating cervix to act as a plug. The incidence of umbilical cord prolapse with a frank breech presentation is approximately 0.5%, which is comparable to the incidence of cord prolapse in vertex presentation which is nearly 0.4%. The incidence of cord prolapse is 5 to 6% with a complete breech presentation and 15 to 18% with a footling breech presentation.

■ MAJOR THREAT TO FETAL LIFE

- Birth trauma
- Prematurity

- Congenital anomalies
  The major threat is to the life of the fetus. Maternal mortality is increased only very slightly because of the greater frequency of cesarean section.

■ BEDSIDE

Quick Look Test

Does the patient appear to be in labor?
If the patient is in active labor, external cephalic version is contraindicated, and therefore a management plan should be made for the delivery of the fetus.

Are there abnormal fetal heart rate patterns suggestive of fetal distress?
If abnormal fetal heart rate patterns suggestive of fetal distress are present on electronic fetal monitoring, prolapse of the umbilical cord should be ruled out.

Does the patient appear to have a premature pregnancy?
If the patient is in labor with a breech fetus and the estimated fetal weight is less than 1500 g, vaginal delivery is not recommended, and cesarean section should be performed if progression of labor cannot be halted.

Vital Signs

Vital signs are usually normal.

Selective History and Chart Review

1. Has the patient had an ultrasound examination during her pregnancy to rule out congenital anomalies and placenta previa?
   Lethal fetal anomalies such as anencephaly must be ruled out by ultrasound examination so that an unnecessary cesarean section is not performed. The diagnosis of placenta previa is a contraindication to vaginal delivery.
2. What is the best estimate of the gestational age of the fetus based on the date of the patient's last menstrual period and ultrasound examinations performed early in pregnancy?
   Knowledge of the gestational age of the fetus is essential for developing a plan for delivery of the fetus with a malpresentation.

Selective Physical Examination

Abdominal   Breech presentation: Round, hard fetal head
                         is palpable high in the fundal region of

the uterus. Fetal heart sounds are heard loudest above the umbilicus.

Transverse lie: Abdomen is wide from one side to the other. Fundal height is low, often extending only slightly above the umbilicus. A hard band is palpable across the front of the abdomen if the fetal back is anterior. Irregular nodular fetal extremities or "small parts" are palpable across the front of the abdomen if the fetal back is posterior.

Oblique lie: Fetal head is palpable in the right or left lower quadrant.

Pelvic	
External genitalia and vagina	Footling breech: Fetal feet can be palpable in the vagina if the cervix is dilated. Transverse lie: Prolapsed arm may be palpable if the cervix is dilated.
Cervix	Frank breech: Fetal buttock is palpable with the anus and both ischial tuberosities forming a straight line. Complete and incomplete breech: Fetal feet or buttock is palpable. Transverse and oblique lie: Early in labor, when the fetus is high in the uterus, no fetal parts or presenting parts are palpable. Later in labor, when the cervix has dilated and the fetus is lower, an arm or shoulder may be palpable. Face presentation: Fetal mouth, nose, orbital ridges, and malar eminences are palpable. The fetal mouth and malar eminences can feel similar to the anus and ischial tuberosities of a breech fetus. The difference is that the mouth and malar eminences form a triangle, whereas the anus and ischial tuberosities form a straight line. Brow presentation: Fetal orbital ridges, root of the nose, and anterior fontanel are palpable. The absence of a palpable mouth or chin distinguishes the brow presentation from the face presentation. Compound presentation: Fetal hand or arm and, less frequently, the fetal feet are palpable along with the vertex or buttock.
Uterus and adnexae	Same findings as abdominal examination.

■ DIAGNOSTIC TESTING

The diagnosis of malpresentation can often be made by abdominal and vaginal examination. Radiographic studies are useful, however, in confirming the diagnosis and providing additional information that is crucial for the management of the patient.

1. **Ultrasound examination**

   Ultrasound examination should be performed to confirm the diagnosis of fetal malpresentation and to rule out congenital anomalies. A fetal anomaly of particular concern is anencephaly, which not only is associated with an increased incidence of breech presentation, but also is a lethal anomaly. Fetal measurements can also be taken to estimate the birth weight. Furthermore, the degree of flexion or extension of the fetal head can also be determined by sonogram. These are all essential to planning the route of delivery of the breech fetus. Unfortunately, ultrasound examination cannot always distinguish between the different types of breech presentations.

2. **Pelvic x-ray**

   Pelvic x-ray not only will confirm the diagnosis of malpresentation but, in the case of breech presentation, will also distinguish between the different types of breech presentations. Furthermore, if vaginal delivery of a breech fetus is being contemplated, pelvimetry can also be performed by pelvic x-ray.

3. **Computed tomography**

   CT can provide all the information provided by pelvic x-ray with less radiation exposure.

■ MANAGEMENT

1. **Previable fetus—Attempt vaginal delivery**

   If the gestational age is <24 to 25 weeks or if the fetus is not viable for other reasons, vaginal delivery should be attempted for all types of malpresentation.

2. **Breech presentation**

   a. **Nonfrank breech at any viable gestational age—Cesarean section**

      The increased incidence of prolapse of the umbilical cord, or delivery of the lower extremities and buttocks through an incompletely dilated cervix, make vaginal delivery of a fetus in the complete and the incomplete breech presentation too risky. Unless imminent vaginal delivery precludes it, cesarean section should be performed.

   b. **Frank breech with fetal weight of <1500 g—Cesarean section**

      The mortality rate for breech fetuses weighing <1500 g is as high as 45% when delivered vaginally, compared with 18% when delivered by cesarean section. If premature labor cannot be treated successfully, cesarean section should be performed.

c. Frank breech with an estimated fetal weight of >1500 g

(1) Vaginal delivery

Vaginal delivery of the frank breech fetus weighing >1500 g has been shown to be safe. However, the following criteria should be met before a vaginal delivery is attempted:

(a) The physician must be experienced in performing a vaginal breech delivery.

(b) Continuous electronic fetal monitoring should be used.

(c) There must be the capability to perform an emergency cesarean section if complications are encountered.

(d) An anesthesiologist or a nurse-anesthetist must be available.

(e) The maternal pelvis should be adequate based on either x-ray or CT scan pelvimetry measurements (Table 10–1).

(f) The estimated fetal weight should be <4000 g.

(g) The fetal head must not be hyperextended and, optimally, should be flexed.

(h) Labor must be progressing normally.

Although studies have shown that the use of oxytocin is safe in patients with a frank breech fetus, this issue remains controversial.

(i) The patient must be counseled in detail concerning the risks of both vaginal delivery and cesarean birth of the breech fetus, and she must consent to the attempt at vaginal delivery.

(2) Cesarean section

If any one of the criteria listed above cannot be met, then a cesarean section should be performed.

(3) External cephalic version

External cephalic version can be attempted if the patient is not in labor and if the gestational age is >36 weeks. Version is usually not recommended before 36 weeks, because of the possibility of spontaneous conver-

Table 10–1 □ **PELVIMETRY MEASUREMENTS OF THE NORMAL PELVIS**

	Anterior–Posterior Diameter (cm)	Transverse Diameter (cm)
Pelvic inlet	≥10.5	≥11.5
Midpelvis	≥11.5	≥10.0

sion to the vertex presentation when remote from term. Successful cephalic version requires the following:

   (a) A physician who is familiar with the technique of external cephalic version.
   (b) Continuous electronic fetal heart rate monitoring during the procedure.
   (c) Ultrasound examination to follow the fetal head during the version.
   (d) Uterine tocolytics to relax the uterus, e.g., **terbutaline 0.25 mg subcutaneously (SC) once or magnesium sulfate 4.0 to 6.0 g IV over 20 minutes once.**

   External cephalic version is successful in 60 to 70% of all cases. Factors that improve the success rate are frank breech presentation, multiparity, adequate amniotic fluid, and fetal back located anteriorly. The most common complication of cephalic version is abnormal fetal heart rate patterns including variable decelerations, tachycardia, and bradycardia. These heart rate patterns are usually the result of cord compression and are in most cases transient. More serious complications are rare and include fetal trauma such as brachial plexus injury and spinal cord transection and fetal–maternal hemorrhage.

3. **Transverse lie**
   a. **External cephalic version**

   A fetus with a gestational age of >25 weeks with a persistent transverse lie cannot usually be delivered vaginally. If the patient is not in active labor, external cephalic version to the vertex presentation can be attempted. Version of a fetus in the transverse lie does not usually need to be attempted until after 39 weeks of gestation because of the high likelihood of spontaneous conversion to a longitudinal lie, either vertex or breech, before 39 weeks. The criteria for cephalic version and the possible complications associated with version are the same as those listed above for cephalic version of the breech fetus.

   b. **Cesarean section**

   If external cephalic version attempted after 39 weeks is unsuccessful or the patient is in active labor at any viable gestational age, then a cesarean section should be performed. Because the fetus is not in the lower uterus, a vertical uterine incision may have to be used instead of the more common low transverse incision.

4. Face presentation

a. Mentum posterior position—Cesarean section

Vaginal delivery is impossible if the fetus is in a persistent mentum posterior position in which the fetal chin is posterior in the maternal pelvis. Cesarean section should be performed in these patients.

b. Positions other than mentum posterior—Attempt vaginal delivery

Vaginal delivery should be attempted if the position is other than mentum posterior. Vaginal delivery is usually successful if the pelvis is not contracted. External continuous electronic fetal heart rate monitoring should be performed. Internal fetal heart rate monitoring with a scalp electrode is not recommended because of the risk of scarring of the face. Face presentation is sometimes caused by a contracted pelvis. Therefore, the need for a cesarean section for arrest of cervical dilatation or arrest of descent of the fetal head is increased in these patients, compared with those with a vertex presentation.

5. Brow presentation—Attempt vaginal delivery

The brow presentation is usually transient. In patients with this presentation, approximately two-thirds will spontaneously convert to either the vertex presentation by flexion of the head or the face presentation by extension of the head. If the brow presentation persists, there is an increased incidence of arrest of cervical dilatation or arrest of descent of the fetal head and, therefore, a greater likelihood that a cesarean section will be needed.

6. Compound presentation

a. Attempt vaginal delivery

The prolapsed fetal extremity, usually the arm, will usually not interfere with labor and therefore should not be manipulated. In many cases, the extremity will spontaneously be pulled back and away from the presenting part.

b. Reduce the extremity

If the prolapsing extremity prevents descent of the fetus during labor, a gentle attempt should be made to reduce it by pushing it upward. If this attempt fails and labor remains obstructed, then a cesarean section should be performed.

11

MASTITIS

■ BACKGROUND AND DEFINITIONS

Mastitis: Infection of the connective tissue of the breast

Endemic mastitis: Mastitis that occurs 2 weeks to several months after delivery due to bacteria in the infant's oropharynx and nose

Epidemic mastitis: Mastitis that occurs in hospitalized women because their infants are infected from contact with infected nursery personnel

■ CLINICAL PRESENTATION

Tender and erythematous breast, usually unilateral
Breast hard and engorged
Fever
Chills and rigor
Malaise
Breast abscess in approximately 10% of patients with mastitis

■ PHONE CALL

Questions

1. How ill does the patient appear?
Breast abscess and, less commonly, septic shock and toxic shock syndrome (TSS) should be considered in the severely ill patient.

Orders

1. Collect breast milk discharge for culture

In the severely ill patient, the following orders should also be given:

2. Start IV
3. Insert Foley catheter
4. Record input and output
5. Obtain a complete blood count (CBC) with differential
6. Obtain chemistry panel
7. Obtain blood cultures
8. Perform urinalysis

Degree of Urgency

Unless the rare complications of septic shock or TSS are encountered, mastitis is not life threatening and the patient does not need to be seen immediately.

■ ELEVATOR THOUGHTS

What causes the most common type of mastitis?

Mastitis is usually caused by transmission of bacteria in the infant's oropharynx and nose into the breast through breast abrasions and fissures that develop from breast feeding.

What bacteria usually cause mastitis?

Staphylococcus aureus
Streptococcus viridans
Group A and B streptococci
Haemophilus influenzae
Haemophilus parainfluenzae

■ MAJOR THREAT TO MATERNAL LIFE

- Septic shock
- Toxic shock syndrome

Both of these life-threatening complications are rare.

■ BEDSIDE

Quick Look Test

Does the patient appear to be severely ill?

Breast abscess, septic shock, and TSS should be considered in severely ill patients.

Vital Signs

Fever is almost always present. Other vital signs are normal unless the patient has developed septic shock or TSS.

Selective History and Chart Review

1. Does the patient have a prior history of breast conditions?
   Other breast diseases such as cancer can mimic mastitis.
2. Is the patient already on antibiotics for other reasons and is she allergic to any antibiotics?

Selective Physical Examination

Dermatological	"Sunburn-like" skin rash with desquamation is suggestive of TSS
Breasts	Tender, hard, engorged, and erythematous breast, usually unilateral; a fluctuant mass would be suggestive of a breast abscess
Abdominal	Normal
Pelvic	Normal

■ DIAGNOSTIC TESTING

The diagnosis of mastitis can usually be made from the patient's history and physical examination. Further testing is usually not necessary unless the diagnosis is unclear or a breast abscess is suspected.

1. **Culture of the breast milk**

   Culturing of the milk may aid in the selection of the appropriate antibiotic to administer, but it is not necessary for making the diagnosis of mastitis if the clinical picture is clear.

2. **Leukocyte and bacterial colony count of the breast milk**

   In patients with mastitis, the breast milk leukocyte count is usually greater than 1 million/ml, and the bacterial colony count is usually greater than 1000/ml.

3. **Ultrasound examination**

   Ultrasound examination of the breast can be used to diagnose breast abscesses that appear as discrete fluid collections within the breast tissue.

■ MANAGEMENT

1. **Ice packs** should be applied to the breast.
2. **Breast support** of some form should be used.
3. **Analgesics and antipyretics** can be used.

   The above measures are used to decrease the amount of pain associated with mastitis.

4. **Breast feeding should be continued** to prevent further breast engorgement.

   If breast feeding is too uncomfortable, the patient should be encouraged to pump her breast.

5. **Antibiotic therapy** is begun.

   Although penicillin and sulfonamides have been used successfully, the following are the antibiotics of choice in the treatment of mastitis:

   a. **Dicloxacillin 125 to 250 mg PO four times per day for 10 days** for penicillin-resistant staphylococci.

b. **Erythromycin 250 mg PO four times per day for 10 days** if the patient is allergic to penicillin.
c. **Vancomycin 250 to 500 mg PO four times per day for 10 days** if a methicillin-resistant staphylococcus is suspected.
d. **Cephalosporins PO for 10 days.**

6. **Surgical incision and drainage** is performed if a breast abscess is present.

12

MECONIUM PASSAGE

■ BACKGROUND AND DEFINITIONS

Meconium: Epidermal cells and fetal hair swallowed by the fetus with amniotic fluid along with mucous and desquamated cells from the fetal intestinal tract

Meconium passage: The passage of meconium from the fetal rectum into the amniotic fluid

Meconium aspiration syndrome: A syndrome caused by either antepartum or intrapartum aspiration of meconium by the fetus; this syndrome is characterized by varying degrees of respiratory distress, caused by both mechanical obstruction of the airways and chemical pneumonitis

Meconium passage can occur in either the antepartum or the intrapartum period. The incidence of intrapartum meconium passage is 1.5 to 18%. Meconium is rarely passed before 34 weeks of gestation. In contrast, the incidence of meconium passage is significantly higher in postdate pregnancies. Intrapartum meconium passage has been associated with a higher incidence of abnormal fetal heart rate tracings, fetal acidosis, and low Apgar scores. This finding is not consistent, however, and some studies have not found this association.

■ CLINICAL PRESENTATION

The amniotic fluid is green or brown; it can be thin and watery or thick and particulate.

■ PHONE CALL

Questions

1. **Is the meconium thin or thick?**
   Meconium aspiration syndrome is caused only by thick meconium, and thin meconium is usually not significant.

Orders

1. Place the patient on external electronic fetal heart rate monitoring
2. Start IV

3. Have available a fetal scalp electrode for internal fetal heart rate monitoring

4. Have available at the delivery a DeLee suction catheter, a neonatal laryngoscope, and an endotracheal tube to allow for endotracheal suctioning of meconium below the vocal cord

5. If delivery is imminent, notify the pediatric team so that they can be present at the delivery

Degree of Urgency

Because meconium passage can be associated with fetal distress, the fetal heart rate tracing should be evaluated immediately. If abnormal heart rate patterns are present, the patient should be seen immediately.

■ ELEVATOR THOUGHTS

What are the causes of meconium passage?
- Fetal acidosis
- Postdate pregnancy
- Idiopathic

■ MAJOR THREAT TO FETAL LIFE

- Fetal meconium aspiration syndrome
- Fetal asphyxia

Meconium passage is not life threatening to the mother, but it can be associated with abnormal fetal heart rate tracings and fetal acidosis that can result in fetal morbidity and mortality.

■ BEDSIDE

Quick Look Test

Is the patient in labor?

Are there abnormal fetal heart rate patterns?

Vital Signs

Vital signs are usually normal.

Selective History and Chart Review

1. What is the gestational age of the fetus based on the patient's last menstrual period and ultrasound examination?
   Meconium is found in up to 44% of postdate pregnancies.

2. Does the patient have any predisposing factors for fetal distress such as intrauterine growth restriction, postdatism, or placental abruption?

Selective Physical Examination

Abdominal	Usually normal
Pelvic	
External genitalia and vagina	Stained green or brown with meconium
Cervix	Normal
Uterus and adnexae	Usually normal

■ DIAGNOSTIC TESTING

The diagnosis of meconium passage is based on physical examination after rupture of the amniotic sac.

■ MANAGEMENT

Management of a patient with meconium passage is twofold.

1. **Monitor the fetus closely for evidence of fetal distress**
   a. **Electronic fetal heart rate monitoring**
      When meconium passage is detected, the fetal heart rate should be monitored electronically. Internal monitoring with a fetal scalp electrode should be considered. If nonreassuring fetal heart rate patterns are present, the following steps, as discussed in Chapter 4, should be taken to improve fetal oxygenation:
      (1) Place the patient in the lateral position to relieve uterine compression of the vena cava and to improve venous return and cardiac output.
      (2) Administer supplemental oxygen at a rate of 8 to 10 L/min via face mask.
      (3) Decrease uterine contractions by either discontinuing oxytocin or administering a tocolytic drug.
      (4) Correct maternal hypotension.
      If the above steps do not result in the resolution of the abnormal fetal heart rate patterns, fetal scalp blood sampling or fetal scalp stimulation testing should be performed to identify the asphyxic fetus.
2. **Prevent meconium aspiration syndrome**
   a. **Suctioning of the fetal oropharynx**
      After delivery of the fetal head but before the delivery of the thorax, the fetal oropharynx should be suctioned, preferably with a DeLee suction catheter. The goal of this

procedure is to suction the oropharynx clear of meconium before the infant can take its first breath and aspirate meconium. If the meconium is thick, endotracheal suctioning under laryngoscopic visualization should be performed, preferably by the pediatric team immediately after the delivery of the infant. Unfortunately, suctioning of the oropharynx, as described above, does not entirely eliminate the risk of meconium aspiration syndrome.

b. **Amnioinfusion**

Room-temperature saline (500 ml) infused by gravity through an intrauterine catheter over 30 minutes

Intrauterine infusion of saline or amnioinfusion has been used to dilute the meconium. This procedure has been shown to decrease the finding of meconium below the vocal cords of the neonate. However, it has not been shown that amnioinfusion decreases the incidence of meconium aspiration.

13

MULTIPLE GESTATION

■ BACKGROUND AND DEFINITIONS

Multiple gestation or multiple pregnancy: Occurs in approximately 1.5% of all births, and most of these are twin gestations. The true incidence of twin gestations is probably higher than 1.5%, because early demise of one of the twins is common. One-third of all multiple gestations are monozygotic, resulting from cleavage of a single fertilized ovum. The incidence of monozygotic twins is independent of maternal race, age, parity, and heredity. Two-thirds of all multiple gestations are dizygotic and are due to the fertilization of two ova. The incidence of dizygotic twins is influenced by maternal race, heredity, age, parity, and the use of ovulation-inducing drugs commonly administered to women with infertility.

The perinatal mortality rate of twin gestations is 50 to 120 per 1000 births, approximately fivefold higher than that of singleton pregnancies. Monozygotic twins have an even higher perinatal mortality rate, because they have a 1% risk of having a monoamniotic sac. This results in a fetal mortality rate of 50% because of umbilical cord entanglement. In triplets, the perinatal mortality rate is 95 to 200 per 1000 births. Even with the widespread use of ultrasonography, approximately 20% of twin gestations are not diagnosed until the patient is admitted to the hospital while in labor. The presentation of both twins will influence the route of delivery.

■ CLINICAL PRESENTATION

Size greater than dates
> Beginning with the second trimester, a patient with a multiple gestation will often appear with a uterus larger than expected for the gestational age. This size–date discrepancy, however, is often unreliable and is not helpful in patients who begin labor having had no prenatal care and/or unclear pregnancy dating. In a similar manner, the palpation of multiple fetuses and the auscultation of multiple fetal heart beats do not diagnose a multiple gestation reliably.

Persistent labor and enlarged uterus after delivery
> A multiple gestation should be suspected in a patient who continues to labor and also has an enlarged uterus after delivery of one fetus.

■ PHONE CALL

Questions

1. **Is the patient in active labor?**
2. **What is the gestational age of the fetus?**

   The gestational age and the presentation of the twins are the two most important factors in the management of the patient who is in labor with twins.

Orders

In the patient who is in labor with a multiple gestation, the following orders should be given:
1. Initiate continuous electronic fetal monitoring of the twins
2. Begin IV
3. Type and crossmatch 2 units of blood
4. Notify the anesthesiologist of the possible need for an emergency cesarean section
5. Notify the pediatrician of the imminent delivery of the twins

Degree of Urgency

Because of the potential for complications to occur during delivery, a patient who presents in labor with a multiple gestation must be seen immediately.

■ ELEVATOR THOUGHTS

What are the fetal complications encountered in a multiple gestation?
- Spontaneous abortion

  The incidence of spontaneous abortion is twofold higher in multiple gestations than in singleton pregnancies. Fewer than 50% of patients diagnosed with twin gestations in the first trimester will actually deliver twins. Some twins will be absorbed without maternal symptoms, whereas other demises will cause vaginal bleeding, uterine contractions, and spontaneous abortion. Occasionally, the dead fetus and placenta will remain as a fetus papyraceus and will be found at the subsequent delivery of the surviving twin.
- Preterm delivery

  The average duration of gestation decreases proportionately as the number of fetuses increases. Nearly 50% of twin gestations will deliver prematurely, before 37 weeks of gestation. Preterm birth is the most common cause of perinatal morbidity and mortality in multiple gestations. Measures taken to prevent preterm birth, including bedrest and the use of prophylactic tocolytic drugs, have not been universally successful.

- Intrauterine growth restriction

    The incidence of intrauterine growth restriction in a multiple gestation is approximately 70% compared with 5 to 10% in singleton pregnancies. Furthermore, the degree of growth restriction increases as the pregnancy approaches term.

- Growth discordancy

    The accepted definition of growth discordancy is a difference of ≥15 to 25% between the two twins. The incidence of growth discordancy is 4 to 23%. The most severe cases of growth discordancy are the results of twin-to-twin transfusion in which there are vascular anastomoses between the two twins in a monochorionic, monoamniotic placenta. The incidence of twin-to-twin transfusion in monochorionic twins is approximately 15%. The perinatal mortality rate increases proportionately with the degree of discordancy. When the degree of discordancy is >25%, the fetal death rate is increased 6.5-fold and the neonatal death rate is increased 2.5-fold.

- Umbilical cord accidents

    The incidence of cord accidents such as cord entanglement is highest with monochorionic, monoamniotic multiple gestations.

- Congenital anomalies

    The frequency of major congenital malformations is approximately 2% in twins, compared with 1% in singletons. The incidence of anomalies in monozygotic twins is twice that found in dizygotic twins.

- Complications at delivery

    Multiple gestation is associated with a higher incidence of fetal malpresentation. Furthermore, after the delivery of the first fetus, premature placental separation may occur before the delivery of the remaining fetus, due to the shrinking uterus. For these reasons, in patients with more than two fetuses, delivery is usually by cesarean section.

- Neurological abnormalities

    Cerebral palsy, microcephaly, and encephalomalacia are encountered more frequently in multiple gestation. The incidence of cerebral necrosis is as high as 14% in fetuses of multiple gestations delivered prematurely.

What are the maternal complications associated with a multiple gestation?

- Hyperemesis gravidarum

    Hyperemesis is probably due to the increased levels of human gonadotropins found in multiple gestation.

- Placental abruption

- Placenta previa
- Preeclampsia

    The incidence of preeclampsia is increased threefold in patients with multiple gestations, compared with that in women with singleton pregnancies. Furthermore, there is also an increase in the severity of the disease in patients with multiple gestations.

- Polyhydramnios

    Polyhydramnios is found in 5 to 8% of patients with multiple gestations and represents one of the causes of preterm labor in these patients.

- Anemia

    Both iron deficiency anemia and folic acid deficiency anemia are more commonly encountered in patients with multiple gestations because of increased fetal demands.

- Postpartum hemorrhage

    The risk of postpartum hemorrhage is increased in patients with multiple gestations because of uterine atony caused by overdistention of the uterus.

- Cholestasis of pregnancy
- Increased risk of cesarean section

    The higher incidences of prematurity and malpresentation contribute to the higher frequency of cesarean sections.

■ MAJOR THREAT TO FETAL LIFE

- Prematurity

    The major threat to life for the fetuses is that of prematurity. This risk of prematurity increases with the number of fetuses.

■ MAJOR THREAT TO MATERNAL LIFE

- Hemorrhage and hypovolemic shock

    Several of the maternal complications in a multiple gestation, such as placental abruption, postpartum hemorrhage, and the increased rate of cesarean section, all increase the risk of hemorrhage and hypovolemic shock.

■ BEDSIDE

Quick Look Test

Are abnormal fetal heart rate patterns present?

    Because of the increased incidence of prematurity, intrauterine growth restriction, and growth discordancy, patients with multiple gestations are at higher risk for developing fetal distress when in labor.

If the first infant has already been delivered, what is its approximate size and gestational age?

In patients with no prenatal care and/or unclear dates, the size and the gestational age of the delivered infant can be useful in the management of the undelivered fetus.

If the first infant has already delivered, is there significant vaginal bleeding?

Heavy vaginal bleeding that occurs between the delivery of the twins may be indicative of premature separation of the placenta. This will usually require immediate delivery, either by operative vaginal delivery or cesarean section.

Vital Signs

Vital signs are usually normal.

Selective History and Chart Review

1. What is the best estimate of gestational age based on early examinations and ultrasound measurements?
2. Has there been appropriate and concordant fetal growth during the pregnancy?
3. If the patient has had prior ultrasound examinations, has a membrane been detected between the twins, thereby ruling out monoamniotic twins (Fig. 13–1)?
4. Has the patient had any complications during her pregnancy such as preeclampsia or polyhydramnios?

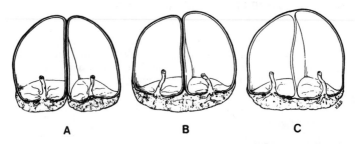

A   **B**   **C**

Figure 13–1 □ Placenta and membranes in twin gestations. *A,* Two placentas, two amnions, and two chorions. *B,* Single placenta, two amnions, and two chorions. *C,* One placenta, one chorion, and two amnions. (From Cunningham FC, MacDonald PC, Gant NF, et al: Williams Obstetrics, 19th ed. Norwalk, Connecticut, Appleton & Lange, 1993, p 892.)

Selective Physical Examination

Abdominal	Patient's uterus appears large for the gestational age
	Uterus still enlarged following delivery of the first twin
Pelvic	
External genitalia and vagina	Normal
Cervix	After delivery of the first twin, fetal parts of the second twin may be palpable through the dilated cervix
Uterus and adnexae	Large for dates
	Uterus still enlarged and contracting after delivery of the first twin

■ DIAGNOSTIC TESTING

1. **Ultrasound examination**

   Ultrasound examination is the quickest test available to determine not only the presence of a multiple gestation, but also the presentation of the fetuses and approximate gestational age. If an ultrasound examination is not possible, a portable abdominal x-ray study should be performed.

■ MANAGEMENT

1. **Continuous electronic fetal heart rate monitoring**
2. **Decision on the route of delivery**

   The route of delivery depends on the presentation, size, and gestational age of the fetuses, the condition of the mother and the twins, the experience of the deliverer, and the availability of an anesthesiologist and pediatrician. A flowchart of intrapartum management of the patient with multiple gestation is presented in Figure 13–2. The most common presentation in twin gestations is vertex–vertex, followed in frequency by vertex–breech. The frequency of presentations in twin gestations is presented in Table 13–1.

   a. **Twin A (vertex)/Twin B (vertex) presentation**

      Vaginal delivery should be attempted in the patient with a vertex–vertex presentation. It is estimated that 70 to 80% of vertex–vertex twins can be delivered safely vaginally. Immediately after the delivery of the first twin, the presentation and heart rate tracing of the undelivered twin should be evaluated. Potential complications encountered in the vaginal delivery of the second twin include premature placental separation, prolapse of the umbilical cord, and abnor-

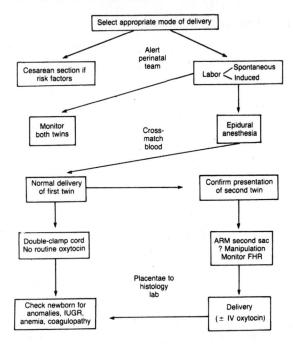

Figure 13–2 □ Intrapartum management of multiple gestation. (From Creasy RK, Resnik R: Maternal-Fetal Medicine: Principles and Practice, 3rd ed. Philadelphia, WB Saunders Co, 1994, p 594.)

Table 13–1 □ **INCIDENCE OF PRESENTATIONS IN TWIN DELIVERIES**

Presentation	Incidence (%)
Vertex–vertex	40
Vertex–breech	26
Breech–vertex	10
Breech–breech	10
Vertex–transverse	8
Miscellaneous	6

From Creasy RK, Resnik R: Maternal-Fetal Medicine: Principles and Practice, 3rd ed. Philadelphia, WB Saunders Co, 1994, p 597.

mal presentation. In the absence of these complications, the time interval between the deliveries of the first and second twins is not critical to the well-being of the second twin.

b. **Twin A (vertex)/Twin B (nonvertex) presentation**

Although cesarean section is often performed for this presentation, an attempt at vaginal delivery is a reasonable alternative if the estimated fetal weight is >1500 g. Vaginal delivery of the breech fetus with an estimated weight of <1500 g is controversial, and some advocate cesarean section for these patients. As an alternative, external cephalic version can be attempted with twin B.

c. **Twin A (nonvertex presentation)**

When twin A has a nonvertex presentation, a cesarean section is usually advisable regardless of the presentation of twin B. External cephalic version of twin A is not technically possible because of the presence of twin B.

3. **Management of the surviving twin after the death of one twin**

The death of a single twin is most common with monochorionic, monoamniotic twins, with an incidence between 0.5 and 6.8%. Early in pregnancy, the twin that has died is usually resorbed. Later in pregnancy, the prognosis for the surviving twin depends on the cause of the death, the gestational age, and the existence of vascular anastomoses between the two twins. Disseminated intravascular coagulation (DIC) can occur in rare cases. Before 34 to 35 weeks, management should be expectant. Fetal surveillance should be performed with either weekly nonstress tests or biophysical profiles. Furthermore, weekly maternal coagulation studies should be obtained. Delivery should be performed if there is evidence of fetal compromise or once fetal lung maturity has been attained. At term, labor should be induced and cesarean section should be performed only for the usual obstetrical indications.

14

PLACENTA PREVIA

■ BACKGROUND AND DEFINITIONS

Placenta previa: Abnormal implantation of the placenta either over or near the internal os of the cervix. The incidence of placenta previa is approximately 1 in 200 to 250 births. It is found more commonly in multiparous patients than in nulliparous patients. The incidence in nulliparous patients is approximately 1 in 1500 births, whereas the incidence in grand multiparous patients, patients who have had ≥5 deliveries, is approximately 1 in 20 births. The incidence of placenta previa has also been found to be increased by as much as five times in patients who have had previous cesarean sections. The risk of recurrent placenta previa in subsequent pregnancies is 4 to 8%. These findings support the theory that placenta previa is caused by defective decidual vascularization or endometrial damage that might occur with each pregnancy, especially when delivered by cesarean section. Placenta previa results in a maternal mortality rate of less than 1% and a perinatal mortality rate of less than 10%. There are four degrees of placenta previa, defined as follows (Fig. 14–1):

Total or complete placenta previa: Placenta covers the entire internal cervical os

Partial placenta previa: Placenta partially covers the cervical os

Marginal placenta previa: Edge of the placenta is at the margin of the internal os

Low-lying placenta: Placenta is implanted in the lower uterine segment, so that the placental edge is near the cervical os but does not actually reach the os

■ CLINICAL PRESENTATION

Painless vaginal bleeding, usually at the end of the second trimester or later

Bleeding often increases with labor

■ PHONE CALL

Questions

1. How much is the patient bleeding?
2. What are the patient's vital signs?

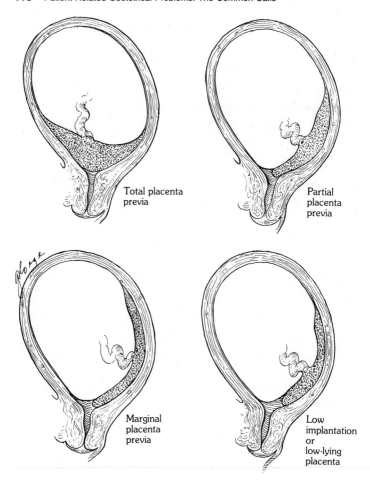

Figure 14–1 □ Degrees of placenta previa. (From Hacker NF, Moore JG: Essentials of Obstetrics and Gynecology, 2nd ed. Philadelphia, WB Saunders Co, 1992, p 156.)

Orders

1. Start a large-bore IV
2. Do not allow anyone to perform a digital or speculum vaginal examination on the patient
3. Obtain a complete blood count (CBC)
4. Type and crossmatch 2 or more units of blood
5. Initiate external electronic fetal monitoring

6. Insert a Foley catheter if the patient appears to be in shock
7. Notify the anesthesiologist and pediatric team of the possible need for an emergency cesarean delivery

Degree of Urgency

Bleeding from a placenta previa can be severe enough to be life threatening. Furthermore, bleeding can become heavier without warning and with no apparent precipitating cause. Patients with bleeding from a suspected placenta previa should be seen immediately.

■ ELEVATOR THOUGHTS

What are other causes of painless vaginal bleeding?
- Mild placental abruption, also referred to as "marginal separation"
- Normal "bloody show" from cervical effacement and dilatation
- Cervical or vaginal lesion

■ MAJOR THREAT TO FETAL LIFE

- Prematurity
   Preterm delivery performed for severe bleeding is the most common cause of perinatal morbidity and mortality.
- Fetal asphyxia
   Severe hemorrhage can result in maternal hypovolemic shock and fetal asphyxia.

■ MAJOR THREAT TO MATERNAL LIFE

- Hypovolemic shock
   Bleeding from placenta previa can be severe enough to result in hypovolemic shock.

■ BEDSIDE

Quick Look Test

Does the patient appear to be in shock?

Is there ongoing bleeding, and if so, how severe is the bleeding?

Does fetal heart rate monitoring suggest the presence of fetal distress?

Is the patient in labor?

Uterine contractions and cervical dilatation will exacerbate bleeding from a placenta previa because they cause further separation of the placenta. Laboring patients can be given tocolytic medications to stop the progression of labor.

Vital Signs

A patient in hypovolemic shock from placenta previa will be hypotensive and tachycardic. The patient might have postural hypotension. Changes in blood pressure (BP) and pulse should be measured when the patient is assisted in sitting or standing from a supine position. A fall in systolic or diastolic BP of >15 mm Hg or a rise in pulse of >15 beats/min is indicative of hypovolemia.

Selective History and Chart Review

1. What is the gestational age of the fetus?

   The gestational age is one of the key factors that influences the management of a patient bleeding from a placenta previa, especially if the bleeding is not severe.

2. Has the patient had an ultrasound examination during the pregnancy?

   A prior sonogram might help to confirm the diagnosis of placenta previa. However, of all patients who are identified as having placenta previa on ultrasound examination performed before 30 weeks of gestation, only ≤5% will have placenta previa at delivery. This is because the placenta in effect moves away from the cervical os as the lower uterine segment develops late in pregnancy. A previous ultrasound examination will also provide information concerning the gestational age.

Selective Physical Examination

Abdominal	Nontender and benign
Pelvic	
External genitalia and vagina	Blood-stained
Cervix	Digital or speculum examination either should not be performed or, if absolutely necessary, should be performed with extreme care in an operation room in case the examination results in severe bleeding. A double-setup is described below.
Uterus and adnexae	Nontender and benign

■ DIAGNOSTIC TESTING

1. Ultrasound examination

Ultrasound examination is the simplest and safest diagnostic test for the localization of the placenta. It has an accuracy rate of approximately 95% in the diagnosis of placenta previa. Distention of the bladder can result in false-positive readings, and therefore, patients who are diagnosed as having placenta previa should have a repeat ultrasound examination after emptying the bladder.

2. Double-setup digital examination

With the availability and resolution of current sonography, there are very few indications for a double-setup examination. However, when ultrasound examination is either equivocal or unavailable, the only way to establish the diagnosis of placenta previa is to digitally palpate the placenta through the cervical os. This type of examination should be performed only if delivery is planned, because heavy bleeding can be caused even by very gentle digital examination. Furthermore, this type of examination should be performed only in an operating room with the patient prepared for both vaginal delivery and cesarean section, so that an immediate cesarean section can be performed if a placenta previa is found. At least 2 to 4 units of blood should be available. A double-setup examination is not indicated if the patient is having bleeding severe enough to require immediate delivery.

■ MANAGEMENT

The management of the patient with placenta previa is dependent on the following factors: (1) presence and severity of the bleeding, (2) gestational age of the fetus, and (3) presence of labor.

1. Minimal or no bleeding, premature gestational age

a. Expectant management

Expectant management consists of the severe restriction of physical activity either in the hospital or at home. The goals of expectant management are (1) attainment of fetal maturity and (2) resolution of the placenta previa. Depending on the gestational age when placenta previa is diagnosed, there is a possibility of resolution as the lower uterine segment develops. Patients followed expectantly at home should be observed in the hospital for approximately 72 hours before discharge, because it has been found that about one-third of these patients will bleed and require delivery within this time. A patient who is managed expectantly at home must be compliant with the restriction of physical activity, including sexual intercourse. Furthermore, she must be attended by an adult and be able to be transported to the hospital immediately if bleeding occurs.

2. **Minimal or no bleeding, mature gestational age**
   a. **Amniocentesis for fetal lung maturity**
   b. **Cesarean section if mature**

   Once the fetus has reached a gestational age of 35 to 36 weeks, little is gained by expectant management, and there remains the risk of sudden unexpected bleeding. Therefore, amniocentesis should be performed and a phospholipid fetal lung profile should be obtained. The fetus should be delivered if the fetal lung profile shows maturity. The route of delivery should in almost all cases be cesarean section. An exception would be for the patient with a low-lying placenta, who could be allowed to labor as long as she is monitored closely for the onset of bleeding. In a patient undergoing cesarean section, blood should be available even if the patient is not actively bleeding, because intraoperative blood loss can be heavy. This is because the placental implantation site is in the lower uterine segment, where there is not the thick uterine musculature found in the uterine fundus that provides for hemostasis through uterine contractions. Furthermore, placenta accreta is commonly associated with placenta previa, occurring in approximately 15% of cases. This is a condition in which the placenta is abnormally attached to the uterine myometrium, resulting in difficult removal and postpartum hemorrhage.

3. **Minimal bleeding associated with premature labor**
   a. **Administration of tocolytic drugs**
   b. **Expectant management if labor is successfully stopped**
   c. **Cesarean section if labor is not stopped and bleeding continues**

   Labor can often precipitate bleeding because progressive cervical dilatation results in further separation of the placenta. The administration of tocolytic drugs such as magnesium sulfate or terbutaline can result in cessation of bleeding in the patient with premature labor and can also be used to temporize with patients who are being prepared for cesarean section.

4. **Severe bleeding, any gestational age**
   a. **Cesarean section**

   Patients who have severe, life-threatening vaginal bleeding should be delivered by cesarean section regardless of the gestational age of the fetus.

15

PLACENTAL ABRUPTION

■ BACKGROUND AND DEFINITIONS

Placental abruption: Separation of a normally implanted placenta before delivery of the fetus, also referred to as abruptio placentae

Placental abruption is one of the common causes of third-trimester bleeding, but it can also occur any time after 20 weeks of gestation. The severity of placental abruption is based on how much of the placenta has undergone separation. Depending on the location of the placenta, bleeding from placental abruption may be concealed, resulting in hypotension out of proportion to the amount of visible bleeding (Fig. 15–1). The incidence of placental abruption is approximately 1 in 150 deliveries, and the perinatal mortality rate associated with this condition is 15 to 20%. Severe abruption may result in Couvelaire uterus or uterine apoplexy, which is a uterus with extravasation of blood into the myometrium, underneath the uterine serosa, and sometimes even

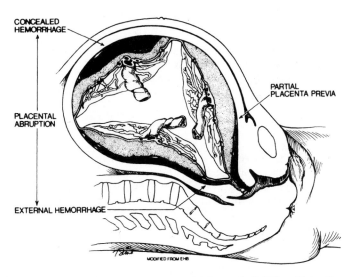

Figure 15–1 □ Concealed hemorrhage in placental abruption. (From Cunningham FC, MacDonald PC, Gant NF, et al: Williams Obstetrics, 19th ed. Norwalk, Connecticut, Appleton & Lange, 1993, p 826.)

into the broad ligament and fallopian tube serosa. This is usually found at the time of cesarean delivery.

■ CLINICAL PRESENTATION

Vaginal bleeding
Hypovolemic shock, often out of proportion to the amount of visible bleeding
Coagulopathy
Uterine pain and tenderness
Uterine irritability
Hypertonic uterine contractions
Back pain
Fetal distress
Fetal demise

A grading system, originally published by Page and colleagues (Page EW, King EB, Merrill JA: Abruptio placentae: dangers of delay in delivery. Obstet Gynecol 1954;3:385) can be used to classify cases of placental abruption depending on maternal and fetal signs and symptoms (Table 15–1).

■ PHONE CALL

Questions

1. **What are the patient's vital signs?**
2. **Does the patient appear to be in pain?**
   Placental abruption commonly results in uterine contractions and/or hypertonus of the uterus, which causes abdominal and back pain.

Orders

1. Start a large-bore IV
2. Initiate electronic fetal heart rate monitoring
3. Obtain a complete blood count (CBC)
4. Obtain coagulation studies: prothrombin time (PT), partial thromboplastin time (PTT), platelet count, fibrinogen, fibrin split products
5. Type and crossmatch blood if bleeding is severe or if the patient is in hypovolemic shock
6. Insert a Foley catheter
7. Record input and output
8. Notify the anesthesiologist and pediatric team of the possible need for an emergency cesarean section

Table 15-1 □ GRADING OF PLACENTAL ABRUPTION

Grade	Concealed Hemorrhage	Uterine Tenderness	Maternal Shock	Coagulopathy	Fetal Distress	Comments
0	–	–	–	–	–	Asymptomatic, based on retrospective examination of placenta
1	–	–	–	–	–	Includes "marginal sinus rupture," bleeding variable
2	+	+	–	Rare	+	Progresses to grade 3 unless delivery is achieved
3	++	+	+	Common	Fetal death	Major maternal morbidity

– = absent; + = present; ++ = severe.
Adapted from Creasy RK, Resnik R: Maternal-Fetal Medicine: Principles and Practice, 3rd ed. Philadelphia, WB Saunders Co, 1994, p 610.

Degree of Urgency

Placental abruption is an obstetrical emergency that can be associated with serious morbidity and even mortality for both the patient and the fetus. The patient should be seen immediately.

■ ELEVATOR THOUGHTS

What factors are associated with placental abruption?
- Pregnancy-induced hypertension
- Chronic hypertension
- Cocaine abuse
- Cigarette smoking
- Trauma
- High parity
- Sudden decompression of the uterus after delivery of the first twin in a multiple gestation
- Short umbilical cord
- Preterm premature rupture of membranes
- Uterine anomaly
- Uterine leiomyomata
- History of placental abruption

■ MAJOR THREAT TO FETAL LIFE

- Fetal demise
    Severe placental abruption can result in fetal asphyxia and fetal death.
- Prematurity
    Preterm delivery performed for severe abruption is a common cause of perinatal morbidity and mortality.

■ MAJOR THREAT TO MATERNAL LIFE

- Hypovolemic shock
- Disseminated intravascular coagulation (DIC)
    Severe abruption can also result in DIC.

■ BEDSIDE

Quick Look Test

Does the patient appear to be in shock?
    Patients with placental abruption may appear to be in shock even in the absence of significant external bleeding because of

concealed retroplacental bleeding. Concealed bleeding is encountered in approximately 10% of all patients with abruption.

Does the fetal heart rate tracing suggest fetal distress?

Significant placental abruption can cause fetal distress and even fetal death. Fetal distress and death can result from placental separation, maternal hemorrhage, fetal hemorrhage, uterine hypertonus, or a combination of these factors. The incidence of fetal distress in the presence of placental abruption is approximately 60%.

Vital Signs

A patient in hypovolemic shock from placental abruption will be hypotensive and tachycardic. The patient might have postural hypotension. Changes in blood pressure (BP) and pulse should be measured when the patient is assisted in sitting or standing from a supine position. A fall in systolic or diastolic BP of >15 mm Hg or a rise in pulse of >15 beats/min is evidence of hypovolemia.

Selective History and Chart Review

1. What is the gestational age of the fetus?

   The gestational age will impact the management of the patient.
2. Has the patient had a prior obstetrical ultrasound examination?

   A prior ultrasound examination will provide an estimate of the gestational age. Furthermore, it can rule out placenta previa, which presents with bleeding similar to that with placental abruption.
3. Does the patient have pregnancy-induced or chronic hypertension?

   Both of these conditions are most commonly associated with placental abruption.

Selective Physical Examination

Abdominal	Uterine fundus hard and tender
Pelvic	
External genitalia and vagina	Blood-stained or negative
Cervix	Blood-stained or negative
Uterus	Fundus hard and tender
	Irritable on palpation

■ DIAGNOSTIC TESTING

1. Ultrasound examination

Ultrasound examination may help confirm the diagnosis of placental abruption if a retroplacental clot is found. Acute hemorrhage is usually hyperechoic and therefore can sometimes be detected between the placenta and the uterine wall. Furthermore, ultrasound examination is helpful in ruling out placenta previa, which can present with signs and symptoms similar to that with placental abruption. A normal ultrasound examination does not exclude placental abruption. Acute hemorrhage can appear isoechoic and therefore be misinterpreted as part of a thick placenta.

The diagnosis of placental abruption is usually made clinically and should be suspected in any patient with bleeding, abdominal pain, uterine tenderness, or uterine irritability.

■ MANAGEMENT

The options in the management of placental abruption are **(1) expectant management** with close monitoring of both the maternal and the fetal status, **(2) induction of labor and vaginal delivery,** or **(3) immediate cesarean section.** The management of placental abruption is dependent on maternal status, fetal status, and gestational age of the fetus. Transfusion of blood, platelets, fresh frozen plasma, or cryoprecipitate may be necessary regardless of the management option chosen. Postpartum hysterectomy may be necessary.

1. Expectant management

Expectant management is appropriate if the following three criteria are met:

a. Degree of placental abruption is mild with minimal bleeding,

b. Maternal status is stable and there is no evidence of hypovolemic shock or severe coagulopathy, and

c. There is no evidence of fetal distress

Expectant management consists of close continuous monitoring of maternal hemodynamic and coagulation status with serial CBCs and coagulation studies. The fetus should also be monitored with electronic fetal heart rate monitoring. Expectant management is especially preferred when the fetus is premature. If it is anticipated that preterm delivery will eventually occur, the administration of steroids to accelerate fetal lung maturation should be considered.

2. Induction of labor and vaginal delivery

Induction of labor is appropriate if the following two criteria are met:

a. Degree of placental abruption is moderate with ongoing bleeding, but the mother is not in immediate jeopardy and there is no evidence of hypovolemic shock or coagulopathy, and

b. There is no evidence of fetal distress

Even when the degree of placental abruption is mild, uterine contractions may be hypertonic and labor may be fast and tumultuous. During labor, the degree of placental separation may increase and result in deterioration of maternal or fetal status, making cesarean delivery necessary. Induction of labor and vaginal delivery is the management of choice for fetal demise when the mother is stable. It is also the best management for the pregnancy with a previable fetus when the degree of placental abruption is severe enough to make delivery necessary. Induction of labor should be attempted with an oxytocin infusion, and amniotomy should be performed as soon as it is safe. As an alternative, in early pregnancies, **20-mg prostaglandin E_2 (dinoprostone) vaginal suppositories** can be used to induce labor.

3. **Cesarean section**

Immediate cesarean section should be performed for any one of the following:

a. Degree of placental abruption is severe with brisk ongoing bleeding,

b. Maternal status is unstable with signs of hypovolemic shock or coagulopathy, or

c. There is evidence of fetal distress

In a patient who is already unstable, cesarean section will almost always result in further deterioration of maternal status. Furthermore, patients with a coagulopathy caused by placental abruption may bleed excessively intraoperatively and postoperatively. Therefore, aggressive efforts to correct anemia, hypovolemic shock, and coagulopathy must be taken before surgery. Red blood cells (RBCs), platelets, fresh frozen plasma (FFP), or cryoprecipitate should be transfused accordingly.

4. **Transfusion of blood products**

a. Red blood cells

RBCs are transfused to increase oxygen-carrying capacity in anemic patients. One unit of packed RBCs and one unit of whole blood have volumes of 250 and 450 ml, respectively. Each unit of RBCs should increase the hematocrit by 3% and hemoglobin by 1 g/dl. Coagulation studies should be obtained after every 5 to 10 units of RBCs transfused.

b. Platelets

Platelets are transfused for a platelet count of <20,000/ mm^3 or, in patients in whom a cesarean delivery is planned, for a platelet count of $<50,000/mm^3$. Each unit of platelets should increase the platelet count by 5000 to $10,000/mm^3$.

c. **Fresh frozen plasma**

FFP is transfused for coagulopathy due to deficiency of clotting factors, usually if PT or PTT is >1.5 times normal. Each unit of FFP will increase any clotting factor by 2 to 3%. The usual initial dose is 2 units, and each unit has a volume of 200 to 250 ml.

d. **Cryoprecipitate**

Cryoprecipitate is transfused for coagulopathy due to deficiency of factor VIII, von Willebrand's factor, factor XIII, fibrinogen, or fibronectin. Cryoprecipitate is concentrated from FFP, and each bag has a volume of 10 to 15 ml. Each bag contains at least 150 mg of fibrinogen.

5. **Postpartum hysterectomy**

Postpartum hysterectomy is performed only if there is severe and persistent uterine bleeding that is not responsive to correction of the coagulopathy or the administration of oxytocin, methergine, or prostaglandin. Before hysterectomy, selective angiographic arterial embolization should be considered. Consideration should also be given to bilateral ligation of the hypogastric arteries, which will decrease pulse pressure enough to allow the patient's coagulation system to decrease blood loss. Bilateral hypogastric artery ligation, however, will preclude the use of angiographic arterial embolization. If the patient has already lost a significant amount of blood or is unstable, supracervical or subtotal hysterectomy should be performed. The presence of Couvelaire uterus is not, by itself, an indication for hysterectomy.

16

POSTPARTUM DEPRESSION

■ BACKGROUND AND DEFINITIONS

Postpartum blues: Also referred to as **maternity blues,** it affects 50 to 70% of postpartum women. This condition develops early in the postpartum period, usually in the first few postpartum days. It is transient and rarely persists beyond 2 weeks.

Postpartum depression: Also known as **postpartum neurotic depression,** it occurs in approximately 10% of postpartum patients. It can develop anytime in the first 6 months of the postpartum period and often lasts for more than 2 weeks.

Postpartum psychosis: Occurs in 1 to 2 of 1000 puerperal women. It most often begins in the first 3 weeks postpartum and rarely begins after 6 weeks postpartum.

■ CLINICAL PRESENTATION

Postpartum blues
- Insomnia
- Weepiness
- Depression
- Fatigue
- Anxiety
- Headaches
- Poor concentration
- Confusion

Postpartum depression
- Symptoms of postpartum blues plus the following:
- Despondency
- Emotional lability
- Apathy
- Listlessness
- Irritability
- Guilt
- Ambivalent feelings toward the infant
- Feelings of inadequacy as a mother
- Anorexia
- Self-derogatory feelings
- Indecisiveness
- Somatic complaints, especially involving the gastrointestinal tract

Postpartum psychosis

> Symptoms of postpartum blues and postpartum depression plus the following:
> Suicidal thoughts or actual attempts
> Threats of violence or actual violence toward the infant
> Delusional and paranoid thoughts
> Cognitive disorders
> Psychomotor retardation or catatonic features
> Motor agitation
> Inappropriate affect
> Hallucinations, especially ones that command her to harm her infant
> Excessive concern over the infant's health
> Delusions that the baby is either dead or defective
> Schizophrenic features
> Manic features

■ PHONE CALL

Questions

1. Does the patient pose a danger to herself or to her infant?

Patients with postpartum psychosis can have suicidal ideations as well as actual suicide attempts. Furthermore, they can exhibit violent behavior toward their infants.

2. When did the patient deliver?

A patient is more likely to have postpartum depression or psychosis, as opposed to the very common postpartum blues, if her symptoms have been present for more than several weeks after her delivery.

Orders

If the patient appears to be potentially harmful to either herself or her infant, she should have an attendant with her and not be left alone. Furthermore, she should not be allowed to leave before being evaluated by a physician.

Degree of Urgency

Patients who appear to have postpartum psychosis should be seen immediately.

■ ELEVATOR THOUGHTS

What factors contribute to postpartum blues?

- Emotional letdown after the long-anticipated labor and delivery
- Fatigue from labor and delivery and from caring for the infant
- Postpartum pain from the delivery process, especially if a cesarean section was performed
- Recovery from complications of the pregnancy and delivery such as infection and blood loss
- Changes in body image after pregnancy

What are predictive factors for postpartum depression?

- Marital difficulties
- Undesired or unplanned pregnancy
- Single or separated marital status
- History of physical violence in the patient's family
- High level of anxiety during pregnancy

What are predictive factors for postpartum psychosis?

- History of bipolar affective disorder
- History of postpartum psychosis
- First-degree relatives with bipolar affective disorders
- First pregnancy
- Cesarean delivery

■ MAJOR THREAT TO INFANT'S LIFE

- Physical violence to infant
  Threat to the life of the infant is a concern only with postpartum psychosis.

■ MAJOR THREAT TO MATERNAL LIFE

- Suicide
  Suicide is a concern only with postpartum psychosis.

■ BEDSIDE

Quick Look Test

Does the patient exhibit motor agitation or catatonic features?
These are symptoms suggestive of psychosis.

Vital Signs

Vital signs are usually normal.

Selective History and Chart Review

1. Does the patient have a past history of postpartum depression or psychosis?

2. Does the patient have any of the predictive factors listed above for postpartum depression or psychosis?

Selective Physical Examination

Physical examination is usually normal.

■ DIAGNOSTIC TESTING

There is no evidence of a direct causative effect of the postpartum physiological and hormonal changes on the incidence of postpartum blues, depression, or psychosis. Therefore, there are no diagnostic laboratory tests available to confirm the diagnosis of these conditions.

■ MANAGEMENT

1. **Postpartum blues**

    No specific treatment is indicated for postpartum blues. The patient should be reassured that her symptoms are very common and transient, rarely persisting for more than 2 weeks. Emotional support, encouragement, and aid and education in the care of the infant can be helpful.

2. **Postpartum depression**
    a. **Psychotherapy**

        Although psychiatric consultation is recommended for severe cases of postpartum depression, more mild cases can be managed by the primary physician if he or she is comfortable dealing with the patient's psychological problems and has the time to provide psychotherapy.
    b. **Antidepressant medication**
        (1) **Imipramine (Tofranil) 75 to 300 mg/day PO**
        (2) **Amitriptyline (Elavil) 75 to 300 mg/day PO**
        (3) **Fluoxetine (Prozac) 20 to 60 mg/day PO**
        (4) **Alprazolam (Xanax) 0.75 to 4 mg/day PO**

        All of the antidepressant medications listed above can be detected in the breast milk of nursing mothers, usually at a level of 10% of that found in maternal serum. Alprazolam has been shown to cause lethargy, weight loss, and impaired temperature regulation in breast-feeding infants. No adverse effects have been found in breast-feeding infants whose mothers use fluoxetine or the two tricyclics imipramine and amitriptyline. Nevertheless, caution is advised in the use of these antidepressant medications in breast-feeding mothers. When in doubt, if the medication is believed to be absolutely necessary, breast feeding should be discontinued.

3. **Postpartum psychosis**
   a. **Psychiatric consultation**
      Patients with postpartum psychosis should be admitted to the hospital and should be seen by a psychiatrist.
   b. **Antipsychotic medication**
      (1) **Chlorpromazine (Thorazine) 400 to 600 mg/day PO or 25 mg IM initially for acute psychosis**
      (2) **Haloperidol (Haldol) 0.5 to 5.0 mg PO two or three times per day or 2 to 5 mg IM initially for acute psychosis**

      Both chlorpromazine and haloperidol are excreted in the breast milk of breast-feeding mothers, and therefore, consideration should be given to cessation of breast feeding.

17

POSTPARTUM FEVER

■ BACKGROUND AND DEFINITIONS

Standard puerperal morbidity: Temperature of 100.4°F or 38.0°C, which occurs in any 2 of the first 10 days postpartum, exclusive of the first 24 hours, taken orally at least four times daily.

Endometritis, endomyometritis, endoparametritis, and metritis with pelvic cellulitis: All are synonymous and defined as uterine infection, the most common cause of a postpartum fever. The incidence of endometritis after vaginal delivery is from 1.3 to 6%. However, the incidence is significantly higher after cesarean section, increasing to 12 to 51%.

■ CLINICAL PRESENTATION

Fever
Chills and rigor
Malaise
Uterine pain and tenderness
Abdominal pain and tenderness
Foul-smelling lochia

■ PHONE CALL

Questions

1. **What are the patient's vital signs?**
2. **How ill does the patient appear?**

Orders

1. Obtain a complete blood count (CBC) with differential
2. Perform urinalysis
3. Obtain blood and urine cultures if the patient appears to be severely ill

Degree of Urgency

Endometritis and other causes of postpartum fever are rarely life threatening, and the patient does not need to be seen immediately.

■ ELEVATOR THOUGHTS

What is the differential diagnosis of postpartum fever?
- Endometritis
- Pyelonephritis
- Mastitis
- Breast engorgement
- Respiratory complications
- Wound infection
    Infection of cesarean section incision
    Infection of episiotomy repair
    Infection of spontaneous obstetrical lacerations
- Thrombophlebitis
    Septic pelvic thrombophlebitis
    Thrombophlebitis of the lower extremities

What are factors that increase the risk for postpartum endometritis?
- Cesarean section
- Prolonged labor
- Prolonged rupture of membranes
- Multiple vaginal examinations
- Use of internal fetal monitoring
- Use of internal uterine monitoring by pressure catheter
- Low socioeconomic status
- Chorioamnionitis
- Bacterial vaginosis
- Anemia
- Major obstetrical trauma of the cervix or vagina

■ MAJOR THREAT TO MATERNAL LIFE

- Sepsis
    Sepsis is a rare complication of endometritis. It is most often caused by *Escherichia coli, Clostridium,* and *Bacteroides.*

■ BEDSIDE

Quick Look Test

Does the patient appear to be severely ill?
   In patients who appear severely ill, sepsis, septic pelvic thrombophlebitis, and pelvic abscess should be considered.

Vital Signs

   Patients are febrile, but otherwise, the vital signs are usually normal. The findings of hypotension and tachycardia are suggestive of sepsis or ruptured pelvic abscess.

Selective History and Chart Review

1. Does the patient have symptoms of a nonpelvic cause of postpartum fever such as pyelonephritis, mastitis, or pneumonia?
2. What was the route of delivery?
    Patients who had cesarean sections are at a much higher risk for endometritis and wound infection.
3. When did the patient give birth?
    Late-onset endometritis is commonly caused by *Chlamydia trachomatis.*
4. If the patient gave birth vaginally, did she have any risk factors for endometritis such as prolonged labor, prolonged rupture of membranes, internal monitoring, or chorioamnionitis?
5. Did the patient have bacterial vaginosis or anemia?

Selective Physical Examination

Breast	Tender, hard, and erythematous in mastitis
Back	Costovertebral angle (CVA) tenderness in pyelonephritis
Abdominal	Tender in uncomplicated endometritis
	Surgical incision erythematous, indurated, and draining purulent fluid in wound infection
	Rigid with rebound tenderness and involuntary guarding in ruptured pelvic abscess
Pelvic	
External genitalia and vagina	Episiotomy or laceration sites tender, erythematous, indurated, and draining purulent fluid in infection
Cervix	Usually normal although a foul-smelling purulent discharge may be present with endometritis
Uterus and adnexae	Tender to palpation in endometritis

■ DIAGNOSTIC TESTING

The diagnosis of endometritis is based on the finding of uterine tenderness, fever, foul-smelling discharge, and malaise. Laboratory tests may be helpful in confirming the diagnosis and in ruling out other causes of fever.

1. CBC with differential
The white blood cell count is elevated in endometritis, as also occurs in other infections.

2. Gram stain and culture of foul-smelling lochia
Cultures may be contaminated with vaginal flora, but they can still be helpful in identifying clostridia, anaerobes, and chlamydia.

3. Ultrasound examination

Ultrasound examination is helpful in detecting a pelvic abscess.

4. Urinalysis

The finding of white blood cell casts is diagnostic of pyelonephritis.

5. Blood cultures

Positive blood cultures can result from any type of infection; cultures are positive in 25% of cases of septic pelvic thrombophlebitis.

6. Computed tomography scan

A CT scan may be helpful in patients who do not respond to antibiotic therapy and who have negative ultrasound examinations, because this test can detect occult abscesses and can also detect the thrombus in septic pelvic thrombophlebitis.

■ MANAGEMENT

1. Endometritis

The organisms usually responsible for endometritis are listed in Table 17–1. Antibiotic regimens are numerous and depend on the organisms suspected.

a. Ampicillin 0.5 to 2.0 g IV every 6 hours plus gentamicin 1.0 to 1.5 mg/kg IV every 8 hours

Table 17–1 ▫ ORGANISMS RESPONSIBLE FOR ENDOMETRITIS

Aerobic organisms

Groups A, B, and D streptococci and
   streptococcus viridans
Staphylococcus aureus
Enterococcus
Escherichia coli
Proteus mirabilis
Klebsiella
Enterobacter
Gardnerella vaginalis

Anaerobic organisms

Bacteroides fragilis, bivius, and *disiens*
Clostridium
Peptococcus
Peptostreptococcus

Miscellaneous

Chlamydia trachomatis
Mycoplasma hominis

This regimen has a cure rate of 70 to 85%, although it does not provide good coverage for anaerobes.

b. **Clindamycin 300 to 600 mg IV every 6 hours or 900 mg IV every 8 hours plus gentamicin 1.0 to 1.5 mg/kg IV every 8 hours**

This regimen has a cure rate of 95%, and most failures are due to poor coverage of enterococcus. A possible adverse effect of clindamycin is diarrhea from pseudomembranous colitis caused by an overgrowth of enterotoxin-producing *Clostridium difficile.* This usually responds to vancomycin or metronidazole and discontinuation of clindamycin.

c. **Clindamycin 300 to 600 mg IV every 6 hours or 900 mg IV every 8 hours plus aztreonam 1.0 to 2.0 g IV every 8 hours**

Aztreonam is a monobactam that provides excellent coverage for aerobic gram-negative organisms. It can be used instead of gentamicin in those patients at risk for aminoglycoside toxicity. Pseudomembraneous colitis as is discussed above is a possible adverse effect of clindamycin.

d. **Beta-lactamase inhibitor combined with penicillin**
   (1) **Ampicillin and sulbactam (Unasyn) 1.5 g (1.0 g ampicillin and 0.5 g sulbactam) to 3.0 g (2.0 g ampicillin and 1.0 g sulbactam) IV every 6 hours**
   (2) **Ticarcillin and clavulanic acid (Timentin) 50 to 75 mg/ kg IV every 6 hours**

e. **Cephalosporins**
   (1) **Cefoxitin (Mefoxin) 1.0 to 2.0 g IV every 6 hours**
   (2) **Cefotetan (Cefotan) 1.0 to 2.0 g IV every 12 hours**
   (3) **Cefoperazone (Cefobid) 0.5 to 1.0 g IV every 6 hours**

With the administration of the appropriate antibiotics, most patients respond within a few days. Antibiotics should be continued until the patient has been afebrile for 24 to 48 hours. There is no need for a course of oral antibiotics to follow the parenteral antibiotics. If a patient fails to respond to antibiotic therapy and nonpelvic sources for fever have been ruled out, septic pelvic thrombophlebitis and pelvic abscess should be considered.

2. **Septic pelvic thrombophlebitis**

Septic pelvic thrombophlebitis has also been referred to as "enigmatic" or "obscure" fever, because fever usually persists after prolonged therapy with multiple antibiotics. It is caused by the extension of endometritis along venous routes, especially the ovarian veins. Patients typically do not appear ill but have multiple fever spikes, giving the temperature curve a "sawtooth" appearance. There is usually either no pain or mild and vague abdominal pain. Findings on pelvic and abdominal examination are vague and unremarkable.

a. **Heparin**
   (1) **Loading dose:** 5000 units IV
   (2) **Maintenance dose:** 1000 to 1500 U/hr IV to achieve PTT of ≥1.5-fold control

Anticoagulation therapy with IV heparin is both diagnostic and therapeutic. Patients with septic pelvic thrombophlebitis respond with rapid defervescence within 2 to 3 days. If there is no such improvement, the diagnosis should be questioned. After successful heparinization, the patient should be placed on oral warfarin therapy. The total duration of anticoagulation therapy should be 10 to 14 days.

3. **Pelvic abscess**

Antibiotic therapy for patients with pelvic abscesses must include agents such as clindamycin, which cover anaerobic bacteria. Pelvic abscesses that do not respond to antibiotics must be drained. This can be performed percutaneously with radiographic guidance if the abscess is accessible. If the abscess is inaccessible or if rupture of the abscess is suspected, exploratory laparotomy is indicated.

18

POSTPARTUM HEMORRHAGE

■ BACKGROUND AND DEFINITIONS

Postpartum hemorrhage: Blood loss of more than 500 ml after delivery

Early postpartum hemorrhage: Postpartum hemorrhage occurring in the first 24 hours after delivery

Late postpartum hemorrhage: Postpartum hemorrhage occurring 24 hours to 6 weeks after delivery

Despite the universal acceptance of the above definition of postpartum hemorrhage, it has been shown that the average blood loss after an uncomplicated vaginal delivery is 550 to 600 ml. The average blood loss after a cesarean section is 1000 ml. Therefore, blood loss of greater than 500 ml after delivery is not necessarily abnormal. The term "postpartum hemorrhage" is therefore used when the estimated blood loss appears to be more than usual. It is important to note that estimated blood loss usually underestimates the actual blood loss by close to 50%.

■ CLINICAL PRESENTATION

Vaginal bleeding
Hypovolemic shock in severe cases

■ PHONE CALL

Questions

1. What are the vital signs?
2. How severe is the bleeding?
3. How long has the patient been bleeding?
4. Is the patient currently receiving intravenous oxytocin?

Orders

1. Start a large-bore IV if the patient does not already have one
2. Obtain a complete blood count (CBC)
3. Obtain coagulation studies: platelet count, prothrombin time (PT), partial thromboplastin time (PTT), fibrinogen, fibrin split products
4. Type and crossmatch blood if the patient has had significant bleeding

5. Insert a Foley catheter to monitor urine output if the patient appears to be in shock

Degree of Urgency

Postpartum hemorrhage is a potentially life-threatening complication that accounts for 4 to 5% of all maternal mortality. Patients should be seen immediately.

■ ELEVATOR THOUGHTS

What are the causes of postpartum hemorrhage?
- Uterine atony
- Lacerations of the vulva, vagina, or cervix
- Retained fragments of placenta
- Retained placenta due to abnormal placental implantation (Fig. 18–1)
    Placenta accreta
    Placenta increta
    Placenta percreta
- Coagulopathy
- Uterine rupture
- Inversion of the uterus (Fig. 18–2)
- Subinvolution of the uterus

■ MAJOR THREAT TO MATERNAL LIFE

- Hypovolemic shock

■ BEDSIDE

Quick Look Test

Does the patient appear to be in shock?
    A patient in hypovolemic shock will usually appear distressed, ill, and apprehensive. She will appear pale and have cold and clammy skin.

Vital Signs

A patient in hypovolemic shock will be hypotensive and tachycardic. Furthermore, the patient might have postural hypotension. Changes in BP and pulse should be measured when the patient is assisted in sitting or standing from a supine position. A fall in

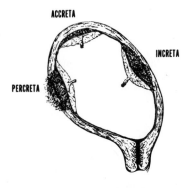

Figure 18–1 □ Placenta accreta, increta, and percreta. (From Breen JL, Neubecker R, Gregori CA, et al: Placenta accreta, increta, and percreta. A survey of 40 cases. Obstet Gynecol 1977; 49:43. Reprinted with permission from The American College of Obstetricians and Gynecologists.)

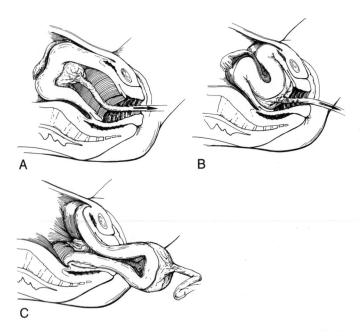

Figure 18–2 □ Uterine inversion secondary to cord traction. *A,* Partial uterine inversion. *B,* Complete uterine inversion. *C,* Complete uterine inversion with prolapse. (From Plauche WC, Morrison JC, O'Sullivan M: Surgical Obstetrics. Philadelphia, WB Saunders Co, 1992, p 219.)

systolic or diastolic BP of >15 mm Hg or a rise in pulse of >15 beats/min is evidence of hypovolemia.

Selective History and Chart Review

1. Did the patient have a prolonged labor?

    A prolonged labor, especially when induced or augmented with oxytocin, is associated with a higher risk of uterine atony.

2. What was the route of delivery?

    Vulvar, vaginal, or cervical lacerations are possible causes of postpartum hemorrhage if the patient had a difficult forceps- or vacuum-assisted delivery. Uterine rupture should be considered if the patient had a vaginal delivery after a prior cesarean section. Retained placental fragments are possible after a vaginal delivery but unlikely after a cesarean section, because the placenta is removed manually under direct visualization.

3. Was the delivery of the placenta difficult?

    Retained placental fragments or abnormal placental implantation should be suspected if the delivery of the placenta was difficult. Furthermore, if excessive traction had been applied to the umbilical cord in an attempt to deliver the placenta, uterine inversion can result.

4. Did the patient have preeclampsia or placental abruption?

    Severe preeclampsia and placental abruption are common causes of coagulopathy in pregnancy.

Selective Physical Examination

Abdominal	Uterine atony: uterine fundus is soft and sometimes difficult to palpate
Pelvic	
External genitalia and vagina	Lacerations or hematomas of the vulva or vagina are easily seen
Cervix	Lacerations are possible after vaginal delivery
Uterus and adnexae	Uterine atony: uterine fundus is soft and sometimes difficult to palpate
	Uterine rupture: hematoma in the broad ligament sometimes detected lateral to the uterus
	Uterine inversion: bleeding mass present in the vagina just inside the introitus
	Subinvolution: uterus large and boggy

■ DIAGNOSTIC TESTING

1. **CBC**
2. **Coagulation studies: platelet count, PT, PTT, fibrinogen, fibrin split products**
3. **Examination of the placenta**
    If examination of the placenta reveals that segments of placenta are absent, retained placental fragments or abnormal placental implantation should be suspected.
4. **Pelvic ultrasound examination**
    If a pelvic mass is palpated lateral to the uterus, ultrasound examination might reveal a broad-ligament hematoma caused by uterine rupture.

■ MANAGEMENT

1. **Uterine atony**
    a. **Massage the uterine fundus vigorously**
    b. **Oxytocin (1 to 2 ampules; 10 IU/ampule) administered IV in 500 to 1000 ml of IV fluid, or oxytocin (1 ampule) IM**
    c. **Methylergonovine (Methergine) 0.2 mg IM or IV if above measures are unsuccessful.**
        Methergine is contraindicated in hypertensive patients.
    d. **15-Methyl prostaglandin $F_{2\alpha}$ (carboprost tromethamine) 0.25 mg IM or by intramyometrial injection**
        This dose can be repeated every 15 to 90 minutes up to a maximum of 8 doses.
    e. **Surgical management: uterine artery ligation, hypogastric artery ligation, or hysterectomy**
        Uterine packing is usually not helpful in treating postpartum hemorrhage from atony, because the uterus is merely distended by the packing. Packing also prevents the postpartum uterus from contracting and can conceal ongoing bleeding. If the medical measures listed above are unsuccessful, several surgical procedures should be considered. Ligation of the anterior branch of the uterine artery is technically the easiest of the surgical procedures to perform (Fig. 18–3). Uterine artery ligation is especially helpful for bleeding from the lower uterine segment. Hypogastric artery ligation decreases the pulse pressure to allow time for the normal clotting mechanisms to function (Fig. 18–4). Hysterectomy should be considered if bleeding is persistent despite all efforts. If the patient is unstable from severe bleeding, subtotal hysterectomy is recommended over total hysterectomy, because it can be accomplished in a shorter amount of time and is associated with less blood loss.

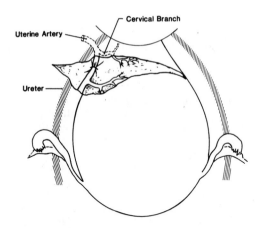

Figure 18–3 □ Ligation of the anterior branch of the uterine artery. (From Creasy RK, Resnik R: Maternal-Fetal Medicine: Principles and Practice, 3rd ed. Philadelphia, WB Saunders Co, 1994, p 882.)

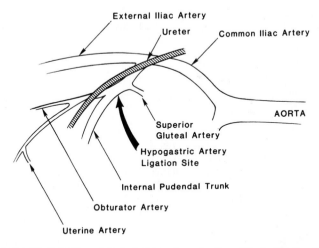

Figure 18–4 □ Site of hypogastric artery ligation. (From Creasy RK, Resnik R: Maternal-Fetal Medicine: Principles and Practice, 3rd ed. Philadelphia, WB Saunders Co, 1994, p 882.)

2. **Lacerations of the vulva, vagina, or cervix**
   a. **Repair of lacerations**
   b. **Evacuation of expanding hematomas**
   c. **Vaginal packing**
   d. **Arterial angiographic embolization**
   e. **Hypogastric artery ligation**

   Stable hematomas do not require surgical intervention. Expanding hematomas, however, should be evacuated, and bleeding vessels should be ligated. Vaginal packing is often helpful and can be used in addition to the repair of vaginal lacerations. If bleeding persists despite these measures, selective arterial angiographic embolization is often successful. Hypogastric artery ligation can also be performed. However, this procedure precludes angiographic embolization.

3. **Retained placental fragments**

   Retained placental fragments can result from abnormal adherence of the placenta. Placental villi are attached to the myometrium in placenta accreta, invade into the myometrium in placenta increta, and penetrate through the entire layer of myometrium in placenta percreta (see Fig. 18–1).
   a. **Manual removal of retained fragments**
   b. **Uterine curettage**

      Uterine curettage should be performed carefully with a large curette to prevent perforation of the postpartum uterus.

4. **Coagulopathy**
   a. **Correct underlying cause of coagulopathy**
   b. **Transfusion with whole blood**
   c. **Transfusion of platelets, initially 6 to 10 units,** or
   d. **Transfusion of fresh frozen plasma, initially 2 bags**

   Severe preeclampsia and placental abruption are common causes of coagulopathy in pregnancy and should be treated appropriately to reverse the coagulopathy. In addition, blood and blood components should be administered. Coagulation studies should be obtained after the transfusion of every 5 to 10 units of blood. Platelets should be transfused in patients with a platelet count of $<20,000/mm^3$. If surgery such as hysterectomy is planned, platelets should be transfused if the platelet count is $<50,000/mm^3$. Each unit of platelets will increase the platelet count by 5000 to $10,000/mm^3$. Fresh frozen plasma should be administered if the PT or PTT are greater than 1.5-times normal.

5. **Uterine rupture**
   a. **Immediate laparotomy with either repair of the rupture site or hysterectomy**

   The incidence of rupture of the uterus is 0.5 to 1.0% with a prior low transverse uterine scar and nearly 5% with a prior vertical uterine scar. Although uterine rupture can occur in an unscarred uterus, most cases occur in women attempting vagi-

nal delivery after a previous cesarean section. Uterine rupture usually occurs during labor but can also appear before labor.
6. **Inversion of the uterus**
   a. **Manual replacement of the uterine fundus with fingers or palm of the hand**
   b. **If manual replacement is unsuccessful, emergency laparotomy with the use of traction sutures to replace the uterine fundus**

Inversion of the uterus occurs at a frequency of 1 in 2100 to 1 in 6400 deliveries and is usually caused by excessive traction on the umbilical cord while the placenta is still implanted in the fundus. Tocolytic drugs such as terbutaline or magnesium sulfate are administered to relax the uterus and facilitate the repositioning. Oxytocin should not be administered until the uterine fundus has been replaced into its normal position. To prevent uterine inversion, manual removal of the placenta should be performed if the placenta does not spontaneously separate (Fig. 18–5).

Figure 18–5 □ Manual removal of the placenta. (From Hacker NF, Moore JG: Essentials of Obstetrics and Gynecology, 2nd ed. Philadelphia, WB Saunders Co, 1992, p 294.)

7. **Subinvolution of the uterus**
    a. **Methylergonovine (Methergine) 0.2 mg PO every 3 to 4 hours for 1 to 2 days**
    b. **Broad-spectrum antibiotics if endometritis is suspected: doxycycline 100 mg PO two times per day or erythromycin 500 mg PO four times per day for 7 days**

    Subinvolution is the delay in involution, the shrinking of the enlarged postpartum uterus back to its normal nonpregnant size. It is the most common cause of late postpartum hemorrhage. Most patients respond to methylergonovine. Endometritis can result in subinvolution. Because up to one-third of cases of late endometritis are caused by *Chlamydia trachomatis*, doxycycline or erythromycin should be administered orally.

19

PREMATURE RUPTURE OF MEMBRANES

■ BACKGROUND AND DEFINITIONS

Premature rupture of membranes (PROM): Rupture of membranes before the onset of labor

Preterm premature rupture of membranes: Rupture of membranes before the onset of labor at a gestational age of less than 37 weeks

Prolonged rupture of membranes: Rupture of membranes for more than 24 hours before delivery

Latency period: Period of time between PROM and the onset of labor

Amniotic fluid is necessary for the normal development of the fetal lungs. Amniotic fluid also protects the fetus from trauma and the umbilical cord from compression. Rupture of membranes and the subsequent loss of amniotic fluid results in the loss of these beneficial effects. Furthermore, rupture of membranes is often followed by labor even at a preterm gestational age. Prolonged rupture of membranes increases the risk of chorioamnionitis, which is associated with increased maternal and neonatal morbidity. The incidence of PROM at term is 8 to 10%. In approximately 25% of all cases of PROM the fetus is preterm.

■ CLINICAL PRESENTATION

Gush of fluid from the vagina followed by persistent leakage of fluid
Chorioamnionitis
Preterm labor

A patient's complaint of a gush of fluid from the vagina followed by ongoing leakage is indicative of rupture of membranes in 90% of cases. In many cases, the patient will have no symptoms until she develops preterm labor or chorioamnionitis. Furthermore, a patient with intact membranes can present with leakage of urine, excessive normal vaginal discharge or mucus, or bloody show associated with labor, all of which may mimic the rupture of membranes.

■ PHONE CALL

Questions

1. **What is the gestational age of the fetus?**
   The gestational age of the fetus is the most critical factor in determining the management of PROM in the patient.
2. **Is the patient in labor?**

Orders

1. Prepare the patient for a sterile speculum examination and have available Nitrazine paper and microscope slides
2. Begin external uterine monitoring
3. Initiate external electronic fetal heart rate monitoring
4. Obtain a complete blood count (CBC) with differential
5. Do not perform digital cervical examination on the patient with preterm PROM who is not in labor

Degree of Urgency

The patient should be seen immediately if she has preterm labor, if she has chorioamnionitis, or if there is a suggestion of fetal distress. Otherwise she should be seen as soon as possible.

■ ELEVATOR THOUGHTS

What conditions are associated with a higher risk of PROM and preterm PROM?
- Local infection
  Patients who are carriers of *Neisseria gonorrhoeae, Chlamydia trachomatis,* group B streptococci, *Trichomonas vaginalis,* and *Gardnerella vaginalis* are at an increased risk for PROM, probably because the local infection results in weakening of the membranes. These patients are also at a greater risk for chorioamnionitis.
- Multiple gestation
- Polyhydramnios
- Incompetent cervix
- Cervical cerclage
- Previous cervical laceration or operation
- Smoking

What are potential complications that can result from PROM?
- Preterm labor
  Preterm PROM is responsible for nearly 30% of all preterm births. This percentage is higher for patients of lower socioeconomic class and patients with sexually transmitted dis-

eases. In cases of PROM at term, 90% of patients are in labor in less than 24 hours. In women with preterm PROM at 28 to 34 weeks of gestation, 50% will be in labor within 24 hours and 80 to 90% will be in labor within 1 week. In women with preterm PROM before 26 weeks, 50% will be in labor within 1 week.

- Maternal chorioamnionitis

    The incidence of chorioamnionitis in all cases of PROM is 0.5 to 1%. In patients with prolonged rupture of membranes, the incidence of chorioamnionitis is 3 to 15%. The incidence of chorioamnionitis is greatest in patients with preterm PROM, ranging from 15 to 25%.

- Fetal infection

    Fetal pneumonia, sepsis, urinary tract infection, or conjunctivitis can occur. Serious neonatal infection is found in 5% of all cases of preterm PROM and in 15 to 20% of cases of maternal chorioamnionitis.

- Fetal distress

    In patients with preterm PROM, the incidence of fetal distress is 8.5%, which represents a nearly sixfold increase over the incidence of fetal distress in patients with preterm labor with intact membranes. This is probably due to the increased frequency of umbilical cord compression when there is no longer adequate fluid to protect the cord. Furthermore, a higher incidence of umbilical cord prolapse, approximately 1.5%, also contributes to the increased risk of fetal distress.

- Fetal deformations

    Preterm PROM at early gestational ages can result in impaired development of the fetal lungs, referred to as pulmonary hypoplasia, which is lethal. Furthermore, early preterm PROM can cause intrauterine growth restriction and compression malformations of the face and limbs. The incidence of these fetal deformations is 3.5% when preterm PROM occurs before 26 weeks of gestational age.

■ MAJOR THREAT TO FETAL LIFE

- Prematurity
- Sepsis
- Fetal distress
- Fetal deformations

■ MAJOR THREAT TO MATERNAL LIFE

- Sepsis secondary to chorioamnionitis

■ BEDSIDE

Quick Look Test

Is the patient in labor?

In the patient with a term pregnancy and PROM, labor is desired, and in the absence of chorioamnionitis and any other pre-existing complications, labor should be managed in the usual manner. However, in the patient with preterm PROM, labor is not necessarily desired despite the potential for chorioamnionitis because of the possibility of prematurity. Furthermore, the appropriate personnel, including the anesthesiologist and pediatrician or neonatologist, should be made aware of the patient's condition. Maternal transport to another medical facility better equipped to care for the premature infant should be considered.

Is there evidence of fetal distress?

Abnormal fetal heart rate patterns suggestive of fetal distress may be caused by umbilical cord compression or prolapse.

Vital Signs

A maternal fever would be suggestive of chorioamnionitis. Otherwise, vital signs are usually normal.

Selective History and Chart Review

1. What is the gestational age of the fetus?

   The gestational age should be established by the patient's last menstrual period, early prenatal examinations, and previous ultrasound examinations.

2. When did rupture of membranes occur?

   The patient should be asked when rupture of membranes occurred. The time of rupture of membranes affects the likelihood of chorioamnionitis, fetal infections, and fetal deformation.

Selective Physical Examination

Abdominal	Uterine contractions may be palpable.
Pelvic	
External genitalia and vagina	Watery discharge is noted externally or in a vaginal pool.
Cervix	Watery discharge may be observed flowing from the cervical os when fundal pressure is applied or the patient performs Valsalva's maneuver.
	Cervical dilatation and effacement

may be noted visually by sterile speculum examination.

Digital cervical examination should not be performed in the patient with preterm PROM who is not in labor.

Uterus and adnexae

Uterine contractions may be palpable. Uterine tenderness is suggestive of chorioamnionitis.

■ DIAGNOSTIC TESTING

1. Tests to document rupture of membranes

If obvious pooling of amniotic fluid in the vagina is not seen on sterile speculum examination, either or both of the following tests should be performed to confirm or rule out rupture of membranes.

a. Nitrazine test for pH of vagina

Nitrazine paper should be used to test the pH of vaginal fluid. This test is performed by swabbing the vagina with a sterile cotton-tipped applicator and then touching a strip of Nitrazine paper. As an alternative, a strip of Nitrazine paper can be applied to the vaginal introitus. The normal vaginal pH is 4.5 to 6.0. Amniotic fluid is more basic and has a pH of 7.1 to 7.3. The color of Nitrazine paper changes from yellow to blue at a pH >6.0. A false-positive Nitrazine test can be caused by contamination of the vagina by semen, blood, vaginal infection, and alkaline antiseptics.

b. Microscope slide test for ferning of vaginal fluid

This test is performed by swabbing the posterior fornix of the vagina with a cotton-tipped applicatior and preparing a smear on a microscope slide. The smear is allowed to dry and is examined under low power with a microscope. A ferning pattern is seen in the presence of ruptured membranes.

2. Ultrasound examination

The gestational age of the fetus should be established by an ultrasound examination if the gestational age is unclear when reviewing menstrual dating, prenatal examinations, and prior ultrasound examinations. Ultrasound examination will also establish the presentation of the fetus. This is especially important in patients with preterm PROM who are not in labor. In these patients, digital examination should not be performed to determine fetal presentation. Ultrasound examination will in some cases help in confirming the diagnosis of PROM by demonstrating a low amniotic fluid index (AFI) (Figs. 19–1 and 19–2).

3. Tests to rule out chorioamnionitis

Figure 19–1 □ Technique for assessing the amniotic fluid index (AFI). (From Creasy RK, Resnik R: Maternal-Fetal Medicine: Principles and Practice, 3rd ed. Philadelphia, WB Saunders Co, 1994, p 621.)

a. **CBC with differential**

An elevated white blood cell count and the presence of bands is suggestive of chorioamnionitis. Unfortunately, the white blood cell count is nonspecific and can be elevated in a patient during normal labor.

b. **Amniocentesis and culture of amniotic fluid**

In patients with preterm PROM who have an adequate amount of fluid, amniocentesis can be performed to confirm or rule out chorioamnionitis. A specimen should be submitted for Gram stain as well as amniotic fluid culture and sensitivity. The frequency of organisms found in the culture of amniotic fluid obtained by amniocentesis is listed in Table 19–1. Because results of amniotic fluid culture can take 24 to 48 hours, amniotic fluid glucose can be measured to possibly diagnose chorioamnionitis sooner. An amniotic fluid glucose concentration of <14 mg/dl is suggestive of chorioamnionitis.

c. **Biophysical profile**

Fetal biophysical profile testing can be used to detect fetal infection (Table 19–2). The loss of fetal heart rate reactivity, fetal movement, fetal tone, and breathing activity are suggestive of fetal infection, although these signs are nonspecific.

d. **Serum C-reactive protein**

An elevated serum C-reactive protein with a level of >0.8

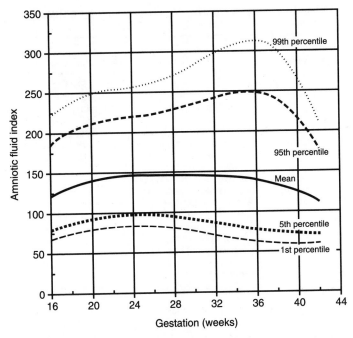

Figure 19–2 ◻ Mean and percentiles for amniotic fluid index. (Redrawn from Moore TR, Cayle JE: Amniotic fluid index in normal human pregnancy. Am J Obstet Gynecol 1990;162:1168.)

Table 19–1 ◻ **COMBINED FREQUENCY OF ORGANISMS CULTURED FROM AMNIOTIC FLUID OBTAINED BY AMNIOCENTESIS IN PATIENTS WITH PRETERM PROM (7 STUDIES)**

Group B streptococci	20%
Gardnerella vaginalis	17%
Peptostreptococcus/Peptococcus	11%
Fusobacteria	10%
Bacteroides fragilis	9%
Other streptococci	9%
Bacteroides species	5%

From Creasy RK, Resnik R: Maternal-Fetal Medicine: Principles and Practice, 3rd ed. Philadelphia, WB Saunders Co, 1994, p 631.

Table 19–2 □ **BIOPHYSICAL PROFILE SCORING: TECHNIQUE AND INTERPRETATION**

Biophysical Variable	Normal Score	Abnormal (Score = 0)
Fetal breathing movements	At least 1 episode of FBM of at least 30-sec duration in 30-min observation	Absent FBM or no episode of ≥30 sec in 30 min
Gross body movement	At least 3 discrete body/limb movements in 30 min (episodes of active continuous movement considered as single movement)	2 or fewer episodes of body/limb movements in 30 min
Fetal tone	At least 1 episode of active extension with return to flexion of fetal limb(s) or trunk; opening and closing of hand considered normal tone	Either slow extension with return to partial flexion or movement of limb in full extension or absent fetal movement with fetal hand held in complete or partial deflection
Reactive FHR	At least 2 episodes of FHR acceleration of ≥15 beats/min and of at least 15-sec duration associated with fetal movement in 30 min	Less than 2 episodes of acceleration of FHR or acceleration of <15 beats/min in 30 min
Qualitative AFV*	At least 1 pocket of AF that measures at least 2 cm in 2 perpendicular planes	Either no AF pockets or a pocket <2 cm in two perpendicular planes

From Creasy RK, Resnik R: Maternal-Fetal Medicine: Principles and Practice, 3rd ed. Philadelphia, WB Saunders Co, 1994, p 345.

FBM = fetal breathing movement; FHR = fetal heart rate; AFV = amniotic fluid volume; AF = amniotic fluid.

*Modification of the criteria for reduced amniotic fluid from <1 cm to <2 cm would seem reasonable.

mg/dl may be indicative of chorioamnionitis, but this test is nonspecific.

4. Cervical cultures

Cultures for *Chlamydia trachomatis, Neisseria gonorrhoeae,* and group B streptococci should be obtained in patients at risk for these sexually transmitted diseases. Patients with positive cultures should be treated with the appropriate antibiotic to decrease the risk of perinatal transmission.

Figure 19–3 □ Amniotic fluid phospholipid levels and gestational age. (From Creasy RK, Resnik R: Maternal-Fetal Medicine: Principles and Practice, 3rd ed. Philadelphia, WB Saunders Co, 1994, p 435. Data from Gluck L, et al: Am J Obstet Gynecol 1974;120:142, and Hallman M, et al: Am J Obstet Gynecol 1976;125:613, as shown in Jobe A: The developmental biology of the lung. In Fanaroff AA, Martin RJ, eds: Neonatal-Perinatal Medicine. St Louis, Mosby–Year Book, 1992, p 792.)

5. **Tests for fetal lung maturity**

Fetal lung maturity is one of the most important factors that is considered in the management of the patient with preterm PROM. Phospholipid analysis of amniotic fluid can be used to document fetal lung maturity. A **lecithin-to-sphingomyelin (L/S) ratio** of >2.0 and the presence of **phosphatidylglycerol (PG)** are very assuring, although they do not provide absolute guarantees of fetal lung maturity. Phospholipid levels as a function of gestational age are illustrated in Figure 19–3.

Unlike lecithin and sphingomyelin, PG is not present in blood, vaginal secretions, or meconium, and therefore, the presence of these contaminants in amniotic fluid will not affect the interpretation of PG levels. The incidence of respiratory distress syndrome is approximately 34% at 33 weeks of gestation, 14% at 34 weeks, 6% at 35 weeks, and 3 to 4% after 35 weeks. Therefore, in the patient with PROM at 33 to 35 weeks of gestation, amniotic fluid should be collected for phospholipid measurements. If there is an adequate vaginal pool, fluid can be collected from the vagina with a sterile syringe and catheter. The presence of PG is indicative of lung maturity at least a week later than the L/S ratio. Therefore, PG determination in vaginal pool fluid should be considered a screening test; if it is absent, amniocentesis should be performed and the

L/S ratio should be determined. Insulin has been shown to interfere with surfactant synthesis. Therefore, the interpretation of the L/S ratio and phospholipid levels is modified in patients with diabetes. An L/S ratio of ≥3.5 and a PG level of ≥3% are required to be assured of fetal lung maturity in the fetus of a patient with diabetes.

An alternative to laboratory measurement of phospholipids is the **foam stability test,** also referred to as the **"shake test,"** which tests amniotic fluid for sufficient surfactant to form a stable foam at the air–surface interface. The steps to perform the shake test are listed in Table 19–3. The presence of a ring of bubbles that persists at the air–fluid interface for 15 minutes is a positive test, verifying fetal lung maturity. A problem with the shake test is the frequency of false-negative tests, because a positive test requires an L/S ratio of 4.0 to 6.0.

■ MANAGEMENT

1. **Patients who present with PROM, along with advanced active labor, chorioamnionitis, or fetal distress, should undergo delivery regardless of gestational age**

   Vaginal delivery should be attempted and cesarean section should be performed only for the usual obstetrical indications. In patients with chorioamnionitis, IV antibiotics should be

Table 19–3 □ STEPS FOR PERFORMING AMNIOTIC FLUID "SHAKE TEST"

Materials needed:	Amniotic fluid recently collected
	95% ethanol (19 parts of absolute alcohol mixed with 1 part of distilled water)
	0.9% saline
	Two 13 × 100-mm glass tubes with Teflon-lined plastic screw cap
Steps of test:	1. Mix 1 ml of amniotic fluid and 1 ml of ethanol in one tube.
	2. Mix 0.5 ml of amniotic fluid, 0.5 ml of saline, and 1 ml of ethanol in the second tube.
	3. Shake both tubes for 15 seconds and place tubes upright.
	4. Wait for 15 minutes and look for a ring of bubbles or foam at the air–liquid interface.
Results:	Positive test: ring of bubbles is observed in both tubes
	Equivocal test: ring of bubbles is observed only in first tube
	Negative test: ring of bubbles is not observed in either tube

given during labor. The choice of antibiotic agents depends on the organisms suspected. Ampicillin, gentamicin, and cephalosporins have been used successfully. There is much more controversy about the optimal management of patients with PROM without chorioamnionitis, advanced labor, or fetal distress, especially if the patient has preterm PROM.

2. **Premature rupture of membranes at term**

   The goal of management of the term patient with PROM is delivery before the development of chorioamnionitis. Fortunately, 90% of patients at term will enter into spontaneous labor within 24 hours of rupture of membranes. Therefore, one of the following two management plans can be used:

   a. **Expectant management**
      (1) Await spontaneous labor
      (2) Avoid digital cervical examinations until the patient is in labor
      (3) Initial intermittent electronic fetal heart rate monitoring
      (4) Perform serial temperature recordings and examinations for clinical signs of chorioamnionitis
      (5) Obtain serial CBCs with differential
      (6) Deliver if chorioamnionitis or fetal distress develops

   b. **Induction of labor immediately**
      (1) Induce labor with IV oxytocin infusion
      (2) Use intracervical prostaglandin E_2 gel for preinduction cervical ripening if the cervix is unfavorable for induction: **prostaglandin E_2 gel 3 mg intracervically every 4 to 6 hours for 2 to 3 doses**

      Immediate induction has been shown in some studies to result in a higher incidence of cesarean section without a decrease in the incidence of chorioamnionitis.

3. **Preterm premature rupture of membranes**

   The major fetal risk that results from preterm PROM is prematurity. Therefore, the goal of the management of a patient with preterm PROM who is not in labor is prolonging the pregnancy as long as there is no evidence of chorioamnionitis or fetal distress.

   There are three management plans commonly used for these patients.

   a. **Expectant management**
      (1) Administer prophylactic antibiotics

         The use of prophylactic antibiotics decreases the risks of perinatal and maternal infection and also increases the latency period by an average of 5 to 7 days. Ampicillin, erythromycin, and the combination of ampicillin, gentamicin, and clindamycin have been used successfully. The use of prophylactic antibiotics is especially important if the patient is a known carrier of group B streptococci.

    (2) Order bedrest

    (3) Avoid digital cervical examinations until the patient is in labor

    (4) Initiate intermittent electronic fetal heart rate monitoring

    (5) Perform serial temperature recordings and examinations for clinical signs of chorioamnionitis

    (6) Obtain serial CBCs with differential

    (7) Deliver if chorioamnionitis or fetal distress develops

b. Selective expectant management

    (1) Expectant management as described above for patients at <32 weeks of gestation

    (2) Obtain vaginal pool amniotic fluid for phospholipid analysis in patients with a gestational age of ≥32 weeks

    (3) Perform amniocentesis for phospholipid analysis and amniotic fluid culture and Gram stain if the vaginal pool amniotic fluid has no PG

    (4) Use an expectant management protocol for patients who have negative amniotic fluid culture and in whom phospholipid analysis shows immature fetal lungs

    (5) Deliver patients who have positive amniotic fluid culture or in whom phospholipid analysis shows mature fetal lungs

c. Tocolysis and corticosteroid therapy followed by delivery

    (1) Treat with either beta-adrenergic drugs or magnesium sulfate, as described in Chapter 20

        Most studies do not show prolongation of the latency period beyond 24 hours in patients with preterm PROM treated with aggressive tocolysis; but fortunately, they also do not show an increased risk of infection.

    (2) Administer corticosteroids to accelerate fetal lung maturity: **Celestone Soluspan solution 2 ml IM, repeat dose in 24 hours** (1 ml of Celestone contains 3 mg of betamethasone sodium and 3 mg of betamethasone acetate)

        In patients with preterm PROM, corticosteroids result in a small reduction in the incidence of neonatal respiratory distress syndrome but also cause a small increase in the risk of infection.

    (3) Because the maximal effects of corticosteroids are seen after 24 hours, tocolysis is continued for 48 hours and then discontinued

    (4) The patient is then managed expectantly as described above or undergoes delivery immediately by induction of labor

4. Preterm premature rupture of membranes at a previable gestational age

When preterm PROM occurs at a gestational age of <25 weeks, there is only a 25 to 40% probability of achieving a viable infant, and there is substantial morbidity for both the infant and the mother. The risk of chorioamnionitis is nearly 40%, and there is a risk of maternal sepsis and even death. Fetal deformation syndromes including pulmonary hypoplasia and intrauterine growth restriction occur at increased frequencies with PROM at extremely early gestational ages. It is often difficult to decide on a management plan. Both parents must be counseled extensively concerning the options and the poor prognosis, so that they are then able to participate fully in deciding on an appropriate management plan. For patients with preterm PROM at a previable gestational age, there are generally two options.

a. **Expectant management**
   (1) Administer prophylactic antibiotics
       As with the patient with preterm PROM at a viable gestational age, a prophylactic antibiotic can be administered, although it is extremely unlikely that a significant prolongation in the latency period will be gained.
   (2) Await spontaneous labor
   (3) Avoid digital cervical examinations until the patient is in labor
   (4) Expectant management can be carried out at home without fetal heart rate monitoring since there is little that can be done for the fetus if fetal distress should occur
   (5) Order bedrest
   (6) Advise against intercourse
   (7) Perform serial temperature recordings and examinations for clinical signs of chorioamnionitis
   (8) Obtain serial CBCs with differential
   (9) Deliver if chorioamnionitis develops

b. **Termination of the pregnancy**
   If the patient elects termination, this can be performed with either an IV oxytocin infusion or prostaglandin E_2 20 mg by vaginal suppository every 4 hours.

5. **Maternal transport**
   The extremely preterm infant who is delivered in a facility with specialized intensive perinatal and neonatal services has both a higher survival rate and lower rates of both short-term and long-term morbidity than the infant who is transported to such a facility after birth. Therefore, if the patient with early preterm PROM is initially admitted to a medical facility where the necessary level of care for the infant cannot be provided, she should be transported before giving birth to the proper facility unless imminent delivery precludes it.

6. **Management of preterm labor after preterm premature rupture of membranes**
   When the patient with preterm PROM begins labor, it should be remembered that preterm labor and delivery are associated

with a higher incidence of complications including fetal distress, malpresentation, and birth trauma. The following steps should be taken:

a. **Initiate continuous electronic fetal heart rate monitoring**
b. **Notify the anesthesiologist and pediatric team of the patient's status**
c. **Provide adequate anesthesia to ensure a controlled delivery**
d. **Consider amnioinfusion**

  Amnioinfusion has been used to decrease the incidence of fetal distress by replacing, at least in part, the amniotic fluid that is lost with PROM and by reducing the risk of umbilical cord compression. **Room-temperature saline (500 ml) is infused by gravity through an intrauterine catheter over 30 minutes.**

e. **Have available the proper personnel and equipment for an emergency cesarean section**
f. **Consider the use of low forceps and an episiotomy to reduce resistance and trauma to the fetal head especially with a prolonged second stage of labor**
g. **Decide on the route of delivery for the preterm fetus by using the same guidelines that would normally apply to the term fetus**

  Cesarean section should be performed for the frank breech infant with an estimated weight of <1500 g because of the increased morbidity associated with vaginal delivery of these infants.

20

PRETERM LABOR

■ BACKGROUND AND DEFINITION

Preterm labor: Onset of labor after 20 weeks of gestation but before the completion of 37 weeks, or 259 days, of gestation. Labor is defined as the presence of documented uterine contractions occurring at a frequency of at least four contractions in 20 minutes or eight contractions in 60 minutes with documented cervical change in dilatation, cervical dilatation of ≥2 cm, cervical effacement of ≥80%, or ruptured membranes. Delivery of a fetus before 20 weeks of gestational age is referred to as an abortion instead of preterm delivery.

The incidence of preterm labor is approximately 10%. Preterm birth accounts for nearly 85% of all neonatal mortality not caused by congenital anomalies. The predicted neonatal survival rates and weekly improvement in survival rates at various premature gestational ages are listed in Table 20–1. The largest weekly improvements in neonatal survival occur at 26 to 28 weeks of gestation. After 30 weeks, survival rates are greater than 90% and improve only slightly weekly. Even if the premature infant survives, there is significant morbidity associated with prematurity, especially from intraventricular hemorrhage and respiratory distress syndrome secondary to immature lungs. Prematurity also results in significant long-term problems including chronic respiratory disease, neurological impairment, seizure disorders, developmental delays, visual impairment, hearing impairment, and cerebral palsy.

Although significant advances have been made in neonatology, resulting in improved survival rates of the preterm neonate, no concomitant advances have been made in the prevention of preterm births. In fact, the rate of premature deliveries has not changed in the past 40 years, despite the significant research efforts made in areas of prevention, early recognition, and treatment of preterm labor. Even routine cervical examinations performed in the late second and early third trimesters and home uterine monitoring have not affected the incidence of preterm births.

■ CLINICAL PRESENTATION

Uterine contractions
Uterine tightening

Table 20–1 □ PREDICTED SURVIVAL BY GESTATIONAL AGE AND WEEKLY IMPROVEMENT IN NEONATAL SURVIVAL

Gestational Age (Weeks)	Survival by Gestational Age (%)	Weekly Improvement in Survival (%)
22	0.0	0.0
23	1.8	1.8
24	9.9	8.1
25	15.5	5.6
26	54.7	39.2
27	67.0	12.3
28	77.4	10.4
29	85.2	7.8
30	90.6	5.4
31	94.2	3.6
32	96.5	2.3
33	97.9	1.4

Adapted from Cooper RL, Goldenberg RL, Creasy RK, et al: A multicenter study of preterm birth weight and gestational age specific mortality. Am J Obstet Gynecol 1993;168:78.

Menstrual-like cramps
Pelvic pressure
Back pain
Rupture of membranes
Watery vaginal discharge
Vaginal spotting

The symptoms of preterm labor are often so vague and subtle that by the time the diagnosis of preterm labor is made, advanced cervical dilatation or rupture of membranes has already taken place. Uterine contractions are frequently painless, and fewer than 50% of patients in preterm labor are aware of their contractions. An increase in vaginal discharge, which is often watery and stained pink, is noticed by 30 to 50% of patients. To make the interpretation of these symptoms even more difficult, many of these symptoms are nonspecific and occur in 5 to 20% of normal patients.

■ PHONE CALL

Questions

1. What is the gestational age of the fetus?
2. Does the patient complain of ruptured membranes?
   Rupture of membranes can be an indication of advanced preterm labor. Furthermore, the treatment of preterm labor

with tocolytic drugs is controversial when there has been rupture of membranes.

3. Is the patient febrile?

   A fever may be caused by chorioamnionitis due to premature rupture of membranes.

Orders

1. Place the patient at bedrest in the lateral decubitus position
2. Begin external uterine monitoring
3. Begin continuous electronic fetal heart rate monitoring
4. Start IV with either 5% dextrose in water or 0.25% normal saline, and hydrate the patient with 500 ml of IV fluid
5. Obtain a clean-catch urine specimen for urinalysis and urine culture and sensitivity

Degree of Urgency

The successful treatment of a patient with preterm labor is more likely if treatment is instituted early, before advanced cervical dilatation or rupture of membranes. Therefore, patients suspected of having preterm labor should be seen and evaluated as soon as possible.

■ ELEVATOR THOUGHTS

What socioeconomic factors are associated with preterm labor?

- Nonwhite race

   Black patients have an incidence of preterm labor of 18.9%, which is almost twice the incidence seen in white patients.

- Low socioeconomic status
- Low maternal age (younger than 20 years of age)
- Advanced maternal age (35 years of age or older)

   The risk is greatest for women who are 35 years old or older at the time of their first delivery.

- Strenuous and physically demanding occupation

   Occupations that require constant standing also appear to increase the incidence of preterm labor.

- Low prepregnancy maternal weight

   Women with weights below their optimal weights at the beginning of pregnancy have a threefold increase in the incidence of preterm labor.

What medical conditions are associated with preterm labor?

- History of preterm delivery

After one preterm birth, the recurrence rate of preterm labor with subsequent pregnancies is 17 to 47%.

- Preterm premature rupture of membranes
- Multiple gestation

  Prematurity is the most common cause of perinatal morbidity and mortality in patients with multiple gestation. Nearly 50% of twin gestations will deliver prematurely. Furthermore, the degree of prematurity increases with the number of fetuses.

- Chorioamnionitis
- Uterine anomaly

  Overall, 5 to 15% of all preterm labor is associated with a uterine anomaly. The risk of preterm labor varies with the specific type of uterine anomaly. A septate uterus is associated with a 4 to 17% incidence of preterm labor. A bicornuate uterus is associated with a 18 to 80% risk.

- Uterine leiomyomata
- Sepsis

  Sepsis from conditions such as acute pyelonephritis or acute appendicitis increases the risk of preterm labor. Endotoxins cause uterine contractions through stimulation of the myometrium.

- Genital infection

  Group B streptococci, *Chlamydia trachomatis, Ureaplasma urealyticum,* and *Trichomonas vaginalis* infections of the lower genital tract have all been associated with an increased risk of preterm labor. Bacterial vaginosis caused by *Gardnerella vaginalis* and multiple anaerobes has also been implicated as a cause of preterm labor.

- Incompetent cervix
- History of second-trimester abortion

  Some studies have also shown an increased risk of preterm labor after multiple first-trimester abortions.

- Placental abruption
- Placenta previa
- Fetal anomalies
- Abdominal surgery during pregnancy

  Abdominal surgery such as for acute appendicitis, cholecystitis, or ovarian neoplasms has been associated with preterm labor.

- Smoking

  The risk of preterm labor appears to be proportionate to the number of cigarettes smoked per day.

- Pregnancy complications

  Certain complications of pregnancy such as severe preeclampsia and intrauterine growth restriction are best treated by early delivery.

What are the causes of neonatal morbidity and mortality associated with prematurity?

- Respiratory distress syndrome (RDS)

    RDS, also referred to as hyaline membrane disease, is the most common neonatal problem associated with prematurity. Its incidence is as high as 93% for infants born at 26 weeks and decreases to 3 to 4% at 36 to 38 weeks of gestation.

- Patent ductus arteriosus (PDA)

    The incidence of PDA is as high as 61% in neonates delivered at 25 weeks and drops to less than 0.5% after 36 weeks of gestation.

- Intraventricular hemorrhage (IVH)

    The incidence of IVH is as high as 30% in infants delivered at 26 weeks and is rarely encountered after 32 weeks of gestation.

- Sepsis
- Necrotizing enterocolitis
- Hyperbilirubinemia
- Hypoglycemia

■ MAJOR THREAT TO FETAL LIFE

- Prematurity

    Preterm delivery is the cause of approximately 85% of all perinatal mortalities, excluding fetuses with congenital anomalies.

■ BEDSIDE

Quick Look Test

A patient who appears to be having painful contractions is likely to be in advanced labor. Depending on the amount of cervical dilatation, treatment of preterm labor in this patient may be futile.

Preterm labor can be associated with vaginal bleeding from placental abruption or placenta previa. In many cases, delivery even at a preterm gestation age is the treatment of choice for these causes of vaginal bleeding.

Vital Signs

Vital signs are usually normal. If the patient is febrile, chorioamnionitis should be suspected.

Selective History and Chart Review

1. What is the estimated gestational age of the fetus, and has the patient had prior ultrasound examinations to confirm the gestational age?
2. Does the patient have any of the socioeconomic factors associated with preterm labor?
3. Had the patient experienced preterm labor in a previous pregnancy?
4. Does the patient have a history of premature rupture of membranes?
5. Does the patient have any medical conditions such as sepsis, chorioamnionitis, uterine anomalies, or multiple gestation that predisposes to preterm labor?

Selective Physical Examination

Abdominal	Uterine tenderness with chorioamnionitis
	Uterine irritability with placental abruption
Pelvic	
External genitalia and vagina	Watery discharge or pooling of fluid in the vagina is suggestive of rupture of membranes.
	Vaginal bleeding is caused by placental abruption or placenta previa or may represent bloody show from cervical dilatation and effacement.
Cervix	Cervical dilatation, effacement, presenting part, and station of the presenting part should be determined.
Uterus and adnexae	Uterine contractions may be palpable.
	Tender with chorioamnionitis
	Tender and irritable with placental abruption

■ DIAGNOSTIC TESTING

All patients suspected of having preterm labor should have the following diagnostic tests performed.

1. **Ultrasound examination**

    An ultrasound examination should be performed to
    a. **Confirm the gestational age**
    b. **Rule out multiple gestation**
    c. **Determine fetal presentation**
        There is a higher incidence of malpresentations at premature gestational ages.
2. **Serial cervical examinations**
    If membranes have not ruptured, serial cervical examinations should be performed, preferably by the same examiner,

to document changes in cervical dilatation and effacement and to confirm the diagnosis of preterm labor. Although treatment of preterm labor is more likely to be successful if initiated early, waiting until there has been cervical change does not jeopardize the efficacy of treatment. The frequency of cervical examinations can be individualized for each patient, based on the strength and the frequency of the uterine contractions and the level of patient discomfort.

3. **Tests to document rupture of membranes**

   If obvious pooling of amniotic fluid in the vagina is not seen on pelvic examination, either or both of the following tests should be performed to determine whether the membranes have ruptured. Testing for rupture of membranes should be performed even if the patient denies symptoms of ruptured membranes, because symptoms can be subtle or even absent.

   a. **Nitrazine test for pH of vagina**

      Nitrazine paper should be used to test the pH of vaginal fluid. This is performed by swabbing the vagina with a sterile cotton-tipped applicator and then touching a strip of Nitrazine paper. As an alternative, a strip of Nitrazine paper can be applied to the vaginal introitus. The normal vaginal pH is 4.5 to 6.0. Amniotic fluid is more basic and has a pH of 7.1 to 7.3. The color of Nitrazine paper changes from yellow to blue at a pH of >6.0. A false-positive Nitrazine test can be caused by contamination of the vagina by semen, blood, vaginal infection, and alkaline antiseptics.

   b. **Microscope slide test for ferning of vaginal fluid**

      This test is performed by swabbing the posterior fornix of the vagina with a cotton-tipped applicator and preparing a smear on a microscope slide. The smear is allowed to dry and is examined under low power with a microscope. A ferning pattern is seen in the presence of ruptured membranes.

4. **External uterine monitoring**

   External uterine monitoring is performed to aid in determining both the presence and the frequency of uterine contractions. Monitoring should be performed even if the patient does not report the presence of uterine contractions. Symptoms of preterm labor can be very subtle, and only approximately 45% of patients with preterm labor report the presence of uterine contractions.

5. **Microscopic urinalysis and culture**

   Because of the high association between urinary tract infections and preterm labor, a urine specimen should be sent for microscopic urinalysis and for culture and sensitivity. Antibiotic and antipyretic therapy should be initiated if there is evidence of a urinary tract infection.

Certain patients suspected of having preterm labor should have the following additional diagnostic tests performed:

6. Cervical cultures

In patients who are at high risk for having a lower genital tract infection, cervical cultures for *Chlamydia trachomatis,* herpes simplex, and bacteria such as group B streptococci, *Gardnerella vaginalis,* and various anaerobes may be indicated. Although the treatment of cervical infections has not been shown to significantly influence the success of treatment of preterm labor, a positive culture could affect management during labor and the route chosen for delivery.

7. Amniocentesis

Amniocentesis can be performed for the following indications:

a. Determination of fetal lung maturity

The incidence of RDS is approximately 13.5% at 34 weeks of gestation, 6.4% at 35 weeks, and 3 to 4% after 35 weeks. Therefore, amniocentesis is an option at 33 to 35 weeks to determine whether the fetal lungs are mature based on phospholipid measurements. A **lecithin-to-sphingomyelin (L/S) ratio** of >2.0 and the presence of **phosphatidylglycerol (PG)** (see Fig. 19–3) are very assuring, although they do not provide absolute guarantees of fetal lung maturity.

Unlike lecithin and sphingomyelin, PG is not present in blood, vaginal secretions, or meconium; and therefore, the presence of these contaminants in amniotic fluid will not affect the interpretation of PG levels. The levels of amniotic fluid phospholipids at various gestational ages are shown in Figure 20–1. Insulin has been shown to interfere with surfactant synthesis. Therefore, the interpretation of the L/S ratio and phospholipid levels is modified in patients with diabetes. An L/S ratio of ≥3.5 and a PG level of ≥3% are required to be assured of fetal lung maturity in the fetus of a patient with diabetes.

An alternative to laboratory measurement of phospholipids is the **foam stability test,** also referred to as the **"shake test,"** which tests amniotic fluid for sufficient surfactant to form a stable foam at the air–surface interface. Although it is inferior to laboratory measurement of phospholipids, the foam stability test can be performed more quickly and inexpensively. The steps taken to perform the shake test are listed in Table 20–2. The presence of a ring of bubbles that persists at the air–fluid interface for 15 minutes is a positive test, verifying fetal lung maturity. A problem with the shake test is the frequency of false-negative tests, because a positive test requires an L/S ratio of 4.0 to 6.0.

Figure 20–1 □ Levels of amniotic fluid phospholipids and gestational age. (From Creasy RK, Resnik R: Maternal-Fetal Medicine: Principles and Practice, 3rd ed. Philadelphia, WB Saunders Co, 1994, p 435. Data from Gluck L, et al: Am J Obstet Gynecol 1974;120:142, and Hallman M, et al: Am J Obstet Gynecol 1976;152:613, as shown in Jobe A: The developmental biology of the lung. In Fanaroff AA, Martin RJ, eds: Neonatal-Perinatal Medicine. St Louis, Mosby–Year Book, 1992, p 792.)

Table 20–2 □ **STEPS FOR PERFORMING AMNIOTIC FLUID "SHAKE TEST"**

Materials needed:	Amniotic fluid recently collected
	95% ethanol (19 parts of absolute alcohol mixed with 1 part of distilled water)
	0.9% saline
	Two 13 × 100-mm glass tubes with Teflon-lined plastic screw cap
Steps of test:	1. Mix 1 ml of amniotic fluid and 1 ml of ethanol in one tube.
	2. Mix 0.5 ml of amniotic fluid, 0.5 ml of saline, and 1 ml of ethanol in the second tube.
	3. Shake both tubes for 15 seconds and place tubes upright.
	4. Wait for 15 minutes and look for a ring of bubbles or foam at the air–liquid interface.
Results:	Positive test: ring of bubbles is observed in both tubes
	Equivocal test: ring of bubbles is observed only in first tube
	Negative test: ring of bubbles is not observed in either tube

b. Tests to confirm chorioamnionitis

Not only is chorioamnionitis a cause of preterm labor, but it is also a contraindication for the use of tocolytic medications to treat preterm labor. It is therefore important to confirm the diagnosis of chorioamnionitis, especially because patients with this infection may be asymptomatic. Although the routine use of amniocentesis has not been established as efficacious in the management of all patients with preterm labor, it can be helpful in patients suspected of having chorioamnionitis, to confirm or rule out the diagnosis. A specimen should be submitted for Gram stain as well as amniotic fluid culture and sensitivity. Because results of amniotic fluid culture can take 24 to 48 hours, amniotic fluid glucose can be measured to help with the detection of chorioamnionitis. An amniotic fluid glucose concentration of <14 mg/dl is suggestive of chorioamnionitis. Patients who have chorioamnionitis should be treated with parenteral antibiotics, and the pediatrician should be notified so that treatment of the infant can be initiated immediately after delivery.

■ MANAGEMENT

1. Bedrest in the lateral decubitus position

The patient should initially be placed at bedrest in the lateral decubitus position while evaluation of the cervix, uterine contractions, and fetal heart rate monitoring are performed.

2. Intravenous fluid hydration

Intravenous hydration should be administered with 500 ml of 5% dextrose in water or 0.25% normal saline. Hydration may successfully treat preterm labor in dehydrated patients but has not been shown to be of benefit in hydrated patients. Because of the possible use of a tocolytic drug and the association between these drugs and pulmonary edema, fluid hydration should not be excessive.

3. Tocolytic medications

Administration of tocolytic drugs has been shown to be more successful in delaying delivery for a few days than in delaying until term. Although these drugs are commonly used, there is no convincing evidence that they significantly affect either neonatal survival or long-term morbidity. Tocolytic medications are used most often to treat preterm labor in patients with a gestational age of less than 34 weeks. Because of the risk of complications associated with the use of tocolytic medication, as well as the cost of not only the drug but also hospitalization, the use of tocolytics is individualized in patients with a gestational age of greater than 34 weeks. After the cervix has dilated beyond 4 to 5 cm, the chances of successfully treating preterm labor with tocolytic medications are very slim. The relative and absolute contraindications to the administration of tocolytic medications are listed in Table 20–3. Comparison studies have shown that tocolytic drugs are comparable with each other in efficacy and that their differences have more to do with side effects and complications associated with their use. Beta-adrenergic agonists and magnesium sulfate are the most commonly used tocolytic drugs. Prostaglandin inhibitors and calcium antagonist are considered third-line drugs, to be used if beta-adrenergic drugs and magnesium sulfate fail to achieve tocolysis.

a. Beta-adrenergic agonists

Beta-adrenergic agonists used to treat preterm labor primarily have beta-2-adrenergic effects, which include the decrease in uterine myometrial activity; they also often have undesired beta-1-adrenergic effects, which include increases in cardiac stroke volume and heart rate.

(1) **Ritodrine (Yutopar) 0.050 to 0.350 mg/min IV** or
5 to 10 mg IM every 2 to 4 hours or
20 mg PO every 2 to 4 hours
(2) **Terbutaline (Brethine) 0.01 to 0.08 mg/min IV** or
0.25 to 0.50 mg IM or SC every 3 to 4 hours or
2.5 to 5.0 mg PO every 2 to 4 hours

The tocolytic beta-adrenergic medication should be administered intravenously with an infusion pump and the dose given should be the lowest recommended. The dose

Table 20–3 □ CONTRAINDICATIONS TO THE USE OF TOCOLYTIC MEDICATIONS

Relative contraindications
  Maternal cardiac disease
  Mild pregnancy-induced hypertension
  Mild vaginal bleeding
  Hyperthyroidism
  Fetal distress
  Nonlethal fetal anomaly
  Mild intrauterine growth retardation
Absolute contraindications
  Fetal maturity
  Severe pregnancy-induced hypertension
  Eclampsia
  Severe vaginal bleeding
  Chorioamnionitis
  Fetal demise
  Lethal fetal anomaly
  Severe intrauterine growth retardation

is then increased every 15 to 30 minutes until uterine contractions are obliterated or until untoward maternal side effects occur. The serum levels of the drugs correlate closely with maternal heart rate. Some have advocated using a maternal pulse rate of 90 to 105 beats/min as an indication of an adequate drug dose. The dose should not be increased once the maternal heart rate has increased to 130 beats/min or once the systolic blood pressure has decreased to below 80. Once the uterine contractions have been halted, the infusion should be continued for 12 to 24 hours. The IV dose should then be decreased and IM or SC therapy started 30 minutes before IV therapy is discontinued. If tocolysis continues to be successful, IM or SC therapy is continued for 12 to 24 hours before changing to oral therapy. If uterine contractions do not return when the patient is on oral therapy, the patient can then be discharged home and allowed to ambulate, although she should be advised to avoid strenuous physical activity and prolonged periods of time on her feet. Because semen contains prostaglandins, which stimulate uterine contractions, and it has been found that uterine contractions occur with orgasm, it is also recommended that patients not engage in sexual intercourse.

(3) Maternal side effects caused by beta-adrenergic tocolytic drugs include the following:
   (a) Nausea
   (b) Emesis
   (c) Restlessness
   (d) Agitation
   (e) Paralytic ileus and dermatitis, which are rare

(4) Potential complications of beta-adrenergic medications include the following:
   (a) Pulmonary edema
      Pulmonary edema is the most common complication. It usually takes place 30 to 60 hours after the initiation of treatment and can occur even after the intravenous route of administration has been discontinued. The cause of pulmonary edema is unclear, but predisposing factors are excessive IV hydration, multiple gestation, persistent maternal heart rate of >130 beats/min, corticosteroid administration, anemia, infection, and underlying maternal cardiac disease.
   (b) Hypotension
   (c) Cardiac insufficiency
   (d) Cardiac arrhythmia
   (e) Myocardial ischemia

      (f) Hyperglycemia

          The administration of beta-adrenergic drugs can cause hyperglycemia, which is usually of no consequence in the nondiabetic patient but can result in ketoacidosis in diabetic patients.

      (g) Hypokalemia

          Hypokalemia is associated with hyperglycemia. Hypokalemia usually results only from intravenous administration of the beta-adrenergic drug and is transient, commonly resolving by 24 hours. Supplemental potassium is rarely needed.

      (h) Maternal death

  (5) Precautionary steps to be taken when a patient is treated with a beta-adrenergic tocolytic include the following:

      (a) Obtain baseline maternal weight

      (b) Obtain baseline laboratory tests

          [1] Serum potassium

          [2] Serum glucose

          [3] Complete blood count (CBC)

          [4] Urinalysis

      (c) Repeat laboratory tests every 6 to 12 hours

      (d) Record intake and output

      (e) Limit fluid intake to 1500 to 2500 ml/24 hr

      (f) Auscultate lungs for evidence of pulmonary edema every 6 to 12 hours

  (6) Contraindications to the use of beta-adrenergic tocolytics, in addition to the contraindications listed in Table 20–3, include the following:

      (a) Maternal cardiac arrhythmia

      (b) Maternal cardiac disease

      (c) Diabetes mellitus

      (d) Uncontrolled hypertension

      (e) Thyrotoxicosis

b. Magnesium sulfate

    Although the mechanism of action is unclear, magnesium sulfate depresses myometrial contractility.

  (1) **Magnesium sulfate 4.0 to 6.0 g IV over 20 minutes as a loading dose and 1.0 to 3.0 g/hr IV as the maintenance dose**

      or

      Magnesium gluconate or magnesium oxide 0.5 to 2.0 g PO every 2 to 4 hours

      Magnesium sulfate should be administered intravenously with an infusion pump, and the initial dose should be the lowest dose recommended. The dose should be increased every 15 to 30 minutes until uterine contractions are obliterated or untoward maternal side effects occur. The optimal dose of magnesium sulfate should be continued IV for approximately 24 hours. The patient should then be placed on an IM or SC beta-adrenergic medication followed by an oral beta-adrenergic tocolytic or oral magnesium gluconate or magnesium oxide. Magnesium has a depressant effect on the central nervous system and also has a competitive antagonistic role with calcium. Inhibition of myometrial contractility takes place at a serum magnesium level of 5 to 8 mg/dl. Loss of deep tendon reflexes occurs at a serum magnesium level of 9 to 13 mg/dl, and respiratory depression takes place at a serum level of ≥14 mg/dl.

(2) Maternal side effects caused by magnesium sulfate include the following:
  (a) Hot flashes
  (b) Headache
  (c) Nausea
  (d) Dizziness
  (e) Nystagmus
  (f) Dryness of the mouth
  (g) Lethargy
  (h) Urticarial eruptions

(3) Potential complications from magnesium sulfate include the following:
  (a) Pulmonary edema
      As is the case with beta-adrenergic tocolytics, the mechanism of pulmonary edema is unclear, and the use of a corticosteroid, often given to accelerate fetal lung maturity, increases the risk of this complication.
  (b) Hypocalcemia
  (c) Hypotension
  (d) Respiratory depression and arrest
  (e) Fetal and neonatal depression
      When the maternal serum level of magnesium is in the therapeutic range, approximately 50% of fetuses will have a nonreactive nonstress test, and 80% will not have sustained respiratory movements on biophysical profile testing.
  (f) Cardiac depression and arrest

(4) Precautionary steps that should be taken when a patient is being treated with magnesium sulfate include the following:
  (a) Obtain baseline maternal weight
  (b) Monitor deep tendon reflexes
  (c) Obtain baseline serum magnesium and calcium
  (d) Repeat laboratory tests every 6 to 12 hours, or as indicated by the clinical status

(e) Record intake and output

Because magnesium is excreted by the kidneys, urine output should be followed as an indicator of renal function.

(f) Limit fluid intake to 1500 to 2500 ml/24 hr

(g) Auscultate lungs for evidence of pulmonary edema every 6 to 12 hours

(h) Keep readily available a 10% solution of calcium gluconate to treat respiratory and cardiac arrest due to magnesium toxicity (calcium gluconate, 10% solution, administer 10 ml [1 g] IV over 3 minutes)

(5) Contraindications to the use of magnesium sulfate for tocolysis, in addition to the contraindications listed in Table 20–3, include the following:

(a) Hypocalcemia

(b) Myasthenia gravis

(c) Renal failure

c. Prostaglandin synthesis inhibitors

Because prostaglandins stimulate myometrial contractility, antiprostaglandin agents can be effective in the treatment of preterm labor.

(1) **Indomethacin, 100-mg rectal suppository, as a loading dose followed by 25 mg PO every 6 hours**

Indomethacin inhibits the synthesis of prostaglandins by inhibiting the enzyme cyclooxygenase. It is not used for more than approximately 48 hours because of the risk of oligohydramnios. This complication is a result of decreased fetal urine output.

(2) Maternal side effects caused by indomethacin include the following:

(a) Nausea

(b) Emesis

(c) Headaches

(d) Dizziness

(e) Depression

(f) Psychosis

(3) Potential complications associated with indomethacin use include the following:

(a) Postpartum hemorrhage

(b) Oligohydramnios

(c) Premature closure of the ductus arteriosus, resulting in pulmonary hypertension in the fetus

(4) Contraindications to the use of indomethacin for tocolysis, in addition to the contraindications listed in Table 20–3, include the following:

(a) Asthma

(b) Oligohydramnios

(c) Coronary artery disease

(d) Renal failure

(e) Hepatitic failure

(f) Gastrointestinal bleeding

d. Calcium antagonists

Calcium channel blockers such as nifedipine inhibit the movement of calcium ions through cell membranes, resulting in inhibition of smooth muscle contractility.

(1) **Nifedipine 10 mg sublingual, repeat after 20 minutes if necessary, and 10 to 20 mg every 4 to 6 hours as the maintenance dose**

(2) Maternal side effects caused by nifedipine include the following:

(a) Vasodilatation

(b) Flushing

(c) Nausea

(d) Headaches

(3) Potential complications associated with nifedipine use include the following:

(a) Hypotension

(b) Liver toxicity

(4) Contraindications to the use of nifedipine for tocolysis, in addition to the contraindications listed in Table 20-3, include the following:

(a) Maternal liver disease

(b) Maternal hypotension

4. Corticosteroids

Antepartum corticosteroid therapy to induce fetal lung maturity should be considered for women in preterm labor with gestational ages of 24 to 34 weeks. The major benefits derived from corticosteroid therapy are reduced incidences of RDS and IVH and decreased neonatal mortality. Although the maximum benefits occur 24 hours after initiation of treatment, some benefits can be gained after less than 24 hours. Therefore, corticosteroid should be administered unless delivery is imminent.

Celestone Soluspan solution 2 ml IM, repeat dose in 24 hours (1 ml of Celestone contains 3 mg of betamethasone sodium and 3 mg of betamethasone acetate)

The effects of treatment last for 7 days; and therefore, a repeat dose should be administered if the fetus remains undelivered and the patient is still undergoing treatment for preterm labor.

5. Maternal transport

The extremely preterm infant who is delivered in a facility with specialized intensive perinatal and neonatal services has a smaller chance of mortality and a lower incidence of both short-term and long-term morbidity than the infant who is transported to such a facility after birth. Therefore, if the patient is initially admitted to a medical facility where these services are not available, she should be transported before delivery to the proper facility as soon as she has been stabilized.

6. **Management during labor**

If efforts to halt preterm labor have failed and delivery is anticipated, management of the patient requires recognition that preterm labor and delivery are associated with a higher incidence of complications including fetal distress, malpresentation, and birth trauma. The following steps should be taken:

a. Initiate continuous electronic fetal heart rate monitoring

b. Notify the anesthesiologist and pediatric or neonatal team of the patient's condition

c. Provide adequate anesthesia to ensure a controlled delivery

d. Have available the proper personnel and equipment for an emergency cesarean section

e. Consider the use of low forceps and an episiotomy to reduce resistance and trauma to the fetal head, especially with prolonged second stage of labor

f. Decide on the route of delivery for the preterm fetus by using the same guidelines that would normally apply to the term fetus

Cesarean section should be performed for the frank breech infant with an estimated weight of <1500 g because of the increased morbidity associated with vaginal delivery of these infants.

21

SHOULDER DYSTOCIA

■ BACKGROUND AND DEFINITION

Shoulder dystocia: An obstetrical emergency that occurs when the anterior shoulder does not deliver either spontaneously or with downward traction and episiotomy after delivery of the head; the incidence of shoulder dystocia is 0.15 to 0.63% or approximately 1 of 300 deliveries.

■ CLINICAL PRESENTATION

Recoil of the fetal chin into the perineum immediately after delivery of the head, also referred to as the "turtle sign."

■ PHONE CALL

Orders

Have the nurse call immediately for assistance from another obstetrician and/or another labor and delivery nurse, an anesthesiologist, and the pediatric or neonatal team.

Degree of Urgency

Shoulder dystocia is an obstetrical emergency, and the patient should be seen immediately.

■ ELEVATOR THOUGHTS

What are factors that contribute to shoulder dystocia?
The best management of shoulder dystocia is prevention. This requires an understanding of the factors that increase the risk of this complication.
- Maternal diabetes mellitus
    Maternal diabetes is associated with fetal macrosomia and an incidence of shoulder dystocia of 2.5 to 16.7%.
- Maternal obesity
    The incidence of shoulder dystocia is 5.1% if the maternal weight is greater than 250 lb.
- Fetal macrosomia

Shoulder dystocia occurs more frequently in infants with birth weights of more than 4000 g (8 lb 13 oz.).
- Postdate pregnancy
- Oxytocin administration
    Fetal macrosomia often causes abnormal labor and requires the administration of oxytocin, which increases the risk of shoulder dystocia.
- Prolonged second stage of labor
    The incidence of shoulder dystocia increases to 4.6% when the second stage of labor is prolonged. A prolonged second stage of labor is defined as more than 2 hours for a nulliparous patient and more than 1 hour for a multiparous patient.
- Mid-pelvic or high-pelvic operative delivery with forceps or vacuum extraction

The above factors are cumulative. The incidence of shoulder dystocia with an infant weighing more than 4000 g and delivered by mid-pelvic operative delivery after a prolonged second stage of labor is 23%.

■ MAJOR THREAT TO FETAL LIFE

- Fetal asphyxia
    The perinatal mortality from shoulder dystocia is as high as 33% and results primarily from asphyxia due to cord compression, which is a result of obstructed delivery.

■ MAJOR THREAT TO MATERNAL LIFE

- Maternal postpartum hemorrhage from uterine atony or lacerations of the cervix, vagina, or vulva

■ BEDSIDE

Quick Look Test

Does the patient appear to have adequate anesthesia?
    The maneuvers used to manage shoulder dystocia can be uncomfortable and, furthermore, may require patient cooperation. Therefore, an anesthesiologist should be called immediately if anesthesia does not appear to be adequate.

Vital Signs

Vital signs are normal.

Selective History and Chart Review

1. Before delivery, a patient's chart should be reviewed to determine if she has any antepartum risk factors for shoulder dystocia, namely, diabetes, fetal macrosomia, excessive maternal weight gain, or postdate pregnancy.
2. The labor records should also be reviewed for intrapartum risk factors such as the use of oxytocin, prolonged second stage of labor, and a high fetal station requiring mid-pelvic operative delivery.

Selective Physical Examination

Pelvic
External genitalia   "Turtle sign" with the fetal chin pulled back
   and vagina   into the perineum after delivery of the fetal head

■ DIAGNOSTIC TESTING

Shoulder dystocia is diagnosed at the time of delivery based on the clinical findings. Unfortunately, there are no diagnostic tests other than the assessment of a patient's risk factors that can be used before delivery to predict which patients will develop shoulder dystocia. Ultrasound examination for estimating fetal weight has not generally been accurate.

■ MANAGEMENT

The management of shoulder dystocia should consist of the following steps performed in the order listed:

1. **Immediate call for additional help**
   Assistance should be requested from another obstetrician or a labor and delivery nurse, an anesthesiologist, and the pediatric or neonatal team.
2. **Cutting of a generous episiotomy**
3. **Sharp flexion of the hips** or **McRoberts maneuver**
   The McRoberts maneuver consists of removing the patient's legs from the stirrups and flexing the hips sharply so that the knees are brought back against the patient's chest. This maneuver straightens the sacrum, rotates the pubic symphysis toward the patient's head, and decreases the angle of

Figure 21–1 □ Rotation of the shoulder to an oblique diameter. (From Plauche WC, Morrison JC, O'Sullivan M: Surgical Obstetrics. Philadelphia, WB Saunders Co, 1992, p 319.)

pelvic inclination. The cephalic rotation of the pelvis will, it is hoped, free the anterior shoulder from behind the pubic symphysis.

4. Suprapubic pressure

An assistant should apply suprapubic pressure with the palm of the hand or a closed fist downward toward the floor, while the delivering physician applies downward traction to the fetal head. The application of suprapubic pressure is performed in an attempt to dislodge the anterior shoulder from behind the pubic symphysis. It is important for the assistant to be elevated on a stand or a lift in order to apply sufficient pressure downward. Furthermore, it is important that the assistant does not apply fundal pressure.

5. Shoulders rotated to an oblique diameter

This maneuver is accomplished by placing a hand behind the anterior shoulder of the fetus and pushing forward toward the anterior surface of the chest, so that the shoulders are now in an oblique orientation instead of an anterior–posterior orientation (Fig. 21–1).

6. Corkscrew maneuver or Woods' maneuver

Woods' maneuver is performed by placing a hand behind the posterior fetal shoulder and pushing forward to rotate the shoulders 180° in a corkscrew fashion (Fig. 21–2). This

Figure 21–2 □ Corkscrew or Woods' maneuver. (From Plauche WC, Morrison JC, O'Sullivan M: Surgical Obstetrics. Philadelphia, WB Saunders Co, 1992, p 319.)

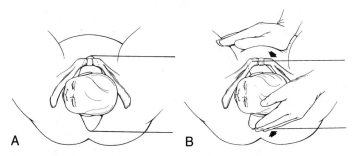

Figure 21–3 □ *A,* The shoulder-to-shoulder diameter is maximal, with the anterior shoulder trapped by the symphysis. *B,* Abduction of the shoulders by Rubin's maneuver. (From Plauche WC, Morrison JC, O'Sullivan M: Surgical Obstetrics. Philadelphia, WB Saunders Co, 1992, p 320.)

maneuver is performed to rotate the anterior shoulder from behind the pubic symphysis.

7. **Delivery of the posterior shoulder**

   To perform this maneuver, the deliverer places a hand along the posterior humerus of the fetus, flexes the fetal arm at the elbow, and sweeps the fetal arm across the fetal chest so that the fetal hand can be grasped. The posterior arm is then delivered, and the shoulders are rotated obliquely to allow delivery of the anterior shoulder.

8. **Abduction of the shoulders** or **Rubin's maneuver**

   Rubin's maneuver is performed by pushing both shoulders toward the fetal chest, resulting in abduction of the shoulders (Fig. 21–3). This decreases the shoulder-to-shoulder diameter and allows the anterior shoulder to be freed from behind the pubic symphysis.

9. **Deliberate fracture of the clavicle**

   This maneuver is performed by pressing the anterior clavicle against the ramus of the pubis. Fracture of the clavicle will then free the anterior shoulder from behind the pubic symphysis. Clavicular fractures heal rapidly without any serious sequelae.

10. **Cephalic replacement** or **Zavanelli's maneuver**

    This maneuver is performed first by administrating terbutaline 0.25 mg SC. The fetal head is then rotated back to an occiput anterior (OA) or occiput posterior (OP) position. The head is then flexed and slowly pushed back into the vagina. Delivery is then accomplished by cesarean section. In some cases, general anesthesia is necessary in order to perform this maneuver because of patient discomfort.

22

TRAUMA IN PREGNANCY

■ BACKGROUND AND DEFINITIONS

Physical trauma: Occurs in approximately 1 of 12 pregnancies. Trauma can be **blunt trauma** or **penetrating trauma.** The most common cause of blunt trauma in pregnant patients is automobile accidents, followed in frequency by falls and direct assaults to the abdomen. Gunshot and knife wounds are the most common types of penetrating trauma. Because of the protective effect of the uterus, gunshot wounds to the abdomen result in injury to other intra-abdominal organs in only 19% of pregnant patients. Trauma to the uterus is rare in the first trimester, because the uterus is still protected by the bony pelvis. Beyond the first trimester, the uterus begins to rise out of the pelvis and is therefore much more vulnerable to trauma.

■ CLINICAL PRESENTATION

The clinical presentation depends on the severity and the type of trauma. If placental abruption has developed, the following signs and symptoms may be present:
Vaginal bleeding
Hypovolemic shock, sometimes out of proportion to the amount of visible bleeding
Coagulopathy
Uterine pain and tenderness
Uterine irritability
Fetal distress
Fetal demise

■ PHONE CALL

Questions

1. What is the type and the severity of trauma sustained by the patient?
2. What is the gestational age of the pregnancy?
3. What are the patient's vital signs

Orders

If the patient has sustained severe trauma, the following should be ordered.

1. Start a large-bore IV
2. Crossmatch 2 to 4 units of blood
3. Displace the uterus off the midline with a hip roll or by turning the patient to one side
4. Obtain a complete blood count (CBC)
5. Perform coagulation studies: prothrombin time (PT), partial thromboplastin time (PTT), platelet count, fibrinogen, fibrin split products
6. Obtain a chemistry panel
7. Perform urinalysis
8. Insert urethral catheter
9. Record intake and output
10. Listen for fetal heart tones and begin continuous electronic fetal monitoring (fetal heart tones are not usually heard until the gestational age is >10 weeks.)
11. Begin electronic uterine monitoring; because of the small size of the uterus early in pregnancy, uterine contractions are not usually detected by uterine monitoring until the gestational age is >16 weeks
12. Keep the patient nothing by mouth (NPO) if surgery is anticipated

Degree of Urgency

Depending on the severity, physical trauma can be life threatening for both the patient and the fetus. In severe cases or if the severity of the trauma is unknown or unclear, the patient should be seen immediately.

■ ELEVATOR THOUGHTS

What are the possible obstetrical complications of trauma?
- Blunt trauma
     Placental abruption
     Uterine rupture
     Direct fetal injury
     Rupture of membranes
- Penetrating trauma
     Uterine trauma
     Direct trauma to the fetus or placenta

■ MAJOR THREAT TO FETAL LIFE

- Direct fetal trauma
- Placental abruption
- Prematurity

■ MAJOR THREAT TO MATERNAL LIFE

- Hypovolemic shock

  Both blunt and penetrating trauma can result in significant intra-abdominal and retroperitoneal hemorrhage. Rupture of the spleen is the most common cause of intraperitoneal hemorrhage after blunt trauma.

- Visceral injuries

  The maternal mortality rate from penetrating trauma is less than 9%. This is lower than the mortality rate for nonpregnant patients, because the pregnant uterus shields other abdominal organs. In contrast, penetrating trauma to the uterus results in a perinatal mortality rate of 41 to 71%.

■ BEDSIDE

Quick Look Test

Does the patient have life-threatening injuries?

Does the patient appear to be in hypovolemic shock?

Does the patient have uterine contractions or uterine tenderness?

Vital Signs

In patients who have suffered severe trauma, bleeding could result in hypovolemic shock with hypotension and tachycardia. Furthermore, the patient might have postural hypotension. Changes in blood pressure (BP) and pulse should be measured when the patient is assisted in sitting or standing from a supine position. A fall in systolic or diastolic BP of >15 mm Hg or a rise in pulse of >15 beats/min is evidence of hypovolemia.

Selective History and Chart Review

1. What is the gestational age of the fetus?

   The gestational age might affect the management of the patient.
2. What is the nature of the trauma sustained by the patient?
3. Has the patient sustained penetrating trauma, and could the uterus have been injured directly?

Selective Physical Examination

Abdominal	Bruising usually seen with blunt trauma
	Uterus tender in placental abruption and uterine rupture
	Uterine contractions and irritability present in placental abruption

Pelvic

External genitalia and vagina	Vaginal bleeding may be present
Cervix	Bleeding may be present
	Pooling of fluid if membranes are ruptured
Uterus and adnexae	Tender in placental abruption and uterine rupture
	Irritable with or without contractions in placental abruption

■ DIAGNOSTIC TESTING

1. **Ultrasound examination**

   Ultrasound examination is useful for determining gestational age, placental location, and fetal viability. Amniotic fluid volume can also be estimated. A very low amniotic fluid volume is found in patients with ruptured membranes. Intra-abdominal fluid caused by bleeding can also be found by ultrasound examination.

2. **Electronic fetal heart rate monitoring**

   Fetal heart rate monitoring is useful in predicting placental abruption secondary to trauma. The finding of fetal tachycardia and/or late decelerations is suggestive of fetal distress secondary to placental abruption. If uterine contractions either are absent or occur at a frequency of less than once every 10 minutes after 4 hours of fetal monitoring, placental abruption is extremely unlikely. Fetal monitoring should be continued if there are uterine contractions, uterine tenderness or irritability, vaginal bleeding, abnormalities in the fetal heart rate tracing, rupture of membranes, or severe maternal injuries. In the absence of these signs and symptoms, fetal monitoring should be performed for approximately 2 to 6 hours.

3. **Peritoneal lavage**

   Open peritoneal lavage is safe and sensitive and can be helpful in diagnosing intraperitoneal hemorrhage. Instead of blind needle insertion, sharp dissection should be performed at the umbilicus and carried down to the peritoneum, which is opened under direct visualization. Peritoneal lavage does not need to be performed if it is obvious that intraperitoneal bleeding is present. Indications for peritoneal lavage include the following findings:

   a. **Unexplained or equivocal abdominal signs or symptoms suggestive of intraperitoneal bleeding**

   b. **Altered sensorium**

   c. **Unexplained shock**

   d. **Major thoracic injury**

   e. **Multiple major orthopedic injuries**

The interpretation of diagnostic peritoneal lavage for blunt trauma in pregnancy is summarized in Table 22–1.

4. Kleihauer–Betke stain of maternal blood

Bleeding from the fetal to maternal circulation occurs in 10 to 30% of trauma cases. The presence of fetal red blood cells in the maternal circulation can be documented by Kleihauer–Betke staining of maternal blood. This test is done by acid elution treatment, after which fetal red blood cells rich in hemoglobin F stain darkly and, in contrast, maternal cells poor in hemoglobin F stain lightly.

■ MANAGEMENT

The initial treatment of trauma in the pregnant patient should be identical to that in the nonpregnant patient. The top priority is the complete assessment and stabilization of the patient. Pregnancy should place very few restrictions in the diagnostic and resuscitative procedures necessary to achieve these goals. There are, however, several important considerations specific to pregnancy.

1. Normal physiological changes of pregnancy

a. Increased blood volume

The pregnant patient normally has a 35 to 40% increase in total blood volume when she is near term. Therefore, the

---

Table 22–1 □ **INTERPRETATION OF RESULTS OF DIAGNOSTIC PERITONEAL LAVAGE* FOLLOWING BLUNT TRAUMA**

Positive†
  Grossly bloody lavage fluid
  RBC count >100,000/mm³
  WBC count >175/dl
  Amylase >175/dl
  Lavage fluid identified in Foley catheter
Indeterminate‡
  RBC count >50,000 but <100,000/mm³
  WBC count >100 but <500/mm³
  Amylase >75 but <175/dl
Negative
  RBC count <50,000/mm³
  WBC count <100/mm³
  Amylase <75/dl

Modified from Rothenberger DA, Quattlesbaum FW, Zabel J, et al: Diagnostic peritoneal lavage for blunt trauma in pregnant women. Am J Obstet Gynecol 129:479, 1977.
*Peritoneal lavage performed with 1 L of Ringer's lactate solution.
†Positive lavage (any one criterion) suggests need for surgical exploration.
‡Recommendations are to repeat lavage.

pregnant patient will have had significantly greater blood loss than the nonpregnant patient for a similar degree of shock. For this reason, larger amounts of blood and fluid will be needed for replacement in pregnant patients.

b. **Increased heart rate**

The heart rate in pregnant patients normally increases by approximately 15%, and therefore, this finding should not be interpreted as a sign of shock.

c. **Decreased blood pressure**

Maternal blood pressure usually falls, in particular in the second trimester, and should not be interpreted as a sign of shock.

d. **Compression of the inferior vena cava, decreasing venous return to the heart**

When the patient is supine, compression of the inferior vena cava by the pregnant uterus decreases blood return to the heart, resulting in hypotension. This can be corrected with lateral displacement of the uterus, by tilting the patient partly to one side with a towel roll or wedge placed underneath the patient's hip.

e. **Displacement of the bowel into the upper abdomen**

As the uterus enlarges, the bowel is pushed up into the upper abdomen. As a result, trauma to the upper abdomen will often injure both small and large intestines. Furthermore, paracentesis or peritoneal lavage is more risky in the patient with an advanced pregnancy.

f. **Decreased gastrointestinal motility and delayed stomach emptying**

Decreased gastrointestinal motility and delayed emptying of the stomach result in a greater risk of aspiration during intubation.

g. **Mild elevation in white blood cell count**

Pregnancy is normally associated with a mild leukocytosis. Therefore, a mild elevation in white blood cells may not be an indication of sepsis in the pregnant patient.

h. **Hypercoagulable state**

Pregnancy is normally a hypercoagulable state. Serum fibrinogen is normally 350 to 400 mg/dl in pregnancy, and therefore, a lower level that would be considered normal in the nonpregnant patient could be an early sign of disseminated intravascular coagulation in the pregnant patient.

2. **Fetal–maternal hemorrhage**

Trauma results in some degree of fetal–maternal hemorrhage in 10 to 30% of cases. However, the amount of the hemorrhage is less than 15 ml in more than 90% of cases. The Kleihauer–Betke stain of maternal blood can be used to estimate the amount of fetal–maternal hemorrhage. To prevent Rh isoimmunization, patients who are Rh negative should receive Rh immunoglobulin if the Rh factor of the father is positive or unknown. One ampule of 300 µg of Rh immunoglobulin should be administered IM for every 30 ml of whole blood that is estimated to have been transfused. Rh immunoglobulin should be administered within 72 hours of fetal–maternal hemorrhage.

3. **Fetal radiation exposure from radiographic procedures**

There is no increase in teratogenesis or risk of childhood malignancy if the fetus is exposed to less than 10 rad (0.1 Gy) of radiation. By using the proper precautions such as shielding of the uterus, most radiological procedures can be performed with a fetal radiation exposure of less than 1 rad. The fetal dose of radiation is approximately the same as the ovarian dose, which has been estimated for common radiological procedures (Table 22–2).

4. **Tetanus toxoid prophylaxis**

Tetanus toxoid prophylaxis should be administered with the same indications as used in nonpregnant patients. If the patient has had a tetanus toxoid booster in the last 10 years, no additional toxoid is needed. If it has been more than 10 years

Table 22–2 □ ESTIMATED OVARIAN RADIATION EXPOSURE FROM COMMON RADIOLOGICAL PROCEDURES*

Procedure	Estimated Ovarian Dose (millirad)	Average Number of Films per Examination
Chest examination		
Radiography	8	1.4
Fluoroscopy	71	
Upper GI series		
Total	558	4.4
Radiography	360	
Fluoroscopy	198	
Barium enema		
Total	805	3.5
Radiography	439	
Fluoroscopy	366	
Intravenous or retrograde pyelography	407	5.0
Abdominal x-rays	289	1.7
Lumbar spine x-rays	275	2.5
Pelvic x-rays	41	1.5

*Ovarian dose approximates fetal exposure.

Adapted from Penfil RL, Brown ML: Genetically significant dose to the United States population from diagnostic medical roentgenology. Radiology 1968;90:209.

since a booster or if the immunization history is unknown, the patient should receive 250 units of tetanus antitoxin IM.

5. Perimortem cesarean delivery

If survival of the pregnant trauma patient is doubtful, perimortem cesarean section should be considered if the pregnancy has reached a viable gestational age, usually greater than 25 weeks. It should be remembered that a cesarean section, and especially the blood loss associated with the operation, will further compromise the patient. After 10 minutes of maternal cardiorespiratory resuscitation, survival of the fetus is unlikely. Therefore, if cesarean section is planned, it should be performed after 4 to 6 minutes of cardiopulmonary resuscitation.

PATIENT-RELATED GYNECOLOGICAL PROBLEMS: THE COMMON CALLS

23

ABNORMAL UTERINE BLEEDING

■ BACKGROUND AND DEFINITIONS

Menorrhagia: Prolonged or excessive bleeding that occurs at regular intervals; also referred to as **hypermenorrhea**

Metrorrhagia: Bleeding that occurs at irregular intervals

Menometrorrhagia: Prolonged or excessive bleeding that occurs at irregular intervals

Polymenorrhea: Bleeding that occurs regularly but at intervals of <21 days

Oligomenorrhea: Bleeding that occurs at intervals of >35 days

Hypomenorrhea: Bleeding that occurs regularly but in small amounts

Dysfunctional uterine bleeding (DUB): Abnormal bleeding from the uterine endometrium that is unrelated to any anatomic lesion of the uterus. More than 80% of all cases of dysfunctional uterine bleeding are due to a disruption of normal ovarian function and anovulation. Therefore, the term **anovulatory bleeding** is used synonymously with dysfunctional uterine bleeding. During anovulatory cycles, the failure of ovulation results in the lack of progesterone production, and therefore, the endometrium is exposed to prolonged unopposed estrogen stimulation. Chronic estrogen stimulation results in an overgrowth of endometrium that then breaks down and bleeds. The remaining 20% of DUB is due to dysfunction of the corpus luteum such as inadequate progesterone production. Bleeding that results from pregnancy, uterine leiomyomata, uterine malignancy, polyps, and coagulopathy is not considered DUB.

The normal menstrual cycle averages 28 days in length with a normal range of 21 to 35 days. The normal duration of bleeding is 4 to 5 days with a normal range of 3 to 7 days. The average blood loss during menses is 35 ml with a normal range of 20 to 80 ml.

■ CLINICAL PRESENTATION

Vaginal bleeding or spotting at times other than when menses is expected or for a longer duration than expected

Heavy bleeding

Passage of blood clots

■ PHONE CALL
Questions
1. **How severe is the patient's bleeding?**
2. **What are the patient's vital signs?**

Orders
1. Obtain a complete blood count (CBC)
2. Perform urine pregnancy test in patients of reproductive age
3. Perform coagulation studies in adolescent patients: platelet count, bleeding time, prothrombin time (PT), partial thromboplastin time (PTT)
4. Start IV if the patient is bleeding heavily or appears to be in hypovolemic shock

Degree of Urgency

The degree of urgency depends on the degree of bleeding. Patients with prolonged heavy bleeding and signs of hypovolemic shock should be seen immediately. Likewise, patients with bleeding and a positive pregnancy test should be seen immediately.

■ ELEVATOR THOUGHTS
What are causes of abnormal uterine bleeding?
- Dysfunctional bleeding
  Anovulatory bleeding
  Dysfunction of the corpus luteum
- Pregnancy complications
  Spontaneous abortion
  Ectopic pregnancy
  Molar pregnancy
- Uterine lesions
  Leiomyomata
  Endometrial polyps
  Atrophic endometrium
  Adenomyosis
  Endometrial hyperplasia
  Endometrial carcinoma
- Lower genital tract lesions
  Cervical polyp
  Cervical carcinoma
  Vaginal malignancy
  Vulvar malignancy
- Infection
  Pelvic inflammatory disease
  Vaginitis

Cervicitis
Endometritis
- Systemic conditions
  Coagulopathies
      von Willebrand's disease
      Thrombocytopenic purpura
  Endocrine disorders
      Thyroid disease
      Adrenal disorders
      Hyperprolactinemia
  Liver disease
      Decreased synthesis of coagulation factors
      Impaired metabolism of estrogen
  Renal disease
      Impaired excretion of both estrogen and progesterone
  Obesity
- Contraceptive complications
  Oral contraceptive pills
  Intrauterine device
  Nonpill hormonal contraception
      Norplant implant system
      Depo-Provera

■ MAJOR THREAT TO LIFE

- Hypovolemic shock
  Abnormal uterine bleeding is rarely severe enough to be life threatening.

■ BEDSIDE

Quick Look Test

Does the patient appear to be in hypovolemic shock?

What are the patient's vital signs?

Vital Signs

Vital signs are usually normal. If the patient has had heavy bleeding, she may have hypotension and tachycardia. The patient might have postural hypotension. Changes in blood pressure (BP) and pulse should be measured when the patient is assisted in sitting or standing from a supine position. A fall in systolic or diastolic BP of >15 mm Hg or a rise in pulse of >15 beats/min is evidence of hypovolemia.

Selective History and Chart Review

1. What is the patient's age?

    Women in the reproductive age group can have bleeding secondary to pregnancy complications. Furthermore, throughout the entire reproductive age range, especially at both extremes, anovulation is a common cause of abnormal uterine bleeding. In adolescent patients with persistent bleeding severe enough to require hospital admission, co-agulopathy accounts for approximately 20% of cases of abnormal bleeding. In postmenopausal patients, abnormal uterine bleeding is commonly caused by hormone replacement therapy. Uterine malignancy and endometrial atrophy are other causes in this age group.

2. What is the nature of the abnormal uterine bleeding?

    The amount, duration, interval, and frequency of the bleeding should be ascertained.

3. When was the patient's last normal menstrual period?

4. Is the patient on any hormonal medication such as hormonal contraception or postmenopausal hormone replacement?

5. If the patient is of reproductive age, is she using contraception; if so, what type?

6. Is the patient pregnant; if so, what is the gestational age of the fetus?

7. Has the patient had bleeding from the gums, prolonged bleeding after minor cuts, or easy bruisability suggestive of a coagulopathy?

8. Does the patient complain of pain in association with the bleeding?

9. Does the patient have a history of any gynecological disorders?

    It should be determined if the patient has a history of fibroid tumors, abnormal cervical cytology, gynecological malignancy, genital infection, and prior episodes of abnormal uterine bleeding.

10. Does the patient have a history of thyroid or hepatic disease?

11. Does the patient engage in strenuous physical activities?

    Rigorous exercise can be a cause of dysfunctional uterine bleeding.

12. Has the patient had significant psychological or emotional stress or suffered from eating disorders?

    These are common causes of dysfunctional uterine bleeding.

13. When did the patient last have a Pap smear?

Selective Physical Examination

General	Obesity often associated with anovulatory bleeding
	Hirsutism and other signs of virilization associated with chronic anovulation
Dermatological	Ecchymotic lesions in patients with coagulopathy
Abdominal	Abdominal mass in patients with uterine leiomyoma
Pelvic	
External genitalia and vagina	Discharge and erythema in patients with vaginitis
	Bleeding lesion in patients with trauma or malignancy
Cervix	Tender with purulent discharge in patients with cervicitis
	Friable cervix that bleeds to the touch in patients with cervicitis
	Bleeding lesion in patients with cervical malignancy
	Cervical os may be dilated with protruding tissue in patients with spontaneous abortion
Uterus and adnexae	Enlarged and often irregular in patients with leiomyomata
	Tender in patients with endometritis
	Adnexal tenderness with palpable mass may be a tubal pregnancy

■ DIAGNOSTIC TESTING

1. **Complete blood count (CBC)**
2. **Urine pregnancy test (hCG)**
   Urine pregnancy test should be performed in all patients of reproductive age.
3. **Coagulation studies: platelet count, bleeding time, PT, PTT**
   Coagulation studies should be obtained, especially in adolescent patients.
4. **Serum prolactin**
   Serum prolactin is often elevated in patients with chronic anovulation.
5. **Serum androgens: testosterone and dehydroepiandrosterone sulfate**
   Serum androgens can be elevated in patients with chronic anovulation and should be obtained especially if there are signs of virilization.
6. **Thyroid function tests**
7. **Liver function tests**

8. **Ultrasound examination**

   Ultrasound examination of the pelvis can detect uterine leiomyomata. Furthermore, the endometrial thickness can be determined by sonography. Endometrial thickness >20 mm is associated with increased risk of endometrial polyps, hyperplasia, and adenocarcinoma.

9. **Cervical culture**

   Cervical cultures should be obtained if cervicitis is suspected.

10. **Cervical Pap smear**

11. **Endometrial sampling**

    Endometrial sampling should be performed in all women with abnormal bleeding, especially postmenopausal women, if premalignant or malignant disease of the endometrium is suspected. Endometrial hyperplasia, especially with atypia, is a premalignant finding, and adenocarcinoma is the most common malignancy of the endometrium. Endometrial sampling can also confirm the diagnosis of dysfunctional or anovulatory bleeding. In these patients, the endometrium is disordered and proliferative, because it has been exposed only to estrogen; secretory endometrium, on the other hand, has been exposed to progesterone that is produced by the corpus luteum after ovulation.

    a. **Endometrial biopsy**

       Endometrial biopsy is performed as an office procedure without the need for anesthesia. However, this procedure provides only a sample of endometrium and not the entire endometrium.

    b. **Office endometrial aspiration**

       Office endometrial aspiration with a small suction curette will usually provide more tissue than endometrial biopsy.

    c. **Dilatation and curettage**

       Dilatation and curettage while under anesthesia can be both diagnostic and therapeutic because of the greater amount of endometrium obtained. This procedure can also be performed along with hysteroscopy.

12. **Hysteroscopy**

    Hysteroscopy is a surgical procedure that provides for direct visualization of the entire endometrial cavity. Furthermore, operative hysteroscopy can be performed to remove lesions such as polyps and submucosal leiomyomata.

■ MANAGEMENT

Anatomic and Medical Causes of Uterine Bleeding

The management of specific anatomical causes of abnormal uterine bleeding, such as spontaneous abortion, ectopic pregnancy, and leiomyomata, is discussed in other chapters. The management of patients with abnormal uterine bleeding due to medical conditions such as thyroid disease, genital tract infection, and liver dysfunction depends on the correction of these medical conditions.

Dysfunctional or Anovulatory Uterine Bleeding

The goals of the management of dysfunctional uterine bleeding are to prevent endometrial hyperplasia and to restore normal menstrual bleeding. This can be accomplished by the following treatment options:

1. **Combination oral contraceptive pills**

   Combination oral contraceptive pills containing 35 μg of estrogen could be administered in the following manner:

   a. 1 pill PO daily starting on day 5 of the menstrual cycle and continued for 21 days, followed by a hiatus of 7 days. This cycle is then repeated.

   For acute and heavy bleeding, the following alternative regimen can be used:

   b. 1 pill PO three times per day for 7 days, followed by a hiatus of 7 days, and then two standard cycles of 1 pill PO each day for 21 days, followed by a hiatus of 7 days

   In both regimens, normal menstrual bleeding is expected during the 7-day hiatus.

2. **Progesterone**

   Progesterone is administered to replace the progesterone that is not produced endogenously because of the absence of ovulation. Progesterone can be administered either orally or intramuscularly. With either route, limited withdrawal bleeding is expected after progesterone administration as a result of progesterone withdrawal.

   a. Medroxyprogesterone 2.5 to 10 mg PO daily for 10 to 14 days each month or

   b. Progesterone, in oil, 50 to 100 mg IM each month

3. **Combination estrogen and progesterone therapy**

   For patients with acute, heavy, and prolonged bleeding, estrogen should be administered to stabilize the endometrium before progesterone is given. Estrogen can be given orally, or for extremely heavy bleeding, it can be administered intravenously.

   a. Conjugated estrogen 1.25 to 2.5 mg PO four times per day or

   b. Conjugated estrogen 25 mg IV every 4 hours

   Either of the above regimens is continued until bleeding subsides. Then, the following oral regimen of estrogen and progesterone is administered to produce withdrawal bleeding:

   c. Conjugated estrogen 2.5 mg PO daily for 3 weeks, fol-

lowed by both conjugated estrogen 2.5 mg PO and me-droxyprogesterone 10 mg PO daily for 7 to 10 days, fol-lowed by a hiatus to allow withdrawal bleeding

The choice of treatment regimen depends on the severity and duration of the bleeding and on the age of the patient, which in turn determines the appropriate maintenance regimen. Younger patients who have chronic and recurrent bleeding of light to moderate amounts and who furthermore desire contraception should have oral contraceptive pills given as described above. After treatment of the bleeding, these patients can be put on a standard regimen of oral contraceptive pills. Patients who have light to moderate bleeding and who do not need contraception should have progesterone alone administered. Patients who have acute and heavier bleeding and who are in the perimenopausal years should be given a combination of estrogen and progesterone therapy. After treatment of bleeding, these patients may continue taking estrogen and progesterone in the usual doses given for postmenopausal hormone replacement.

24

BARTHOLIN'S ABSCESS

■ BACKGROUND AND DEFINITIONS

Bartholin's gland: Bilateral round, lobulated glands, approximately 1 cm in diameter, located in the posterior lateral aspect of the vestibule. Also referred to as **major vestibular glands,** the glands secrete lubrication during intercourse, but their major function is unclear.

Bartholin's cyst: This cyst results from obstruction and subsequent distention of the duct of the Bartholin's gland secondary to trauma and/or infection.

Bartholin's abscess: An abscess that develops from an infection of Bartholin's cyst. It is more accurately referred to as **Bartholin's duct abscess.**

■ CLINICAL PRESENTATION

Vulvar enlargement, usually unilateral
Acute vulvar pain
Dyspareunia
Difficulty sitting or walking

Bartholin's cysts without the formation of an abscess are usually asymptomatic unless they are significantly enlarged. The cysts can range from 1 to 8 cm in diameter and are usually unilateral.

■ PHONE CALL

Questions

1. **Does the patient appear to be seriously ill?**
2. **What are the patient's vital signs?**
   Bartholin's abscesses can result in cellulitis, and in rare cases, synergistic bacterial gangrene and sepsis can occur.

Orders

1. Have available the equipment necessary for an incision and drainage procedure
   At the minimum, this would include a scalpel, local anes-

thetic, a hemostat or a similar clamp, and a catheter such as a Word catheter.
2. Have available the material needed to culture the abscess fluid

Degree of Urgency

Uncomplicated Bartholin's abscess is rarely life threatening, but because of the intense discomfort that is associated with this condition, the patient should be seen as soon as possible. If sepsis or bacterial gangrene is suspected, the patient should be seen immediately.

■ ELEVATOR THOUGHTS

What is the differential diagnosis of Bartholin's abscess?
- Vulvar hematoma
- Sebaceous cyst
- Epithelial inclusion cyst
- Mesonephric cyst
- Gartner's duct cyst
- Skene's duct cyst
- Perineal hernia
- Enterocele
- Ischiorectal abscess
- Hydrocele of the round ligament
- Lipoma
- Fibroma
- Adenocarcinoma of Bartholin's gland
- Metastatic carcinoma

■ MAJOR THREAT TO LIFE

- Synergistic bacterial gangrene
- Sepsis

■ BEDSIDE

Quick Look Test

How ill does the patient appear?

Does the patient appear to be having pain?
Significant discomfort is associated with Bartholin's abscess, ischiorectal abscess, and vulvar hematoma, whereas other conditions in the differential diagnosis are not associated with excessive pain.

Vital Signs

Vital signs are usually normal. The patient may have a fever if she has extensive cellulitis. A patient with septic shock will be hypotensive and tachycardic.

Selective History and Chart Review

1. Has the patient had a prior Bartholin's abscess on the same side?

   Bartholin's abscesses can be recurrent. Furthermore, a recurrent abscess in a postmenopausal patient should raise suspicion for adenocarcinoma of Bartholin's gland.

2. Has the patient had any recent trauma, especially "saddle injuries," in the area affected?

   A vulvar hematoma should be suspected if there is a positive history of local trauma.

3. Does the patient have a history of diabetes mellitus?

   Diabetes mellitus is associated with a higher risk of bacterial gangrene.

Selective Physical Examination

Pelvic

External genitalia and vagina	Unilateral, tense enlargement of the vulva
	Severe tenderness
	Diffuse erythema
	Yellow-green or bronze discoloration with crepitation in bacterial synergistic gangrene
Cervix	Normal
Uterus and adnexae	Normal

■ DIAGNOSTIC TESTING

The diagnosis of Bartholin's abscess can usually be made based on the physical examination. Usually, no specific diagnostic tests are necessary.

■ MANAGEMENT

1. **Incision and drainage**

   Incision and drainage is the initial step in the management of all Bartholin's abscesses and symptomatic Bartholin's cysts. This procedure can be performed easily if the abscess is pointing. If the abscess is not pointing, the patient can be instructed to use warm compresses on the abscess and to return in 1 to 2 days. An incision should then be made where the abscess is pointing, by using a no. 11 scalpel; the abscess should then be drained by both manual expression and the use of a sterile clamp to break up any loculations within the abscess cavity. The abscess fluid should be sent for culture and sensitivity. Organisms most commonly recovered are listed in Table 24–1. Any patient with a positive culture should be treated with the appropriate antibiotics. Incision and drainage alone are usually not adequate management. Bartholin's abscesses treated this way have a recurrence rate of 68 to 75%. Therefore, initial incision and drainage should be accompanied by one of the following procedures.

2. **Placement of an indwelling catheter**

   The goal in the placement of an indwelling catheter into the abscess cavity is to develop a permanent fistula between the duct and the vaginal mucosa. A Word catheter is commonly used. This catheter has an inflatable balloon at the distal tip to keep the catheter in the abscess cavity. After incision and drainage, the catheter is placed into the abscess cavity, and the balloon is filled, by syringe, with 2 to 3 ml of saline in a way similar to the filling of a Foley catheter balloon. The catheter should be kept in place for a minimum of 3 weeks before removal to allow the fistula tract to become epithelialized. The patient should be seen weekly during this time, and if necessary, additional saline can be infused into the balloon if it appears to be deflating spontaneously. To decrease the risk of the catheter's falling out prematurely, the initial incision into the abscess cavity should be less than 2 cm long. The recurrence rate after use of an indwelling catheter is 3 to 17%.

3. **Marsupialization**

   As with the placement of an indwelling catheter, the goal of marsupialization is the development of a permanent communication, in this case a stoma, between the duct and the vaginal mucosa. Marsupialization should not be performed in the presence of acute inflammation, and therefore it should not be

Table 24–1 □ ORGANISMS COMMONLY RECOVERED FROM BARTHOLIN'S ABSCESSES

Organisms	
Escherichia coli	*Proteus* spp.
Neisseria gonorrhoeae	*Pseudomonas* spp.
Chlamydia trachomatis	*Klebsiella* spp.
Bacteroides spp.	*Clostridium* spp.
Enterococcus spp.	*Staphylococcus aureus*

used for an acute Bartholin's abscess. Instead, it can be used in the patient with an uninfected Bartholin's cyst or in the patient with a chronic or recurrent Bartholin's abscess. The initial incision should be made in the vagina and should be made long enough to ensure patency of the stoma. After drainage of the cyst, the inner lining of the cyst is everted and approximated to the vaginal mucosa with interrupted sutures of 2-0 absorbable suture. This creates a "buttonhole" appearance. The recurrence rate after marsupialization is 10 to 24%.

4. **Excision of the cyst**

   Total removal of the cyst is rarely necessary. As with marsupialization, this procedure is usually performed on patients with symptomatic and uninfected cysts or chronic or recurrent abscesses, but not on patients with acute abscesses. Excision of the cyst is indicated in the postmenopausal patient with a recurrent cyst, especially with induration of the base of the cyst, because of the risk of adenocarcinoma of Bartholin's gland. Excision of Bartholin's cyst is usually accompanied by significant blood loss and should be performed in the operating room.

25

ECTOPIC PREGNANCY

■ BACKGROUND AND DEFINITIONS

Ectopic pregnancy: Pregnancy that implants outside of the endometrial lining of the uterus

Tubal pregnancy: Ectopic pregnancy that implants in the fallopian tube, usually in the ampullary portion of the tube

The incidence of ectopic pregnancy is increasing. Ectopic pregnancies occur at a rate of approximately 17 per 1000 reported pregnancies or 1 of every 60 pregnancies. This incidence is a fourfold increase over that reported in 1970. It is fortunate that earlier detection of ectopic pregnancies has resulted in a steady decrease in the mortality rate, which is now fewer than 5 deaths per 10,000 cases. Although there are several implantation sites for ectopic pregnancies, nearly 98% of all ectopic pregnancies implant in the fallopian tubes (Fig. 25–1). **Interstitial** or **cornual pregnancies** are the second most common type of ectopic pregnancies and are caused by implantation of the embryo in the interstitial or intramyometrial portion of the fallopian tube. **Cervical** and **ovarian pregnancies** are rare. **Abdominal pregnancies** are the rarest of ectopic pregnancies and are believed to be caused by tubal abortion in which the embryo is aborted into the peritoneal cavity and reimplantation occurs on the gastrointestinal tract or

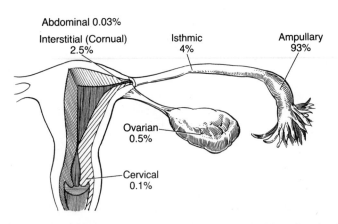

Figure 25–1 □ Sites for ectopic pregnancy implantation. (From Copeland LJ: Textbook of Gynecology. Philadelphia, WB Saunders Co, 1993, p 244.)

pelvic side wall. Because the incidence of these ectopic pregnancies is so low compared with tubal pregnancies, the terms "tubal pregnancy" and "ectopic pregnancy" are often used synonymously.

■ CLINICAL PRESENTATION

Abdominal pain
Pelvic pain
Vaginal bleeding
Palpable adnexal mass
Hypovolemic shock

The classic presentation is the triad of abdominal or pelvic pain, vaginal bleeding, and the finding of an adnexal mass.

■ PHONE CALL

Questions

1. **What are the patient's vital signs?**
2. **Does the patient appear to be in hypovolemic shock?**
   Intra-abdominal bleeding from a ruptured tubal pregnancy must be ruled out in any patient of reproductive age who presents with hypovolemic shock.
3. **Is the patient having heavy vaginal bleeding?**
   Patients with tubal pregnancies usually do not have heavy vaginal bleeding. Vaginal hemorrhage is more suggestive of spontaneous abortion.

Orders

1. Obtain a complete blood count (CBC)
2. Obtain a rapid urine qualitative pregnancy test
3. Measure serum quantitative human chorionic gonadotropin (hCG)
4. Test for the blood type and Rh factor
5. Type and crossmatch 2 units of blood if the patient appears to be in hypovolemic shock
6. Start IV infusion
7. Insert urethral catheter
8. Record intake and output
9. Place patient at bedrest, and give nothing by mouth (NPO)

Degree of Urgency

Because intra-abdominal bleeding from a ruptured tubal pregnancy is life threatening, the patient should be seen immediately.

■ ELEVATOR THOUGHTS

What are risk factors for tubal pregnancy?

- History of salpingitis

    Of those patients who conceive after salpingitis, 4 to 5% will have an ectopic pregnancy.
- Tubal reconstruction surgery

    Up to 20% of pregnancies occurring after tubal reconstructive surgery are tubal pregnancies.
- Tubal sterilization

    Up to 75% of pregnancies resulting from failure of tubal sterilization are tubal pregnancies.
- Reversal of tubal sterilization
- History of infertility
- Use of intrauterine device (IUD)

    Unless complicated by salpingitis, use of the IUD does not increase the risk of tubal pregnancy. However, if an IUD user becomes pregnant, that pregnancy has a greater chance of being a tubal pregnancy than it would in a non-IUD user. This is because the IUD offers better protection against intrauterine pregnancy than it does against tubal pregnancy. Up to 10% of pregnancies that occur in IUD users are tubal.
- Previous tubal pregnancy

    Patients with one tubal pregnancy have a recurrence rate of up to 15 to 20%.
- History of ruptured appendix
- In utero exposure to diethylstilbestrol (DES)
- Use of ovulation-inducing drugs
- In vitro fertilization and embryo transfer

■ BEDSIDE

Quick Look Test

Does the patient appear to be in hypovolemic shock?

The patient who is in hypovolemic shock and who is suspected of having a tubal pregnancy must undergo immediate surgical intervention even if all diagnostic tests have not been performed.

Vital Signs

A patient in hypovolemic shock from a ruptured tubal pregnancy will be hypotensive and tachycardic. The patient might have postural hypotension. Changes in blood pressure (BP) and pulse should be measured when the patient is assisted in sitting or standing from a supine position. A fall in systolic or diastolic

BP of >15 mm Hg or a rise in pulse of >15 beats/min is evidence of hypovolemia.

Selective History and Chart Review

1. When did the patient's last menstrual period begin?

   Almost all patients with tubal pregnancies will present in the first trimester of pregnancy.

2. Has the patient had any recent episodes of syncope or light-headedness?

   Such episodes would suggest hypovolemia from bleeding.

3. Has the patient had unilateral abdominal or pelvic pain?

   Pain is one part of the triad that represents the classic presentation of ectopic pregnancy.

4. Has the patient passed any tissue through the vagina?

   Although patients with tubal pregnancies can pass decidual tissue (also referred to as a **decidual cast**) through the vagina, patients who pass a significant amount of tissue should be suspected of having a spontaneous abortion.

5. Does the patient have any of the risk factors listed above?

Selective Physical Examination

Abdominal	Tenderness, usually unilateral
	Distended, if there is a significant hemoperitoneum
Pelvic	
External genitalia and vagina	Normal, except for vaginal bleeding
Cervix	Bleeding through the cervical os
	Cervical os usually closed
Uterus and adnexae	Uterus is of normal size or is slightly enlarged
	Unilateral adnexal tenderness
	Unilateral adnexal mass

■ DIAGNOSTIC TESTING

1. **Rapid urine pregnancy test**

   The currently available rapid urine pregnancy tests are monoclonal enzyme–linked immunoassays that are sensitive in the range of 15 to 25 mIU/ml.

2. **Serum human chorionic gonadotropin**

   Serum hCG rises exponentially in the first trimester of normal intrauterine pregnancies (Fig. 25–2). The interpretation of

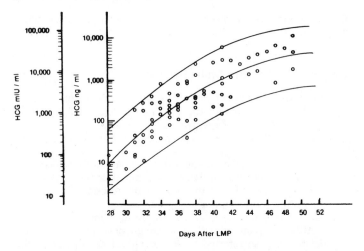

Figure 25–2 □ Rise in serum hCG in normal intrauterine pregnancies. (Modified from Pittaway DE, Reish RL, Wentz AC: Doubling times of human chorionic gonadotropin in early viable intrauterine pregnancies. Am J Obstet Gynecol 1985;152:299.)

serum hCG is complicated by the existence of two reference standards, the Second International Standard (Second IS) and the International Reference Preparation (IRP). The use of serum hCG in the diagnosis of ectopic pregnancies is based on the following two principles:

a. **When serum hCG values reach a certain level defined by the discriminatory zone, a gestational sac should be detectable by ultrasound examination in a normal intrauterine pregnancy.**

   When the serum hCG exceeds 6500 mIU/ml (IRP), a gestational sac should be detectable by transabdominal ultrasound examination. If transvaginal ultrasound examination is performed, a gestational sac should be detected when the serum hCG exceeds 2000 mIU/ml (IRP) or 1000 mIU/ml (Second IS).

b. **Because ectopic pregnancies are abnormal pregnancies, they produce an abnormal rise in serum hCG.**

   In the early first trimester of normal intrauterine pregnancies, serum hCG doubles every 1.5 to 3.5 days. In the first trimester, serum hCG should rise by ≥66% every 48 hours. If serial measurements of serum hCG demonstrate either an abnormal rise or a fall, either an ectopic pregnancy or an abnormal intrauterine pregnancy should be suspected.

3. Ultrasound examination

Ultrasound examination will rarely confirm the diagnosis of a tubal pregnancy. The finding of a complex adnexal mass is suggestive, although not diagnostic, of a tubal pregnancy. The only ultrasound finding that is diagnostic of a tubal pregnancy is the finding in the adnexa of a fetus with cardiac activity. In most cases, ultrasound examination is useful because it rules out the presence of a normal intrauterine pregnancy, based on the hCG discriminatory zone and ultrasound findings listed in Table 25–1.

4. Serum progesterone

A single serum progesterone level of $\geq$25 ng/ml is highly suggestive of a normal intrauterine pregnancy. Of women with spontaneous abortions or ectopic pregnancies, 85 to 90% have a progesterone level of <10 ng/ml. Therefore, a serum progesterone level of <5 ng/ml is a strong indication of an abnormal pregnancy. Unfortunately, this test cannot distinguish between an ectopic pregnancy and an abnormal intrauterine pregnancy.

5. Culdocentesis

Culdocentesis is performed to detect blood in the peritoneal cavity. A 20- or 22-gauge spinal needle attached to a 20-ml syringe is placed transvaginally through the posterior vaginal fornix into the posterior cul-de-sac (Fig. 25–3). A positive culdocentesis is defined by the finding, on aspiration, of free-flowing and nonclotting blood. This is an indication of intraperitoneal bleeding or hemoperitoneum, but it does not determine the cause of the bleeding. In addition to a tubal pregnancy, a hemorrhagic corpus luteum cyst is a common gynecological cause of a positive culdocentesis. A negative culdocentesis is defined by the finding of straw-colored peritoneal fluid. If no fluid is obtained, the test is nondiagnostic.

Table 25–1 □ SONOGRAPHIC FINDINGS IN NORMAL FIRST TRIMESTER PREGNANCIES

Ultrasound Finding	Gestational Age at Detection (weeks)	
	Transabdominal Examination	Transvaginal Examination
Gestational sac	6	5
Yolk sac	6	5
Fetus	7	6
Fetal cardiac activity	7	6

Blood in the
cul-de-sac

Figure 25–3 □ Technique of culdocentesis. (From Hacker NF, Moore JG: Essentials of Obstetrics and Gynecology, 2nd ed. Philadelphia, WB Saunders Co, 1992, p 432.)

6. **Dilatation and curettage**

   When serum hCG rises abnormally or falls, dilatation and curettage is helpful in distinguishing between an abnormal intrauterine pregnancy and a tubal pregnancy. If chorionic villi are seen by direct visual inspection of the specimen or are found on pathological evaluation, an intrauterine pregnancy is confirmed. This finding virtually precludes the diagnosis of tubal pregnancy, although the incidence of coexistent intrauterine and tubal pregnancy is actually much higher than was once thought and may be as high as 1 in 3000 pregnancies.

7. **Diagnostic scheme**

   Early diagnosis of tubal pregnancy not only decreases mortality and morbidity, but also allows for more conservative management that preserves tubal function. A diagnostic scheme for ectopic pregnancy is illustrated in Figure 25–4. The following are key points of the diagnostic scheme:

   a. **Any patient suspected of having an ectopic pregnancy should first have a rapid urine pregnancy test.**

      A negative urine pregnancy test rules out the diagnosis of ectopic pregnancy.

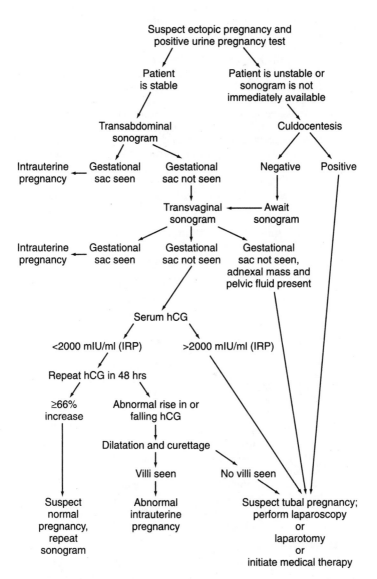

Figure 25–4 □ Diagnostic scheme for ectopic pregnancy.

b. **If the patient has a positive urine pregnancy test but is hemodynamically unstable or if an ultrasound examination is not immediately available, culdocentesis should be performed.**

If the culdocentesis is positive, the patient should undergo either laparotomy or laparoscopy immediately.

c. **If the patient has a positive urine pregnancy test and is hemodynamically stable, ultrasound examination should be performed.**

Transabdominal ultrasound examination should be performed first. If an intrauterine gestational sac is not found, then a transvaginal ultrasound examination should be performed. The finding of an intrauterine gestational sac excludes the diagnosis of ectopic pregnancy. On the other hand, the finding of a complex adnexal mass and fluid in the pelvic cavity is highly suggestive of a tubal pregnancy with a hemoperitoneum, and either surgical or medical treatment should be initiated.

d. **If an intrauterine gestational sac is not found on transvaginal ultrasound examination, serum hCG should be obtained to determine if the patient is in the discriminatory zone.**

If the serum hCG exceeds 2000 mIU/ml (IRP) or 1000 mIU/ml (Second IS), an ectopic pregnancy or abnormal intrauterine pregnancy should be suspected.

e. **If the serum hCG is below the discriminatory zone, it should be repeated in 48 hours.**

If there has been at least a 66% increase in serum hCG, a repeat ultrasound examination should be planned and the patient can be followed expectantly. If a 66% increase has not been achieved or if the serum hCG falls, then either an ectopic pregnancy or an abnormal intrauterine pregnancy should be suspected.

f. **Dilatation and curettage can be used to distinguish between an abnormal intrauterine and an ectopic pregnancy.**

If villi are seen on visual examination of the specimen, an abnormal intrauterine pregnancy is confirmed. If villi are not seen, then frozen-section examination can be performed by a pathologist. If villi are still not detected, the patient should be treated for an ectopic pregnancy.

■ MANAGEMENT

The management of a patient with a tubal pregnancy can be conservative, with the goal of preserving tubal function, or nonconservative, in which tubal function is sacrificed. The type of management used depends on the patient's desire to preserve fertility, the status of the affected fallopian tube, and the status of the contralateral tube. Conservative management may not be possible in a patient with active hemorrhage from a ruptured fallopian tube. A greater attempt at conservative management should be made if the contralateral tube has already been removed or if it is severely damaged in a patient who desires to maintain her fertility. In a patient who has a tubal pregnancy after undergoing tubal sterilization, conservative management is not appropriate. Conservative management can be either surgical or medical. Both conservative and nonconservative surgical management can be performed via laparoscopy. Laparoscopy has the advantages of a shorter hospitalization and a faster postoperative convalescence for the patient, compared with laparotomy.

1. **Conservative management**
   a. **Surgical management**
      (1) Segmental tubal resection or partial salpingectomy
         The segment of fallopian tube containing the ectopic pregnancy is removed, with an attempt made to preserve as much of the uninvolved tube as possible. Partial salpingectomy can be performed via laparotomy (Fig. 25–5) or via laparoscopy (Fig. 25–6). This allows for the possibility of tubal reanastomosis to restore tubal patency at a future time.
      (2) Linear salpingostomy
         With this procedure, on the antimesenteric surface

Figure 25–5 □ Segmental resection of tubal pregnancy via laparotomy. *A,* Kelly clamps are placed across the fallopian tube and the mesosalpinx. *B,* The tube and mesosalpinx are sutured. (From Keye WR, Chang RJ, Rebar RW, Soules MR: Infertility, Evaluation and Treatment. Philadelphia, WB Saunders Co, 1995, p 489.)

A

B

Figure 25–6 □ Segmental resection of tubal pregnancy via laparoscopy. *A,* The tube is elevated and a pretied suture is looped around the ectopic pregnancy. *B,* The segment of fallopian tube containing the pregnancy is excised and removed, leaving the two stumps secured by the suture. (From Keye WR, Chang RJ, Rebar RW, Soules MR: Infertility, Evaluation and Treatment. Philadelphia, WB Saunders Co, 1995, p 491.)

over the tubal pregnancy, an opening in the tube is made using a scalpel, electrocautery, or laser beam, and then the embryo is removed (Fig. 25–7). A vasoconstrictive agent is often used before the salpingostomy. A dilute solution of 20 units (1 ml) of vasopressin in 50 ml of injectable saline can be injected with a spinal needle into the serosa of the fallopian tube at the planned incision site. After the salpingostomy and removal of the embryo, bleeding sites are coagulated and the incision is left to heal by secondary intention.

b. Medical management with methotrexate therapy

Medical therapy with methotrexate is successful when treating the patient who is stable and in whom the diagnosis of tubal pregnancy has been made early. Methotrexate is a folic acid antagonist that interferes with the synthesis of DNA. Trophoblastic tissue is sensitive to methotrexate because of its rapid growth. The drug can be administered on an outpatient basis. The advantages of medical therapy include decreased cost, the lack of surgical and anesthetic risks, reduced tissue trauma, and less adhesion formation than results from surgery.

(1) Criteria for the use of methotrexate therapy in the patient with a tubal pregnancy are as follows:

(a) Desire for preservation of fertility
(b) Patient is stable with no active bleeding
(c) Tubal pregnancy is unruptured
(d) Size of tubal pregnancy is <3.5 cm in diameter
(e) Absence of fetal cardiac activity by ultrasound examination
(f) Peak value of hCG is <15,000 mIU/ml (IRP)

(2) A suggested protocol for methotrexate therapy is as follows:

(a) Obtain baseline laboratory studies.
[1] Complete blood count (CBC)
[2] Platelet count
[3] Blood urea nitrogen (BUN)
[4] Serum creatinine

Figure 25–7 □ Linear salpingostomy via laparoscopy. *A,* After the fallopian tube is secured with a Babcock clamp, an incision is made in the antimesenteric border of the tube over the ectopic pregnancy. *B,* The pregnancy is then removed with the forceps. *C,* The incision is left open to heal. (From Keye WR, Chang RJ, Rebar RW, Soules MR: Infertility, Evaluation and Treatment. Philadelphia, WB Saunders Co, 1995, p 488.)

A

B

C

Figure 25–8 □ Total salpingectomy via laparoscopy. (From Keye WR, Chang RJ, Rebar RW, Soules MR: Infertility, Evaluation and Treatment. Philadelphia, WB Saunders Co, 1995, p 491.)

   [5] Serum glutamic-oxaloacetic transaminase (SGOT)
  (b) Administer methotrexate 50 mg/m² IM (day 1).
  (c) Obtain serum hCG on day 4 and repeat on day 7.
  (d) If there is not a 15% decrease in hCG between day 4 and day 7, repeat a dose of methotrexate 1 week after the first dose.
  (e) Repeat serum hCG weekly until the level falls to <15 mIU/ml.
  (f) Repeat course of methotrexate if hCG plateaus or increases.
      Patients should be warned that there is a 20% incidence of lower abdominal pain approximately 5 to 10 days after treatment and that 5 to 15% of patients may suffer rupture of the fallopian tube, making surgery necessary. Side effects such as stomatitis, gastritis, dermatitis, pleuritis, bone marrow suppression, and elevation in liver enzymes occur in fewer than 5% of cases.
 (3) Contraindications to methotrexate therapy are as follows:
  (a) Poor patient compliance
  (b) History of active liver or renal disease
  (c) Active peptic ulcer disease
  (d) White blood cell count <30,000
  (e) Platelet count <100,000
  (f) Abnormal serum creatinine
  (g) Abnormal serum SGOT

2. Nonconservative management
  a. Total salpingectomy
    This procedure removes the entire fallopian tube and therefore precludes future tubal function (Fig. 25–8). Total salpingectomy is appropriate management if the patient does not want to preserve tubal function or if the extent of damage to the tube makes normal function extremely unlikely. Total salpingectomy should also be considered if the patient had a previous tubal pregnancy in the same tube.

26

GONORRHEA AND CHLAMYDIAL INFECTIONS

■ BACKGROUND AND DEFINITIONS

Gonorrhea: Infection caused by *Neisseria gonorrhoeae*, a gram-negative diplococcus that has a predilection for columnar and pseudostratified epithelieum of the genital tract. This infection involves primarily the endocervical canal and transformation zone of the cervix. In 80% of infected women, the urethra is also infected. Approximately 15 to 20% of women with gonorrhea will develop pelvic inflammatory disease (PID) (discussed in Chapter 28). In women who have undergone a hysterectomy, the urethra is the primary site of infection. Skene's glands or the paraurethral glands and Bartholin's glands can also become infected. In pediatric and postmenopausal patients, gonorrhea can also cause vaginitis. Gonorrhea in pregnant women has been associated with a higher risk of spontaneous abortion, premature rupture of membranes, chorioamnionitis, and preterm delivery. Nongenital gonorrheal infections in women include pharyngeal infection and disseminated gonorrhea.

The incubation period of gonorrhea is 3 to 5 days, and transmission is primarily by sexual contact. Women are more vulnerable to infection than men. The risk of transmission from an infected male to a female after a single sexual contact is 80 to 90%, whereas the risk of transmission from an infected female to a male is 20 to 25%. Forty to 60% of women with gonorrhea are asymptomatic. Nearly 50% of gonorrhea isolates are resistant to penicillin, tetracycline, and spectinomycin.

Disseminated gonorrhea: Has two stages, (1) an initial bacteremic stage manifested by systemic symptoms and skin lesions from gonococcal emboli, and (2) a later, arthritis stage usually involving the knees, ankles, or wrist joints.

Chlamydial infections: The most prevalent sexually transmitted infection in the United States, caused by *Chlamydia trachomatis*, an obligatory intracellular bacterium. The prevalence of this infection is 3% in asymptomatic women to as high as 33% in women who present to sexually transmitted disease clinics. There have been 15 serotypes of *Chlamydia trachomatis* identified. Serotypes D, E, F, G, H, I, J, and K are responsible for urethritis, cervicitis, infection of Bartholin's gland, endometritis, PID, perihepatitis, and perinatal infections; and serotypes L1, L2, and L3 are responsible for lymphogranuloma venereum (discussed in Chapter 35).

The incubation period is 6 to 14 days. As is the case with gonorrhea, many women are asymptomatic. Approximately 40 to 60% of women with gonorrhea have concomitant chlamydial infection.

■ CLINICAL PRESENTATION

The clinical presentations of gonorrhea and chlamydial infections are similar:
Mucopurulent cervical and vaginal discharge
Dysuria
Abnormal vaginal bleeding
Erythema of the cervix
Cervical friability
Pelvic discomfort
Pharyngitis
Symptoms associated with PID:
     Abdominal pain
     Pelvic pain
     Fever and chills
     Perihepatitis or Fitz-Hugh–Curtis syndrome
     Nausea
     Vomiting
     Anorexia

Clinical presentation associated with disseminated gonococcal infection:
Fever and chills
Skin lesions characterized by erythematous macules that become pustules with hemorrhagic base and necrotic center, most commonly found on the fingers and palm of the hand
Tenosynovitis
Polyarthralgias
Hepatitis
Myocarditis
Pericarditis
Meningitis

■ PHONE CALL

Questions

What are the patient's vital signs?

What symptoms does the patient have?
The presence of fever and severe pain is suggestive of PID, tubo-ovarian abscess (TOA), or disseminated gonorrhea.

Orders

1. Obtain a complete blood count (CBC) with differential
2. Obtain erythrocyte sedimentation rate (ESR)
3. Start IV in the severely ill patient
4. Insert urethral Foley catheter in the severely ill patient
5. Record intake and output in the severely ill patient
6. Obtain urine pregnancy test if the patient has missed a menstrual period or is unsure of her last menses

Degree of Urgency

Most cases of sexually transmitted disease caused by *Neisseria gonorrhoeae* and *Chlamydia trachomatis* are uncomplicated and are not life threatening. However, the severely ill patient should be seen immediately because of the possibility of ruptured TOA or disseminated gonorrhea.

■ ELEVATOR THOUGHTS

What are the risk factors for gonorrhea and chlamydial infections?
- Young age; highest incidence in women aged 20 to 24 years
- Lower socioeconomic class
- Young age at time of first intercourse
- Multiple sexual partners
- Partner with multiple sexual partners
- Failure to use barrier-method contraception

■ MAJOR THREAT TO LIFE

- Ruptured TOA
- Gonococcal meningitis
- Gonococcal endocarditis

Gonorrhea and chlamydial infections are rarely life threatening. However, overwhelming sepsis from a ruptured TOA and certain complications of disseminated gonorrhea can be fatal.

■ BEDSIDE

Quick Look Test

Does the patient appear severely ill?
PID, TOA, or disseminated gonorrhea should be suspected in patients who appear to be extremely ill.

Vital Signs

Vital signs are usually normal in a patient with uncomplicated gonorrhea or chlamydial infection. The finding of a fever suggests PID or disseminated gonorrhea. Hypotension with a systolic blood pressure of <60 mm Hg and tachycardia are usually found in the patient with a ruptured TOA.

Selective History and Chart Review

1. How long has the patient had symptoms of a sexually transmitted infection?
2. What risk factors does the patient have for gonorrhea or chlamydial infection?
3. Has the patient had a prior gonococcal or chlamydial infection?
4. Is the patient sexually active, and if so, what does she use for contraception?
5. Does the patient's sexual partner have any symptoms suggestive of a sexually transmitted infection?
6. When was the patient's last menstrual period?

Selective Physical Examination

Dermatological	Erythematous macules with a diameter of 1 to 5 mm that become pustules with a hemorrhagic base and a necrotic center, most commonly found on the fingers and palm of the hand in a patient with disseminated gonorrhea
Abdominal	Tender to palpation, sometimes with guarding and rebound tenderness in PID
	Rigid and board-like with ruptured TOA
Pelvic	
External genitalia and vagina	Mucopurulent discharge
Cervix	Mucopurulent discharge through the cervical os
	Tender to cervical motion
	Erythematous
	Friable and bleeding
Uterus and adnexae	Adnexal tenderness in PID
	Adnexal mass if TOA is present
Extremities	Tenosynovitis and arthritis, most commonly involving the knees in patients with disseminated gonorrhea

■ DIAGNOSTIC TESTING

Diagnostic tests for uncomplicated gonorrhea and chlamydial infections are listed below. Diagnostic tests for patients suspected of having PID or TOAs are discussed in Chapter 28.

1. **Gonorrhea**
   a. **Endocervical culture**
      An endocervical culture using selective media containing antibiotics has a sensitivity of 80 to 90% from a single culture.
   b. **Gram stain**
      A Gram stain showing gram-negative intracellular diplococci has a sensitivity of 50 to 70% and a specificity of 97%. A Gram stain can also be performed on joint effusion in patients with disseminated gonorrhea.
   c. **Blood culture**
      A blood culture is positive in approximately 25% of patients with disseminated gonorrhea.
   d. **Aspiration and culture of joint effusion**
      A culture of joint effusion is positive in 20 to 30% of patients with disseminated gonorrhea.
2. **Chlamydial infection**
   a. **Endocervical culture**
      A specimen of as many cervical epithelial cells as possible should be obtained to optimize the sensitivity of the culture. A rayon- or cotton-tipped applicator with either a plastic or a metal shaft should be used.
   b. **Enzyme-linked immunosorbent assay**
      Enzyme-linked immunosorbent assays (ELISAs) such as Chlamydiazyme have a sensitivity of 90% and a specificity of 97%.
   c. **Fluorescence-labeled monoclonal antibody testing**
      Detection tests, such as MicroTrak, that use monoclonal antibodies have a sensitivity of 89% and a specificity of 98%.

■ **MANAGEMENT**

1. **Uncomplicated gonorrhea in nonpregnant patients**
   Administer one of the following antibiotics:
   Ceftriaxone 250 mg IM once or
   Cefixime 400 mg PO once or
   Ciprofloxacin 500 mg PO once or
   Ofloxacin 400 mg PO once or
   Spectinomycin 2 g IM once
   Because of the high frequency of a coexistent chlamydial infection, also administer
   Doxycycline 100 mg PO two times per day for 7 days
2. **Uncomplicated gonorrhea in pregnant patients**
   Administer one of the following antibiotics:
   Ceftriaxone 250 mg IM once or
   Cefixime 400 mg PO once or
   Spectinomycin 2 g IM once

Because of the high frequency of a coexistent chlamydial infection, also administer

> **Erythromycin base 500 mg PO four times per day for 7 days**

3. **Gonococcal bacteremia and arthritis**
   a. **Single-agent therapy**
      Ceftriaxone 1 g IV daily for 7 to 10 days
   b. **Double-agent therapy**
      Administer one of the following antibiotics:
      Ceftriaxone 1 g IV daily for 2 to 3 days or
      Ceftizoxime 1 g IV every 8 hours for 2 to 3 days or until improved or
      Cefotaxime 1 g IV every 8 hours for 2 to 3 days or until improved
      Also administer the following:
      Cefixime 400 mg PO two times per day to complete 7 to 10 days of total therapy or
      Ciprofloxacin 500 mg PO two times per day to complete 7 to 10 days of total therapy

4. **Gonococcal meningitis**
   Ceftriaxone 2 g IV daily for at least 10 days or
   Penicillin G at least 10 million units IV daily for at least 10 days or
   Chloramphenicol 4 to 6 g IV daily for at least 10 days or

5. **Gonococcal endocarditis**
   Ceftriaxone 2 g IV daily for at least 3 to 4 weeks or
   Penicillin G at least 10 million units IV daily for at least 3 to 4 weeks

6. *Chlamydia trachomatis* **in nonpregnant patients**
   Azithromycin 1 g PO once or
   Doxycycline 100 mg PO two times per day for 7 days or
   Erythromycin 500 mg PO four times per day for 7 days or
   Ofloxacin 300 mg PO two times per day for 7 days or

7. *Chlamydia trachomatis* **in pregnant patients**
   Erythromycin 500 mg PO four times per day for 7 days or
   Amoxicillin 500 mg PO three times per day for 10 days or
   Sulfisoxazole 500 mg PO four times per day for 10 days

8. **Lymphogranuloma venereum** (see Chapter 34)
   Doxycycline 100 mg PO two times per day for 21 days or
   Erythromycin 500 mg PO four times per day for 21 days

27

MOLAR PREGNANCY

■ BACKGROUND AND DEFINITIONS

Gestational trophoblastic neoplasia (GTN): A spectrum of diseases that result from the abnormal proliferation of trophoblastic tissue associated with pregnancy. GTN includes diseases ranging from benign hydatidiform mole to malignant choriocarcinoma (Table 27–1). All forms of GTN are associated with abnormally high serum levels of human chorionic gonadotropin (hCG).

Hydatidiform mole: The benign and most common form of GTN. Approximately 85 to 90% of all GTNs are hydatidiform moles, also referred to as molar pregnancies. The incidence of molar pregnancies ranges from 1 in 1500 to 1 in 2000 pregnancies among white women in the United States, to 1 in 800 among Asian women in the United States, to 1 in 85 to 200 among Asian women in Asia. Molar pregnancies appear grossly as multiple vesicles that have the appearance of a bunch of grapes. Hydatidiform moles do not metastasize, but embolization or deportation of vesicles can occur, most commonly to the lungs.

Complete moles: Make up the majority (60 to 75%) of molar pregnancies and have a 46 XX karyotype. In complete moles, there is an absence of fetal tissue, except in the rare instance of a twin pregnancy in which one of the twin gestations is a molar pregnancy.

Partial moles or incomplete moles: Make up 25 to 40% of molar pregnancies and are distinguished by the coexistence of a pregnancy confirmed by the presence of normal villi or products of conception. When a fetus is present, fetal demise usually occurs. Most partial moles have a triploid karyotype, usually 69 XXY; the next most common karyotype is trisomy, most commonly trisomy 16. After treatment by surgical evacuation, both complete and partial moles can result in persis-

Table 27–1 □ CLASSIFICATION OF GESTATIONAL TROPHOBLASTIC NEOPLASIA

Benign disease
   Hydatidiform mole
      Complete mole
      Partial mole or incomplete mole
Malignant disease (may be metastatic or nonmetastatic)
   Invasive mole or chorioadenoma destruens
   Choriocarcinoma

tent GTN in the form of invasive mole or choriocarcinoma. The risk of persistent GTN is 15 to 20% with complete moles and decreases to 5 to 7% with partial moles.

Invasive moles or **chorioadenoma destruens:** A form of GTN that is locally invasive into the myometrium of the uterus. Approximately 5 to 10% of all GTNs are invasive moles. Invasive moles can cause rupture of the uterus and hemorrhaging by penetrating through the entire thickness of the myometrium. The diagnosis of invasive mole is usually made by pathological evaluation of the uterus after hysterectomy is performed for continued bleeding or persistently elevated serum hCG. Metastasis to the vagina and the lungs can occur.

Choriocarcinoma: The malignant form of GTN. Approximately 3 to 5% of all GTNs are choriocarcinomas. Of all patients who develop choriocarcinoma, 50% have had a preceding molar pregnancy, 15% have had a preceding term pregnancy, and 25% have had a preceding spontaneous abortion, therapeutic abortion, or ectopic pregnancy. Choriocarcinoma progresses rapidly and metastasizes hematogenously to the brain, lungs, liver, kidneys, gastrointestinal tract, and lower genital tract (Table 27–2).

■ CLINICAL PRESENTATION

- Complete hydatidiform mole

  Vaginal bleeding, initially painless, in the first or early second trimester of pregnancy

  Uterine contractions

  Passage of vesicles

  Excessive nausea or hyperemesis gravidarum

  Pelvic pain from theca-lutein cysts

  Symptoms of preeclampsia before 24 weeks of gestational age in 5 to 10% of patients:

  Hypertension

  Edema

  Proteinuria

  Central nervous system (CNS) symptoms: headache, mental confusion, dizziness, drowsiness

Table 27–2 □ **SITES AND FREQUENCY OF METASTATIC CHORIOCARCINOMA**

Site	Frequency (%)
Lungs	60–90
Vagina	40–50
Vulva or cervix	10–15
Brain	5–15
Liver	5–15

Visual symptoms: blurred vision, scotomata, flashes of light, diplopia, blindness

Gastrointestinal symptoms: epigastric pain, vomiting, hematemesis

Renal symptoms: anuria, oliguria, hematuria

Symptoms of hyperthyroidism in 2 to 7% of patients:

Nervousness

Tremulousness

Anorexia

Uterus large for dates in 50% of patients

Absence of fetal heart tones or palpable fetal parts

Dyspnea in patients with pulmonary embolization of vesicles

- Partial hydatidiform mole

Same as the presentation for complete mole except:

Uterus large for dates in only 11% of patients

Uterus small for dates in 66% of patients

Fetal heart tones and fetal parts may be present

Symptoms usually present later than with complete moles, often in the late first trimester and in the second trimester

- Invasive mole or chorioadenoma destruens

Hemorrhage

Sudden onset of heavy vaginal or intra-abdominal bleeding may result from penetration through the myometrium and rupture of the uterus

Symptoms of metastasis:

Vaginal bleeding from vaginal metastasis

CNS symptoms from brain metastasis

- Choriocarcinoma

Most patients with choriocarcinoma have symptoms of metastasis:

Vaginal bleeding from vaginal metastasis

Symptoms of lung metastasis:

Hemoptysis

Cough

Dyspnea

Symptoms of brain metastasis:

Headaches

Dizziness

Syncopal episodes

■ PHONE CALL

Questions

1. **Is the patient bleeding, and if so, how heavily?**
2. **What are the patient's vital signs?**

3. **Does the patient appear to be short of breath or dyspneic?**

Orders

1. Keep patient (NPO) in preparation for surgical evacuation
2. Obtain a serum hCG
3. Obtain a complete blood count (CBC) with differential
4. Perform coagulation studies: platelet count, prothrombin time (PT), partial thromboplastin time (PTT)
5. Perform thyroid function tests: total thyroxine (T_4), triiodothyronine (T_3) resin uptake, and thyroid-stimulating hormone (TSH)
6. Type and crossmatch blood
7. Obtain chest x-ray, posteroanterior and lateral
8. Obtain an electrocardiogram (ECG)
9. Start IV
10. Record input and output

Degree of Urgency

Patients who have heavy vaginal bleeding or who are suspected of having intra-abdominal hemorrhage should be seen immediately. Patients with severe preeclampsia or hyperthyroidism also should be seen immediately.

■ ELEVATOR THOUGHTS

What is the differential diagnosis of molar pregnancy?
- Spontaneous abortion
- Ectopic pregnancy

What are risk factors for molar pregnancy?
- Young maternal age (<15 years)
- Advanced maternal age (>40 years)
- Prior molar pregnancy
- Prior spontaneous abortion
- Diet with vitamin A deficiency
- Asian ethnicity

■ MAJOR THREAT TO LIFE

- Hemorrhage
- Metastatic disease

- Complications of preeclampsia
  Disseminated intravascular coagulation (DIC)
  Eclampsia
  Stroke

■ BEDSIDE

Quick Look Test

Does the patient appear to be in hypovolemic shock?
Hypovolemic shock can result from blood loss due to either vaginal bleeding or intra-abdominal bleeding.

Does the patient appear to have any respiratory difficulties?
Dyspnea and hemoptysis are suggestive of either pulmonary metastasis or embolization of vesicles.

Does the patient appear to be hyperthyroid?
Hyperthyroidism is found in 2 to 7% of patients and results either from the high levels of hCG, which has thyroid-stimulating activities, or from an elevated level of T_4, which is found in 25 to 50% of patients.

Vital Signs

Hypotension and tachycardia can occur in a patient with significant blood loss. Postural hypotension may be present. Changes in blood pressure (BP) and pulse should be measured when the patient is assisted in sitting or standing from a supine position. A fall in systolic or diastolic BP of >15 mm Hg or a rise in pulse of >15 beats/min is evidence of hypovolemia. Tachycardia alone may result from hyperthyroidism.

Selective History and Chart Review

1. Has the patient had a normal pregnancy recently?
   GTN that develops after a normal pregnancy is almost always a choriocarcinoma and not a hydatidiform mole or an invasive mole.
2. Has the patient had an episode of syncope or lightheadedness?
3. When was the patient's last menstrual period?
4. Has the patient had a prior molar pregnancy?
5. Has the patient had a previous ultrasound examination demonstrating the presence of fetal parts or a viable fetus?
   This finding would be diagnostic of a partial mole. The

finding of a viable fetus is an indication for amniocentesis for karyotype determination of the fetus.

Selective Physical Examination

General	Tremulousness, diaphoresis, anxiety, and nervousness if the patient is hyperthyroid
Pulmonary	Wheezing and rhonchi may be present due to embolization of vesicles
Abdominal	Enlarged uterus
	Absence of fetal parts on palpation or fetal heart tones on auscultation unless there is a partial mole with a viable fetus
Pelvic	
External genitalia and vagina	Vaginal bleeding usually present
	Spontaneous passage of vesicles sometimes present
	Polypoid vaginal lesion may be present if there has been vaginal metastasis from choriocarcinoma
Cervix	Cervix may be dilated, with bleeding and protruding vesicles
Uterus	Uterus is large for dates in one-half of patients with complete moles but may be appropriate or even small for dates with partial moles
Adnexae	Bilateral ovarian theca-lutein cysts may be present

■ DIAGNOSTIC TESTING

1. **Ultrasound examination**

   Ultrasound examination is the diagnostic test of choice for hydatidiform moles. The finding of a "snowstorm" pattern in a gestation of more than 14 weeks is diagnostic of a hydatidiform mole. This ultrasound finding in a pregnancy of less than 14 weeks of gestation may also be consistent with a spontaneous abortion. Ultrasonography can detect bilateral theca-lutein cysts, which are found in nearly 25% of patients with hydatidiform moles and are caused by stimulation of the ovaries by elevated hCG levels. The concurrent finding of fetal parts or a viable fetus is diagnostic of a partial mole.

2. **Serum human chorionic gonadotropin**

   Serum hCG levels are elevated above the levels obtained in normal pregnancies (Table 27–3). A level above 100,000 mIU/ml is highly suggestive of a molar pregnancy.

Table 27–3 □ hCG LEVELS IN NORMAL PREGNANCIES

Gestational Age (weeks)	Serum hCG (mIU/ml)
4	100
6	1000–10,000
7	10,000–50,000
9	50,000–100,000
20	10,000–20,000

3. Thyroid function tests

In 25 to 50% of patients, T_4 is elevated above the normal levels found in pregnancy.

4. Chest x-ray

A chest x-ray may detect embolization of vesicles in patients with hydatidiform moles and lung metastasis in patients with either invasive mole or choriocarcinoma.

5. Electrocardiogram

An ECG may reveal cardiac rhythm abnormalities such as supraventricular tachycardia associated with hyperthyroidism.

■ MANAGEMENT

Management of patients with hydatidiform moles is threefold, as follows: (1) Treatment of medical complications such as preeclampsia and hyperthyroidism, (2) surgical evacuation of the uterus, and (3) posttreatment surveillance of hCG levels.

1. Treatment of medical complications

    a. Preeclampsia

        The definitive treatment for preeclampsia is evacuation of the uterus. Before this, management of preeclampsia includes prevention of eclamptic seizures by the administration of magnesium sulfate and treatment of severe hypertension.

        (1) Magnesium sulfate 2 to 4 g IV over 5 minutes as a loading dose, followed by 1.0 g/hr IV as the maintenance dose or

        (2) Magnesium sulfate 2 to 4 g IV over 2 to 4 minutes, concurrently with 10 g IM as the loading dose, followed by 5 g IM every 4 hours

        Side effects of magnesium sulfate include flushing and nausea. More serious complications resulting from magnesium toxicity include respiratory depression and cardiac arrest. If respiratory or cardiac arrest develops, the magnesium sulfate infusion should be discontinued and calcium gluconate should be administered as follows:

Calcium gluconate (10% solution): administer 10 ml (1 g) IV over 3 minutes

b. **Hyperthyroidism**

The treatment of hyperthyroidism consists of antithyroid drugs such as propylthiouracil or methimazole and a beta-adrenergic blocker such as propranolol.

(1) Antithyroid medication

(a) **Propylthiouracil (PTU) 100 to 150 mg PO every 8 hours** or

(b) **Methimazole (Tapazole) 20 to 30 mg PO every 12 hours**

(2) Beta-adrenergic blocker

(a) **Propranolol (Inderal) 10 to 40 mg two to three times per day**

2. **Surgical evacuation of the uterus**

a. **Suction dilatation and curettage**

Suction dilatation and curettage should be performed in an operating room with a 10- to 12-mm curette. Intravenous oxytocin should be administered after the procedure has begun. Severe blood loss may necessitate blood transfusion. After suction curettage, sharp curettage should be performed to ensure that all tissue has been evacuated. The major complications of the procedure are uterine perforation and hemorrhage. If the uterus is larger than 14 weeks' size, the use of ultrasound guidance should be considered to decrease the risk of uterine perforation. In patients with a partial mole and a dead fetus of more than 13 weeks' gestation, dilatation and evacuation may be required in addition to suction curettage.

b. **Hysterotomy**

Hysterotomy may be indicated if equipment or training for suction dilatation and curettage and/or dilatation and evacuation is lacking.

c. **Hysterectomy**

In certain patients who do not desire future fertility, abdominal hysterectomy may be considered.

3. **Posttreatment surveillance of hCG levels**

After surgical evacuation, patients should have serum hCG drawn weekly until the hCG level is negative for 3 consecutive weeks. Then serum hCG should be drawn monthly for 6 to 12 months. Figure 27–1 shows the normal regression curve for hCG after evacuation of a hydatidiform mole. During the period of surveillance, the patient must use contraception, preferably oral contraceptive pills. Otherwise, it will be impossible to distinguish between hCG from the new pregnancy and that

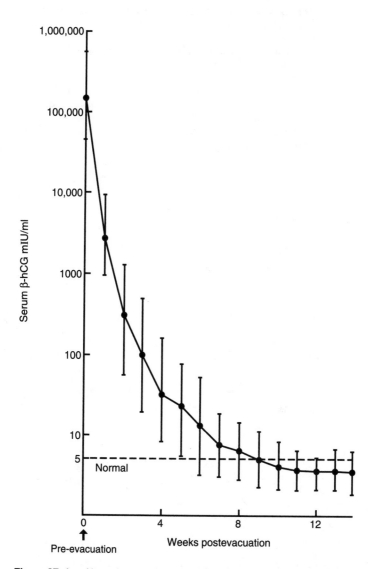

Figure 27–1 □ Normal regression curve of hCG following surgical evacuation of hydatidiform mole. (From Morrow CP, Kletzky OA, DiSaia PJ, et al: Clinical and laboratory correlates of molar pregnancy and trophoblastic disease. Am J Obstet Gynecol 1977;128:424.)

from persistent and possibly metastatic disease. Approximately 80 to 85% of patients will have spontaneous regression and achieve a negative hCG. Approximately 15 to 20% of patients will demonstrate a plateau or rise in hCG. In these patients, a new pregnancy must first be ruled out. Then, staging and a metastatic workup should be performed. Patients with no metastatic disease should be treated with single-agent chemotherapy with methotrexate. Patients with metastatic disease will require combination therapy. MAC therapy, which includes methotrexate, actinomycin D, and cyclophosphamide, is a commonly used regimen.

28

PELVIC INFLAMMATORY DISEASE

■ BACKGROUND AND DEFINITIONS

Pelvic inflammatory disease (PID): Nonspecific term that refers to inflammation of the upper genital tract, which includes the uterus, the fallopian tubes, and the ovaries. This is in contrast to inflammation of the lower genital tract, which includes the cervix, the vagina, and the vulva. The term pelvic inflammatory disease can be used to refer to inflammation of the fallopian tubes (**salpingitis**), ovaries (**oophoritis**), uterine myometrium (**myometritis**), endometrium (**endometritis**), or broad ligament (**parametritis**). However, pelvic inflammatory disease is most commonly used to refer to **salpingitis.**

Pyosalpinx: A collection of pus in the fallopian tube, often encountered in acute salpingitis

Hydrosalpinx: A collection of sterile fluid in the fallopian tube, an end stage of pyosalpinx

Tubo-ovarian abscess (TOA): An abscess complex involving the tubes, the ovaries, and often the intestines. In a TOA, inflammation involves the stroma of the ovary, often resulting in destruction of the ovary.

There has been a steady increase in both the incidence of PID and the number of hospital admissions for PID. It is estimated that more than 1 million women are treated for PID each year in the United States. PID almost always results from infection ascending from the lower genital tract. It is usually a polymicrobial infection caused by *Neisseria gonorrhoeae, Chlamydia trachomatis, Escherichia coli, Peptococcus* spp., *Peptostreptococcus* spp., *Bacteroides fragilis,* other *Bacteroides* species, and less commonly *Mycoplasma hominis* and *Ureaplasma urealyticum.*

The most serious immediate complication resulting from PID is formation of a TOA. The incidence of TOA formation in patients with PID is approximately 15%. The presence of a TOA may require surgical intervention if the abscess does not respond to antibiotic therapy or if the abscess ruptures. Rupture of a TOA constitutes a life-threatening emergency and has a mortality rate of 5 to 10%. The major long-term sequelae resulting from PID include chronic pelvic and abdominal pain, infertility, tubal pregnancy, and recurrent PID. The incidence of chronic pelvic and abdominal pain after PID is approximately 20%. The incidence of tubal factor infertility is close to 12% after one episode of PID, increases to 25% after two episodes, and is approximately 50 to 60% after three episodes of PID. There is an increase of four- to eightfold in the risk of tubal pregnancy among patients with a history of PID. Approximately 50% of tubal pregnancies occur in tubes previously damaged by salpingitis. Recurrent PID is encountered in 15 to 25% of women with a history of PID.

■ CLINICAL PRESENTATION

Abdominal pain
Pelvic pain
Vaginal discharge
Abnormal vaginal bleeding
Fever
Chills
Nausea
Vomiting
Anorexia
Urinary symptoms

The frequencies of the above symptoms of PID are listed in Table 28–1.

■ PHONE CALL

Questions

1. **What are the patient's vital signs?**
2. **Does the patient appear to be in shock?**
   The most serious complication resulting from PID is rupture of a TOA. These patients appear severely ill and can present in septic shock.

Orders

1. Obtain a complete blood count (CBC) with differential
2. Obtain erythrocyte sedimentation rate

Table 28–1 □ FREQUENCIES OF SYMPTOMS FOUND IN PATIENTS WITH PID

Symptom	Frequency (%)
Lower abdominal or pelvic pain	99
Vaginal discharge	70
Irregular vaginal bleeding	40
Fever or chills	35
Urinary symptoms	20
Nausea or vomiting	10
Anorexia	10

3. Start IV in the severely ill patient
4. Insert a urethral Foley catheter in the severely ill patient
5. Record intake and output in the severely ill patient
6. Perform a urine pregnancy test if the patient has missed a menstrual period or is unsure of when her last menses began

Degree of Urgency

PID is usually not life threatening unless it is complicated by ruptured TOA. The patient suspected of having this complication should be seen immediately.

■ ELEVATOR THOUGHTS

What are the risk factors for PID?
- Younger age, <25 years
  Approximately 75% of all PID cases occur in women younger than 25 years old.
- Young age at first intercourse
- Multiple sexual partners
  The risk of PID is increased fivefold in patients with multiple sexual partners.
- Partner with multiple sexual partners
- Single marital status
- Frequent intercourse with multiple partners
  The risk of PID is not increased with frequent intercourse with a single monogamous partner.
- Use of an intrauterine device (IUD)
  Women who have an IUD have a two- to threefold increase in the risk of PID, especially in the first 3 months after IUD insertion.
- Transcervical instrumentation
  Any procedure that requires penetration of the cervical mucus barrier increases the risk of PID. Common procedures are dilatation and curettage, pregnancy termination, hysterosalpingogram, and IUD insertion. The incidence of PID after first-trimester pregnancy termination is approximately 1 in 200 cases.

What is the differential diagnosis of PID?
- Cervicitis
- Tubal pregnancy
- Adnexal mass with rupture or torsion
- Endometriosis
- Appendicitis
- Diverticulitis

■ MAJOR THREAT TO LIFE

- Sepsis from ruptured TOA
  This complication has a mortality rate of 5 to 10%.

■ BEDSIDE

Quick Look Test

How ill does the patient appear?
  A patient who appears severely ill, with signs and symptoms of septic shock, should be suspected of having a ruptured TOA.

Vital Signs

Approximately 35% of patients with PID will present with a fever. Hypotension with systolic blood pressure of <60 mm Hg and tachycardia is usually found in patients with sepsis from a ruptured TOA.

Selective History and Chart Review

1. What risk factors does the patient have for PID?
2. Has the patient had prior episodes of PID?
3. How long has the patient had symptoms of PID?
4. Is the patient sexually active, and if so, what does she use for contraception?
5. Does the patient's sexual partner have symptoms of a sexually transmitted disease?
6. When was the patient's last menstrual period?

Selective Physical Examination

Abdominal	Tenderness to palpation
	Guarding
	Rebound tenderness
	Rigid and board-like with ruptured TOA
Pelvic	
External genitalia and vagina	Purulent vaginal discharge
Cervix	Tender to cervical motion
	Purulent discharge through the cervical os
Uterus and adnexae	Adnexal tenderness
	Adnexal mass or fullness if TOA or hydrosalpinx is present

■ DIAGNOSTIC TESTING

1. **Laparoscopy**

   Laparoscopy is the most accurate diagnostic procedure for PID. In patients with uncomplicated PID, the fallopian tubes will appear erythematous, indurated, and edematous. An exudate is usually seen on the tubal surface or at the fimbriated end of the tube. A pyosalpinx or hydrosalpinx may be observed. Laparoscopy will also confirm or rule out the presence of a TOA. Furthermore, laparoscopy will help in ruling out an adnexal mass and appendicitis, both of which are part of the differential diagnosis for PID. In practice, PID is usually diagnosed based on clinical presentation, with confirmation of the diagnosis by less invasive tests. Laparoscopy is usually reserved for the patient who has an unclear diagnosis or who fails to respond to antibiotic therapy.

2. **Ultrasound examination**

   Ultrasound examination is crucial in detecting a TOA. Furthermore, ultrasonography will also detect a pyosalpinx and hydrosalpinx, although it cannot distinguish between the two. Therefore, ultrasound examination is often helpful when pelvic examination reveals an adnexal mass or when a patient has too much tenderness to permit an adequate pelvic examination.

3. **Laboratory tests**

   The following laboratory tests can be helpful in confirming the diagnosis of PID, but all of these tests are nonspecific:

   a. **Vaginal wet smear with normal saline**

      Microscopic examination of a wet smear of vaginal discharge will reveal the presence of multiple white blood cells.

   b. **Gram stain of cervical discharge**

      The finding of >30 white blood cells per high-power field is highly suggestive of cervicitis. Furthermore, the presence of gram-negative intracellular diplococci is suggestive of *Neisseria gonorrhoeae* infection. However, Gram stain has only a 50 to 60% sensitivity for *Neisseria gonorrhoeae* infection.

   c. **White blood cell count**

      Leukocytosis is defined by a white blood cell count of >10,000 cells/mm^3. Fewer than 50% of patients with PID have leukocytosis.

   d. **Erythrocyte sedimentation rate**

      An elevated sedimentation rate of >20 mm/hr is found in nearly 75% of patients with PID.

   e. **C-reactive protein**

      An elevated C-reactive protein of >2 mg/dl, like the white blood cell count and sedimentation rate, is a nonspecific indicator of infection and is only slightly more sensitive than the sedimentation rate.

f. **Testing for *Neisseria gonorrhoeae* and *Chlamydia trachomatis***

Cervical culture is the best test for detecting *Neisseria gonorrhoeae,* and rapid antigen detection tests such as Chlamydiazyme or MicroTrak are the most readily available tests for *Chlamydia trachomatis.* Positive testing may be helpful in supporting the diagnosis of PID. However, cervical cultures are diagnostic only for cervicitis.

g. **Culdocentesis**

Although it is nonspecific, culdocentesis can help to confirm the diagnosis of PID if purulent peritoneal fluid is obtained. In patients with PID, the white blood cell count of peritoneal fluid is usually >30,000 cells/mm^3.

h. **Endometrial biopsy**

An endometrial biopsy will allow for the pathological diagnosis of endometritis. However, this test is not able to distinguish between endometritis alone and endometritis with salpingitis.

4. **Clinical criteria for the diagnosis of PID**

Because of the nonspecific nature of diagnostic tests other than laparoscopy, the following clinical criteria for the diagnosis of PID should be used:

Patients must have all three of the following:

a. **Abdominal tenderness**
b. **Cervical motion tenderness**
c. **Adnexal tenderness**

plus one or more of the following:

d. **A positive Gram stain for gram-negative intracellular diplococci**
e. **A fever (>38°C or 100.4°F)**
f. **An elevated white blood cell count (>10,000 cells/mm^3)**
g. **Purulent fluid obtained from the peritoneal cavity by culdocentesis or laparoscopy**
h. **A pelvic abscess detected by either pelvic examination or ultrasonography**

■ MANAGEMENT OF PELVIC INFLAMMATORY DISEASE

PID can be treated with antibiotics on either an inpatient or an outpatient basis. Early and aggressive treatment can decrease the incidence of long-term sequelae such as infertility (Table 28–2).

1. **Indications for hospitalization and treatment with parenteral antibiotics include the following:**
   a. Failure of outpatient therapy
   b. Nulliparity, especially in a young patient
   c. Pregnancy

Table 28–2 □ INCIDENCE OF LONG-TERM SEQUELAE OF PID

Sequelae	Incidence (%)
Chronic pelvic pain	20
Infertility	
One episode of PID	12
Two episodes of PID	25
Three episodes of PID	50–60
Tubal pregnancy	6–13
Recurrent PID	15–25

   d. Presence of TOA
   e. Presence of gastrointestinal symptoms
   f. Peritonitis in the upper abdominal quadrants
   g. Presence of IUD
   h. Inability to rule out surgical emergencies such as appendicitis and ectopic pregnancy
   i. Patient is severely ill
   j. Patient is unreliable, and noncompliance with outpatient therapy and follow-up is suspected
   k. Patient intolerance of outpatient therapy
   l. Unclear diagnosis
2. **Inpatient treatment regimen for uncomplicated PID**
   Cefoxitin 2 g IV every 6 hours or Cefotetan 2 g IV every 12 hours plus
   Doxycycline 100 mg IV or PO every 12 hours
   An alternative inpatient regimen is:
   Clindamycin 900 mg IV every 8 hours plus
   Gentamicin 2 mg/kg IV loading dose followed by 1.5 mg/ kg IV every 8 hours
   Either of the above regimens is continued for at least 48 hours after there has been clinical improvement. After discharge, the patient is placed on the following:
   Doxycycline 100 mg PO two times per day for 10 to 14 days or
   Clindamycin 450 mg PO four times per day for 10 to 14 days
3. **Outpatient treatment regimen for uncomplicated PID**
   Cefoxitin 2 g IM with probenecid 1 g PO or Ceftriaxone 250 mg IM plus
   Doxycycline 100 mg PO two times per day for 10 to 14 days or
   Tetracycline 500 mg PO four times per day for 10 to 14 days or
   Erythromycin 500 mg PO four times per day for 10 to 14 days
4. **Alternative outpatient regimen**

Ofloxacin 400 mg PO two times per day for 14 days plus
Clindamycin 450 mg PO four times per day for 14 days or
Metronidazole 500 mg PO two times per day for 14 days

■ MANAGEMENT OF PELVIC INFLAMMATORY DISEASE WITH TUBO-OVARIAN ABSCESS

Initial management of a patient with a TOA is the administration of IV antibiotics including an agent that provides anaerobic coverage such as clindamycin or metronidazole. Patients with an abscess larger than 8 cm in diameter have a higher incidence of treatment failure. Patients in whom antibiotic therapy fails will require either drainage or surgical excision.

1. **Antibiotic therapy**
   a. **Inpatient antibiotic regimen**
      Clindamycin 900 mg IV every 8 hours plus
      Gentamicin 2 mg/kg IV loading dose followed by 1.5 mg/kg IV every 8 hours
   b. **Alternative inpatient antibiotic regimen**
      Metronidazole 15 mg/kg IV loading dose over 1 hour followed by 7.5 mg/kg IV every 6 hours plus
      Gentamicin 2 mg/kg IV loading dose followed by 1.5 mg/kg IV every 8 hours

   Either of the above regimens is continued for at least 48 hours after there has been clinical improvement. After discharge, the patient is treated as follows:

   c. **Postdischarge antibiotic regimen**
      Doxycycline 100 mg PO two times per day for 10 to 14 days or
      Clindamycin 450 mg PO four times per day for 10 to 14 days

2. **Drainage of abscess**
   If there is no clinical improvement after 72 hours of IV antibiotics, surgical drainage should be considered.
   a. **Posterior colpotomy**
      Transvaginal drainage of a TOA can be considered if the abscess fulfills the following three requirements:
      (1) Abscess is midline
      (2) Abscess should dissect the rectovaginal septum and be adherent to the cul-de-sac peritoneum
      (3) Abscess must be fluctuant and cystic
   b. **Radiographically guided drainage**
      Fluoroscopically guided drainage can be performed by interventional radiologists. An indwelling catheter can be left in the abscess cavity for irrigation and continued drainage.

3. **Surgical excision**

   In patients in whom antibiotic therapy and attempts at drainage fail or who have a rupture of a TOA, laparotomy is indicated with excision of the abscess.

   a. **Unilateral salpingo-oophorectomy**

   If preservation of fertility is desired, conservative surgery with unilateral salpingo-oophorectomy is indicated.

   b. **Total abdominal hysterectomy with bilateral salpingo-oophorectomy**

   If preservation of fertility is not desired or if the severity of the infection makes conservative surgery ill-advised, total hysterectomy and bilateral salpingo-oophorectomy should be performed. In a patient with a ruptured TOA, the case should be considered contaminated and the surgical incision should be left open.

29

PELVIC MASS

■ BACKGROUND AND DEFINITIONS

The adnexae comprise the fallopian tubes, ovaries, and round ligaments. Pelvic masses commonly arise from the adnexae and are referred to as **adnexal masses.** Pelvic masses can also arise from the uterus as well as from organs other than the reproductive organs such as the bladder and the gastrointestinal tract. The differential diagnosis of an adnexa mass is vast and depends on the patient's age. Adnexal masses are uncommon in the premenarchal and postmenopausal patient, and when they are encountered, malignancy should be suspected. In contrast, adnexal masses are commonly found in women in the reproductive age range because of the frequency of **functional** or **physiological cysts.** These cysts result from the process of ovulation and usually resolve spontaneously. A large variety of nonneoplastic and neoplastic ovarian masses, both benign and malignant, are found in women of all age groups. The most common pelvic masses not involving the adnexa are **leiomyomata,** or **fibroids.** Leiomyomata are benign tumors that originate from smooth muscle cells in the myometrium of the uterus. Approximately 10 to 25% of white women and 30 to 50% of black women have leiomyomata.

■ CLINICAL PRESENTATION

Pelvic pain
Abdominal pain
Abdominal distention
Dyspareunia
Vaginal bleeding
Urinary frequency
Gastrointestinal symptoms
    Nausea
    Dyspepsia
    Obstipation
    Painful bowel movements

■ PHONE CALL

Questions

1. How much pain is the patient experiencing?
In patients with severe pain, torsion of an adnexal mass,

tubal pregnancy, hemorrhagic ovarian cyst, and tubo-ovarian abscess should be suspected.
2. **What are the vital signs, and is the patient unstable?**
    A ruptured tubo-ovarian abscess or a ruptured tubal pregnancy with intra-abdominal bleeding should be suspected in the patient who is unstable and has a pelvic mass.

Orders

1. Obtain a complete blood count (CBC) with differential
2. Perform a urine pregnancy test for patients of reproductive age
3. Start IV in the patient who appears severely ill
4. Have the patient keep her bladder full for ultrasound examination
5. Keep the patient NPO (nothing by mouth) if surgery is anticipated

Degree of Urgency

In most cases, a pelvic mass is not life threatening. If the patient is in severe pain, has a positive pregnancy test, or is unstable, she should be seen immediately.

■ ELEVATOR THOUGHTS

What is the differential diagnosis of the pelvic mass?
    Table 29–1 lists the differential diagnosis of the pelvic mass.
1. **Ovarian masses**
    a. **Functional or physiological cysts**
        (1) Follicular cysts
            Follicular cysts are the most common cystic masses found in the ovary. They result from either failure of the mature follicle to ovulate or failure of an immature follicle to resorb or undergo atresia. Most follicular cysts are asymptomatic and range in size from several millimeters to 8 cm in diameter.
        (2) Corpus luteum cysts
            Corpus luteum cysts are approximately 4 cm in diameter and result from hemorrhage into the corpus luteum 2 to 3 days after ovulation. Because these cysts may rupture and result in intra-abdominal bleeding, they can mimic tubal pregnancies. Rupture usually occurs late in the menstrual cycle and is associated with acute pain, which usually lasts less than 24 hours but may be present for up to 1 week.
        (3) Theca-lutein cysts
            Theca-lutein cysts develop from overstimulation of

Table 29–1 □ **DIFFERENTIAL DIAGNOSIS OF THE PELVIC MASS**

	Ultrasound Characteristics	
Source	**Cystic**	**Solid or Complex**
Ovaries	Functional cyst Endometrioma Neoplasm 　Benign 　Malignant	Neoplasm 　Benign 　Malignant
Fallopian tubes	Hydrosalpinx Tubo-ovarian abscess Pyosalpinx Paratubal cyst	Neoplasm Tubo-ovarian abscess Tubal pregnancy
Uterus		Intrauterine pregnancy Uterine anomaly Leiomyoma Adenomyosis Sarcoma
Bowel	Ileus	Appendiceal abscess Diverticular abscess Neoplasm Stool
Bladder and kidneys	Distended bladder	Pelvic kidney

the ovaries by human chorionic gonadotropin (hCG). They are encountered in patients with molar pregnancies and in those who had undergone ovulation induction for infertility.
  b. **Endometriomas**
     Endometriomas can develop in patients with endometriosis involving the ovaries. These cysts are filled with old blood that has the appearance of chocolate, and therefore, endometriomas are also called "chocolate cysts."
  c. **Ovarian neoplasms** (Table 29–2)
     (1) Benign neoplasms
     (2) Malignant neoplasms
2. **Tubal masses**
  a. **Tubal pregnancy**
  b. **Pyosalpinx**
  c. **Hydrosalpinx**
  d. **Tubo-ovarian abscess**
  e. **Paratubal cyst**
     Paratubal cysts are found adjacent to the fallopian tubes. They are predominantly cystic and are asymptomatic unless they undergo torsion. Paratubal cysts found at the fimbriated ends of the tube are also referred to as hydatid cysts of Morgagni.

Table 29–2 □ HISTOGENETIC CLASSIFICATION OF OVARIAN NEOPLASMS

Origin	Frequency	Tumor Types
Celomic epithelium	75–80%	Serous tumor Mucinous tumor Endometrioid tumor Clear cell or mesonephroid tumor Brenner tumor Carcinosarcoma or mixed mesodermal tumor Undifferentiated carcinoma
Germ cell	10–15%	Teratoma 　Mature teratoma 　　Solid adult teratoma 　　Dermoid cyst 　　Struma ovarii 　　Malignant neoplasm arising from mature cystic teratoma 　Immature teratoma Dysgerminoma Embryonal carcinoma Endodermal sinus tumor Choriocarcinoma Gonadoblastoma
Specialized gonadal stroma	3–5%	Granulosa–theca cell tumors 　Granulosa cell tumor 　Thecoma Sertoli-Leydig cell tumors 　Arrhenoblastoma 　Sertoli cell tumor Gynandroblastoma Lipid cell tumor
Nonspecific mesenchyme	≤1%	Fibroma Hemangioma Leiomyoma Lipoma Lymphoma Sarcoma
Metastatic to ovary	4–8%	Gastrointestinal tract (Krukenberg's tumor) Breast Uterine endometrium Lymphoma

3. **Uterine masses**
   a. **Leiomyomata**
   b. **Intrauterine pregnancy**
   c. **Adenomyosis of the uterus**
   d. **Uterine sarcoma**
   e. **Congenital anomaly of the uterus**
      (1) Bicornuate uterus
      (2) Rudimentary uterine horn
      (3) Didelphic uterus
4. **Masses from the gastrointestinal tract**
   a. **Appendiceal abscess**
   b. **Diverticular abscess**
   c. **Stool or gas in the sigmoid colon**
5. **Masses from the kidneys and the urinary tract**
   a. **Distended bladder**
   b. **Pelvic kidney**
6. **Miscellaneous masses**
   a. **Abdominal wall abscess, seroma, or hematoma**
   b. **Retroperitoneal neoplasm**

What are potential complications associated with an adnexal mass?

1. **Torsion**

   An adnexal mass that is freely mobile on a pedicle can undergo spontaneous torsion. Torsion can be intermittent, resulting in crampy colicky pain that is episodic. Torsion can also compromise the vascular supply and cause ischemic damage to the ovary or fallopian tube.

2. **Rupture of cyst**

   Rupture can result in resolution of the cyst. However, in certain cysts, rupture can lead to further complications such as intraperitoneal dissemination of disease with malignant ovarian cysts and chemical peritonitis with a dermoid cyst. Rupture of a tubo-ovarian abscess causes peritonitis and sepsis and is life threatening.

3. **Hemorrhage**

   Bleeding into a cyst will result in distention of the cyst and increased pain. Rupture of the cyst and intraperitoneal bleeding severe enough to lead to hypovolemic shock can result. This is most commonly found in a ruptured hemorrhagic corpus luteum cyst. Bleeding from an adnexal mass may also be caused by a ruptured tubal pregnancy, as discussed in Chapter 25.

■ MAJOR THREAT TO LIFE

- Hypovolemic shock from rupture and hemorrhage of an adnexal mass

- Sepsis secondary to ruptured tubo-ovarian abscess
- Sepsis secondary to ruptured abdominal abscess from appendicitis or diverticulitis
- Ovarian malignancy

■ BEDSIDE

Quick Look Test

Does the patient appear to be severely ill?

Rupture of a tubal pregnancy, a hemorrhagic cyst, or a tubo-ovarian abscess should be suspected in patients who appear to be severely ill with either severe pain or unstable vital signs.

Vital Signs

Vital signs are normal unless the patient is in shock from rupture of a tubal pregnancy, a hemorrhagic cyst, or a tubo-ovarian abscess. A patient in hypovolemic shock will be hypotensive and tachycardic and might have postural hypotension. Changes in blood pressure (BP) and pulse should be measured in the supine, sitting, and standing positions. A fall in systolic or diastolic BP of >15 mm Hg or a rise in pulse of >15 beats/min when the patient is assisted into the sitting or standing position from the supine position is evidence of hypovolemia.

Selective History and Chart Review

1. Does the patient have a history of a chronic pelvic mass?

   Chronic pelvic masses include leiomyomata, hydrosalpinges, and endometriomas.
2. Is the patient premenarchal or postmenopausal?

   Adnexal masses are more likely to be malignant in these patients, compared with women in the reproductive age group.
3. If the patient is of reproductive age, when was her last menstrual period?

   Women who have missed a menstrual period should have intrauterine and ectopic pregnancies ruled out.
4. Is the patient using oral contraceptive pills?

   Oral contraceptive pills suppress ovulation, and therefore, functional cysts are less likely although not totally precluded in pill users. Women who use contraceptive pills are also less likely to have either an intrauterine or ectopic pregnancy, although neither is totally excluded.
5. Does the patient have a history of pelvic inflammatory disease (PID)?

The patient with a history of PID and who has a pelvic mass should be suspected of having a pyosalpinx, a hydrosalpinx, or a tubo-ovarian abscess.

6. Does the patient have a history of pelvic endometriosis?

An endometrioma should be suspected in these patients.

7. Does the patient have a history of weight loss and vague abdominal symptoms such as anorexia, dyspepsia, distention, nausea, and dull pain or discomfort?

These symptoms can be caused by ovarian malignancy.

8. Does the patient have abnormal vaginal bleeding?

Abnormal bleeding in a patient with a pelvic mass is suggestive of intrauterine pregnancy, ectopic pregnancy, uterine leiomyoma, and uterine sarcoma.

Selective Physical Examination

Abdominal	Mass with or without tenderness may be palpable
	Distention from the mass or hemorrhage
	Ascites may be present in ovarian malignancy
Pelvic	
External genitalia and vagina	Vaginal bleeding in ectopic pregnancy, intrauterine pregnancy, uterine fibroids, or sarcoma
Cervix	Cervical motion tenderness may be present with PID or tubo-ovarian abscess
Uterus	Enlarged with or without tenderness in leiomyomata, sarcoma, or intrauterine pregnancy
Adnexae	Mass may be palpable, either unilateral or bilateral, with or without tenderness
	Fixed and nonmobile adnexa is suggestive of endometrioma, PID, or ovarian malignancy

■ DIAGNOSTIC TESTING

1. **Ultrasound examination**

Ultrasound examination will confirm the presence of a pelvic mass and furthermore will provide information concerning the size, bilaterality, origin, and consistency of the mass, whether cystic, solid, or complex. Ultrasonography is the method of choice in the radiological evaluation of an ovarian mass.

2. **Computed tomography**

A computed tomography (CT) scan can sometimes supplement the information obtained by ultrasound examination. CT scan of the pelvis should be performed with contrast to opacify and therefore delineate the bowel. A CT scan is especially helpful in the evaluation of masses in the pelvic side wall. A CT scan is also helpful in staging pelvic malignancies, detecting peritoneal implants, and delineating pelvic abscesses during drainage procedures.

3. **Magnetic resonance imaging**

    Magnetic resonance imaging (MRI) provides soft-tissue contrast resolution that is superior to that obtained by ultrasound examination or CT scan. It is especially helpful in the assessment of conditions that result in uterine enlargement such as congenital anomalies of the uterus, leiomyomata, and adenomyosis. MRI can provide information on the size, number, and location of leiomyomata.

4. **Intravenous pyelogram**

    An intravenous pyelogram (IVP) will provide information concerning the kidneys and the bladder. A pelvic kidney can be diagnosed by IVP. Furthermore, displacement of the pelvic ureters by a pelvic mass is usually found by IVP, and this information is critical in patients about to undergo surgery.

5. **Complete blood count with differential**

    A CBC with differential should be obtained to help with the diagnosis of masses associated with PID, such as a pyosalpinx or tubo-ovarian abscess. It can also detect anemia in those patients with intraperitoneal bleeding from any source.

6. **Rapid urine pregnancy test**

    A pregnancy test should be obtained in all patients of reproductive age to rule out either intrauterine or ectopic pregnancy.

7. **Serum cancer antigen-125**

    Cancer antigen-125 (CA-125) is a tumor marker for ovarian epithelial cancers. Unfortunately, CA-125 is nonspecific and is also elevated in adenocarcinoma of the uterus and colon, endometriosis, PID, inflammatory bowel disease, pregnancy, and hepatitis.

8. **Serum human chorionic gonadotropin and alpha-fetoprotein**

    Serum hCG and alpha-fetoprotein (AFP) are tumor markers in germ cell tumors of the ovaries. These tumors make up nearly 20% of all ovarian neoplasms, and most occur in young women.

■ MANAGEMENT OF THE ADNEXAL MASS

Management of patients with tubal pregnancies and tubo-ovarian abscesses is discussed in Chapter 25 and Chapter 28, respectively. Management of ovarian masses and other adnexal masses depends on the age of the patient, the severity of pelvic pain, and the consistency of the mass as demonstrated by radiographic examination.

1. **Expectant management**

    Expectant management should be considered in patients in the reproductive age group with a painless cystic mass less than 8 cm in diameter. These cysts are likely to be functional or physiological, and most will resolve spontaneously within 2 months. Patients can be treated with oral contraceptive pills to inhibit ovulation and possibly encourage earlier resolution.

2. **Surgical management**

    a. **Laparoscopy and laparotomy**

    Surgical intervention with laparoscopy or laparotomy should be considered in the following clinical situations:

    (1) Persistent mass in any age group

    (2) Solid or complex mass in any age group

    (3) Cystic mass greater than 3 cm in diameter in postmenopausal and premenarchal patients

    (4) Mass associated with severe pain

    (5) Mass associated with significant and persistent intraabdominal bleeding

    (6) Mass suspected of being malignant based on symptoms, physical findings, radiological findings, and serum tumor markers.

■ **MANAGEMENT OF LEIOMYOMATA**

The management of the patient with leiomyomata depends on the severity of symptoms such as bleeding and pain, the desire for fertility, and the size of the leiomyomata.

1. **Expectant management**

    Expectant management should be used in asymptomatic patients with an overall uterine size of 12 weeks of gestation or less and slow growth. Expectant management should be attempted even if the patient desires fertility because leiomyomata of this size rarely jeopardize fertility or result in spontaneous losses. Conservative management can also be used in asymptomatic patients who have an overall uterine size of more than 12 weeks if there is slow growth and the patient does not desire fertility.

2. **Medical management**

    a. **Gonadotropin-releasing hormone (GnRH) agonist**

    The administration of a GnRH agonist such as the following results in a hypoestrogenic state similar to that found in menopause: **leuprolide acetate (Lupron) 3.75 mg IM each month.** GnRH administration results in a median reduction in uterine size of 50%. Unfortunately, within 12 weeks of cessation of therapy, there is often rapid regrowth of the leiomyomata. Patients treated with GnRH agonist should be warned to expect hypoestrogenic symptoms such as hot flashes and atrophic vaginitis. Furthermore, the risk of osteoporosis from the hypoestrogenic state limits the duration of treatment to 3 to 6 months. For these reasons, GnRH is not considered to be a primary treatment method for leiomyomata. GnRH treatment is used for the following purposes:

(1) To decrease the symptoms of leiomyomata, especially bleeding, while the patient is awaiting surgery

(2) To decrease the size of the leiomyomata to allow for greater ease of surgery and less intraoperative blood loss

(3) To decrease the size and symptoms of leiomyomata in the perimenopausal patient with the hope that when menopause is reached, this decrease in uterine size and symptoms will be permanent

3. Surgical management

a. Myomectomy

The major advantage of myomectomy is the preservation of fertility. This procedure can be performed via laparotomy, hysteroscopy, or laparoscopy. Myomectomy should be considered in any patient who has symptomatic or enlarging leiomyomata and who also wants to preserve her uterus. Myomectomy is indicated especially in patients in whom the leiomyomata are believed to be a cause of infertility or recurrent pregnancy losses.

b. Hysterectomy

Hysterectomy is the definitive treatment of leiomyomata in the patient who does not desire to preserve her fertility. Indications for hysterectomy include the following:

(1) An asymptomatic leiomyoma that is large or is growing rapidly

(2) Excessive bleeding caused by the leiomyoma

(3) Pelvic or abdominal pain caused by the leiomyoma

30

PELVIC PAIN

■ BACKGROUND AND DEFINITIONS

Dysmenorrhea: Painful menstruation; the pain is located in the lower abdomen and is frequently described as a painful, crampy sensation that is often accompanied by nausea, vomiting, headaches, swelling, sweating, fatigue, and lightheadedness. The symptoms typically appear at or just before the onset of menses and can persist for days. Fifty to 75% of women have dysmenorrhea, although only 10 to 15% have dysmenorrhea that is severe enough to require bedrest and that interferes with routine daily life.

> **Primary dysmenorrhea:** Applies to women with no obvious pathological condition
>
> **Secondary dysmenorrhea:** Applies to women with pathological conditions that cause dysmenorrhea

Dyspareunia: Painful intercourse

Dyschezia: Painful bowel movements

Endometriosis: The presence and growth of endometrial glands and stroma in locations outside the endometrial cavity of the uterus. Endometriosis most often involves the ovaries, the cul-de-sac, the uterosacral ligaments, the rectosigmoid, and the posterior cervix. The classic symptoms of endometriosis include dysmenorrhea, dyspareunia, dyschezia, and infertility. The incidence of endometriosis in women of reproductive age is 10 to 15% and increases to 30 to 45% in women with infertility.

Adenomyosis: The presence and growth of endometrial glands and stroma in the uterine myometrium at a depth of ≥ 2.5 mm from the basal layer of the endometrium. The classic symptoms of adenomyosis include dysmenorrhea and menorrhagia, although some patients are asymptomatic. It is usually found in women 35 to 50 years old, and it has an incidence as high as 60% in this age group.

Pelvic congestion syndrome: Syndrome caused by pelvic varicosities that result in pelvic pain or heaviness that is worse during the premenstrual period, after prolonged standing, and after intercourse

■ **CLINICAL PRESENTATION**

Sharp, dull, colicky, crampy, or pressure-like pain
Localized or general pain
Pain with menses or ovulation
Associated symptoms include:
    Vaginal bleeding
    Gastrointestinal symptoms
        Nausea
        Vomiting
        Obstipation
        Dyschezia
        Anorexia
    Abdominal distention
    Fever
    Back pain
    Urinary symptoms such as frequency, urgency, and dysuria

■ **PHONE CALL**

Questions

1. **What are the patient's vital signs?**
2. **Is the patient having vaginal bleeding?**
   Patients of reproductive age who present with pain and vaginal bleeding should be suspected of having a tubal pregnancy or spontaneous abortion.

Orders

1. Obtain a complete blood count (CBC) with differential
2. Obtain an erythrocyte sedimentation rate
3. Perform a rapid urine pregnancy test if the patient is of reproductive age
4. Obtain a urinalysis
5. Start an IV if the patient appears to be severely ill or the vital signs are unstable
6. Keep the patient NPO (nothing by mouth) if surgery is anticipated

Degree of Urgency

Unless associated with a ruptured tubo-ovarian abscess, a ruptured tubal pregnancy, or intraperitoneal bleeding from a hemorrhagic cyst, pelvic pain is usually not life threatening. However, patients with significant pelvic pain or unstable vital signs should be seen immediately.

■ ELEVATOR THOUGHTS

What are causes of pelvic pain?

- Pelvic mass (see Chapter 29)
    - Functional cyst of the ovary
    - Ovarian neoplasm, benign or malignant
    - Paratubal cyst
    - Adnexal masses—cause pain by distention of the ovary, torsion, or rupture
- Endometriosis
- Adenomyosis
- Pelvic inflammatory disease (PID) (see Chapter 28)
    - Uncomplicated salpingitis
    - Pyosalpinx
    - Tubo-ovarian abscess
- Endometritis
- Cervicitis
- Uterine leiomyomata
- Pelvic adhesions
    - Prior pelvic surgery
    - Prior PID
- Tubal pregnancy (see Chapter 25)
- Spontaneous abortion (see Chapter 32)
- Pelvic congestion syndrome
- Dysmenorrhea
    - Primary
    - Secondary
- Pelvic congestion syndrome
- Urological disorder
    - Urinary tract infection
    - Urethral syndrome
    - Renal calculus
- Gastrointestinal disorder
    - Appendicitis
    - Diverticulitis
    - Inflammatory bowel disease
    - Irritable colon
    - Bowel obstruction
    - Bowel neoplasm, benign or malignant
- Musculoskeletal disorder
- Psychogenic disorder

■ MAJOR THREAT TO LIFE

- Hypovolemic shock
    - Ruptured tubal pregnancy
    - Intra-abdominal bleeding from hemorrhagic ovarian cyst
- Sepsis from ruptured tubo-ovarian abscess

■ BEDSIDE

Quick Look Test

Does the patient appear to be unstable or in severe pain?
The patient who is unstable and in severe pain should be suspected of having a ruptured tubo-ovarian abscess, intra-abdominal bleeding from a ruptured tubal pregnancy, or a hemorrhagic ovarian cyst.

Vital Signs

Vital signs are usually normal unless the patient has had significant bleeding or is in septic shock. This patient may be hypotensive, may be tachycardic, and may have postural hypotension. Changes in blood pressure (BP) and pulse should be measured when the patient is in the supine, sitting, and standing positions. A fall in systolic or diastolic BP of >15 mm Hg or a rise in pulse of >15 beats/min when the patient is assisted in sitting or standing from a supine position is evidence of hypovolemia. A patient with a fever should be suspected of having an infectious process such as PID, appendicitis, or diverticulitis.

Selective History and Chart Review

1. What is the quality, intensity, and location of the pain?
2. How long has the pain been present, and has there been any prior workup performed?
3. When was the patient's last menstrual period?
   If the patient has missed a menstrual period, either intra-uterine or ectopic pregnancy should be suspected.
4. What is the relationship between the pain and the menstrual cycle?
   Pain that is correlated with menses is suggestive of endometriosis, adenomyosis, or primary dysmenorrhea.
5. Is the pain exacerbated by intercourse, bowel movements, urination, or increased physical activity?
   Pain that is worse with intercourse and bowel movements is suggestive of endometriosis.
6. Is the pain associated with abnormal vaginal bleeding?
   Pain associated with vaginal bleeding is suggestive of leiomyomata or adenomyosis. If the patient is pregnant, tubal pregnancy or spontaneous abortion should be ruled out.
7. Is there a history of PID?
   Pelvic adhesions or hydrosalpinx can result from PID. Approximately 20% of patients with a history of PID will have chronic pelvic pain.
8. Is there a history of infertility?

A history of infertility is consistent with endometriosis or pelvic adhesions from prior PID.

9. Has the patient had pelvic or abdominal surgery?

Previous surgery can result in pelvic pain from pelvic adhesions.

10. Is there a history of gastrointestinal or urological disease?

Selective Physical Examination

Abdominal	Tender to palpation
	Mass may be palpable
	Guarding may be present
	Rebound tenderness is suggestive of peritonitis
Pelvic	
External genitalia and vagina	Usually normal unless there is bleeding
Cervix	Tenderness to cervical motion and the presence of a purulent discharge is suggestive of PID
	Bleeding from the cervix in tubal pregnancy and spontaneous abortion
	Dilated with or without tissue protruding in spontaneous abortion
Uterus	Enlarged and irregular in patient with leiomyomata
	Uniformly enlarged and globular, tender around the time of menses in patients with adenomyosis
	Uterus often retroverted and fixed, with tenderness and scarring posterior to the uterus in patients with endometriosis. Tender nodularity of the uterosacral ligaments is often palpable on rectovaginal examination.
	Tenderness in the parametrial area and pain on elevation of the uterus is suggestive of pelvic congestion syndrome.
Adnexae	Tender to palpation
	Mass may be palpable

■ DIAGNOSTIC TESTING

1. **Complete blood count with differential**

A CBC with differential will help diagnose infection. Severe anemia is suggestive of bleeding from a ruptured tubal pregnancy or from a hemorrhagic ovarian cyst.

2. **Urinalysis**
3. **Urine pregnancy test**
4. **Ultrasound examination**

Ultrasound examination will detect pelvic masses such as uterine leiomyomata and adnexal masses as well as abdominal masses. Ultrasonography will not detect pelvic adhesions or pelvic endometriosis.

5. **Computed tomography**

A computed tomography (CT) scan may provide additional information or clarify the ultrasound examination. Contrast should be used to opacify and identify the bowel. A CT scan is helpful in the evaluation of masses in the pelvic side wall. A CT scan can also detect pelvic abscesses and peritoneal implants and aid in the staging of pelvic malignancies.

6. **Magnetic resonance imaging**

Magnetic resonance imaging (MRI) provides greater soft-tissue contrast resolution than either ultrasound examination or CT scan. Therefore, MRI is helpful in the diagnosis of conditions that cause pelvic pain and uterine enlargement such as leiomyomata and adenomyosis. MRI can detect the size, number, and location of leiomyomata.

7. **Intravenous pyelogram**

An intravenous pyelogram (IVP) is helpful in evaluating the kidneys and the urinary tract. An IVP will diagnose pelvic kidneys.

■ MANAGEMENT

Management of patients with pelvic pain depends on the severity and duration of the pain and on the physical, laboratory, and radiographic findings. Patients who have no physical, laboratory, or radiographic findings and who complain of only mild pain with recent onset should be followed conservatively. Patients who have severe pain or pain of prolonged duration or are suspected of having pelvic pathology may require surgical intervention.

1. **Conservative management**
   a. **Nonsteroidal anti-inflammatory agents**
      (1) **Ibuprofen (Motrin, Nuprin, Advil) 600 to 800 mg three to four times per day with a maximum dosage of 3200 mg/day**
      (2) **Naproxen (Naprosyn, Anaprox) 500 mg two times per day with a maximum dosage of 1000 mg/day**
         Nonsteroidal anti-inflammatory agents are especially helpful in patients with primary or secondary dysmenorrhea.
   b. **Oral analgesics**
   c. **Oral contraceptive pills**
      Oral contraceptive pills are helpful in treating patients with dysmenorrhea and endometriosis. Pills will also suppress the formation of functional ovarian cysts by inhibiting ovulation.
   d. **Gonadotropin-releasing factor (GnRH) agonist**

Administration of GnRH agonist results in the suppression of ovulation and in the establishment of a hypoestrogenic state similar to that found in menopause. GnRH agonist can be used in patients with pelvic pain secondary to endometriosis, adenomyosis, and uterine leiomyomata. Because ovulation is suppressed, the formation of functional ovarian cysts is also suppressed. Patients receiving GnRH agonist should be cautioned to expect hypoestrogenic symptoms such as hot flashes and atrophic vaginitis. Furthermore, the risk of osteoporosis from the hypoestrogenic state limits the duration of treatment to 3 to 6 months.

   (1) **Leuprolide acetate (Lupron) 3.75 mg IM each month**
   (2) **Nafarelin acetate (Synarel) 200-μg intranasal spray two times per day** (patients who do not achieve amenorrhea can be placed on 400 μg two times per day)

2. Surgical management

a. Laparoscopy

Laparoscopy is the definitive diagnostic test for evaluating patients with pelvic pain. In addition to providing a diagnosis, laparoscopy often allows certain therapeutic procedures to be performed, such as lysis of adhesions, cauterization or laser vaporization of endometrial implants, excision of ovarian or paratubal cysts, salpingostomy for removal of a tubal pregnancy, and even salpingo-oophorectomy. In patients with chronic pelvic pain, laparoscopy will reveal no significant abnormalities in approximately 30% of cases.

b. Laparotomy

Laparotomy is indicated when the degree of pathology makes surgical treatment by laparoscopy unsafe or technically difficult. Hysterectomy for a large, fibroid uterus or excision of a large ovarian mass is usually performed by laparotomy. Patients with severe pelvic adhesions secondary to endometriosis or PID are often appropriate candidates for laparotomy. Laparotomy is indicated for patients with pelvic malignancies. Laparotomy is also indicated for patients with endometriosis who are undergoing presacral neurectomy or uterosacral nerve ablation.

3. Psychological evaluation and counseling

Patients with chronic pelvic pain and a negative workup after extensive diagnostic testing and diagnostic laparoscopy may benefit from psychological evaluation and counseling. A positive correlation has been found between a history of sexual abuse and chronic pelvic pain. Management of such patients is often most effective if it is provided by a multidisciplinary team comprising a gynecologist, a psychiatrist or psychologist, and an anesthesiologist who specializes in pain management.

31

SEXUAL ASSAULT

■ BACKGROUND AND DEFINITIONS

Sexual assault: Also referred to as **rape,** sexual assault is defined as any sexual act performed by one person on another without consent and with force, the threat of force, or the inability of the victim to give appropriate consent. Sexual assault accounts for approximately 6% of all violent crimes. It has been determined that as many as 44% of women have been victims of sexual assault or attempted sexual assault. Furthermore, sexual assault is one of the most underreported crimes, and it has been estimated that only 10 to 20% of rapes are reported. Women of all ages, ethnic origins, and socioeconomic classes can be victims of sexual assault. Younger women, older women, and women with mental or physical handicaps are especially vulnerable. Nearly 75% of victims know the assailant.

Spousal rape: Sexual assault that occurs in a marriage

Date rape: Sexual assault that occurs during a date. Date rape is not usually reported, because the victim feels that she is partially responsible for the assault or that she even encouraged it.

Statutory rape: Sexual intercourse with a female under a certain age, as specified by the particular state, regardless of whether consent is given.

Only a minority of victims of rape present immediately after the assault. If a victim seeks help, she does so a longer time after the incident.

■ CLINICAL PRESENTATION

The clinical presentation of the victim of rape is highly variable. The patient can appear calm and in control or she may appear with the complete loss of emotional control. She might appear to have depression, anxiety, or lability of mood. The patient might present with generalized complaints such as vague aches and pain, insomnia, and eating disturbances. She might also present with specific complaints referable to the genital area such as vaginal or rectal pain, itching, and discharge. Furthermore, as many as 40% of victims of sexual assault also suffer nongenital injuries, and approximately 1% of these injuries require hospitalization. The extent and severity of these physical injuries are also highly variable.

■ PHONE CALL

Questions

1. **How severe are the patient's physical injuries?**
2. **When did the alleged assault occur?**
   The amount of time that has passed between the alleged assault and when the patient presents determines how successful the effort to recover evidence for legal purposes will be and also determines the appropriate tests to obtain to screen for sexually transmitted diseases.

Orders

1. Provide the patient with a private examination room
2. Notify the appropriate social service worker or experts trained specifically to work with rape victims
3. Notify the police of the alleged assault
4. Obtain a urine pregnancy test to rule out pre-existing pregnancy
5. Obtain a Venereal Disease Research Laboratory (VDRL) test
6. Keep the patient from washing, to preserve evidence

If the patient has suffered severe physical trauma, the following orders should be given:

1. Start a large-bore IV
2. Type and crossmatch for 2 units of blood
3. Obtain a complete blood count (CBC)
4. Perform coagulation studies: platelet count, PT, PTT, fibrinogen, and fibrin split products
5. Obtain a chemistry panel
6. Perform a urinalysis
7. Place a urethral catheter
8. Keep the patient NPO (nothing by mouth) if surgery is anticipated

Degree of Urgency

The patient should be seen as soon as possible. If she has sustained severe physical trauma, she should be seen immediately.

■ ELEVATOR THOUGHTS

What are the components of the "rape trauma" syndrome?

The **rape trauma syndrome** described by Burgess and Holmstrom (Burgess AW, Holmstrom LL: Rape trauma syndrome. Am J Psychiatry 1974;131:981) is divided into two phases.

- **Disorganization** or **acute phase:** Lasts several days to many weeks and is composed of the following:
    Fear of injury or death
    Fear of being assaulted again
    Humiliation and embarrassment
    Guilt
    Depression
    Anger
    Irritability
    Difficulties in concentration
    Anxiety
    Thoughts of revenge
    Generalized pain
    Eating and sleeping disturbances
    Vaginal pain, discharge, or itching
    Rectal pain
- **Reorganization** or **delayed phase:** Lasts several months to years and is composed of the following:
    Sexual aversion
    Inability to attain orgasm
    Vaginismus
    Flashbacks
    Nightmares
    Insomnia
    Paranoia
    Phobias toward men and sex
    Nonspecific gynecological and menstrual complaints

What are common misconceptions of rape?
- Rape is a crime of passion and the assailant is usually over-sexed or sexually frustrated.
    Rape is not a crime of passion but rather is an act of violence in which the assailant wants to abuse, degrade, and control the victim.
- Rape is an indication of the victim's promiscuity.
    Rape victims are not more promiscuous than nonvictims. Furthermore, promiscuity does not justify rape.
- Certain victims deserve to be sexually assaulted because of their behavior, their manner of dress, or their state of intoxication.
    No one deserves to be raped, regardless of the circumstances. Victims do not encourage sexual assault.

■ MAJOR THREAT TO LIFE
- Physical trauma
    As many as 40% of rape victims also suffer nongenital trauma. Approximately 1% will require hospitalization for the trauma, and 0.1% will have fatal injuries.

■ BEDSIDE

Quick Look Test

Does the patient appear to have sustained severe physical trauma?

What is the patient's state of mind?

One of the key aspects of sexual assault is that the victim has lost control to the assailant. One of the critical goals of health care providers is to restore control to the patient. This requires allowing the patient and her state of mind to dictate the pace of the history taking and the performance of the physical examination.

Vital Signs

Vital signs are usually normal. The patient with signs of hypovolemic shock such as hypotension and tachycardia should be suspected of having intra-abdominal hemorrhaging secondary to trauma.

Selective History and Chart Review

1. What was the time and the date of the assault?
2. What was the number of assailants?
3. What was the nature of the assault, and what acts were committed?
4. Did ejaculation occur, and if so, where did it occur?
5. Was there any nongenital trauma?
6. Was there oral, vaginal, or rectal penetration?
7. Were any foreign objects used in the assault?
8. Has the patient already bathed or cleansed herself, changed her clothes, or brushed her teeth?
9. Does the patient have any pre-existing gynecological or medical conditions?
10. When was the patient's last menstrual period?
11. Is the patient using contraception?
12. When was the patient's last consensual intercourse?

Selective Physical Examination

General	Cuts, bruises, abrasions, and bite marks may be signs of extragenital trauma
Abdominal	Distention and tenderness are suggestive of intra-abdominal bleeding secondary to trauma
Pelvic	
External genitalia and vagina	Edema, erythema, lacerations may be present in the areas of the urethra, vulva, rectum, or vagina

	Deep lacerations in the vagina and into the abdominal cavity may be present, especially if foreign objects were used in the assault
Cervix	Lacerations may be present from foreign objects
Uterus and adnexae	Usually normal, unless there is extensive trauma due to the use of foreign objects resulting in uterine laceration and broad ligament hematomas

■ DIAGNOSTIC TESTING

1. **Rapid urine pregnancy test**
   Pre-existing pregnancy should be ruled out.
2. **Testing for *Chlamydia trachomatis* (see Chapter 26)**
   Chlamydia is the sexually transmitted disease most likely to be acquired from sexual assault. Although culturing is the most sensitive test for chlamydia, it is expensive, time consuming, and not always available. Therefore, testing for chlamydia can be done by rapid antigen detection tests such as Chlamydiazyme or MicroTrak. Testing should be repeated in 3 to 4 weeks.
3. **Cultures for *Neisseria gonorrhoeae* (see Chapter 26)**
   A rape victim's risk of acquiring gonorrhea is 6 to 12%. Oral and rectal cultures may be appropriate, in addition to cervical cultures, if there has been penetration of those orifices. Cultures should be repeated in 3 to 4 weeks.
4. **Vaginal smear for *Trichomonas vaginalis* (see Chapter 35)**
   A vaginal wet smear with normal saline should be performed to rule out *Trichomonas vaginalis*. The diagnosis of this sexually transmitted infection is easily made because of the finding of the motile *Trichomonas* protozoans. The organism has an ovoid body and a visible posterior flagellum, and it is usually found moving in circles in a jerky fashion. The vaginal smear should be repeated in 3 to 4 weeks.
5. **Venereal disease research laboratory (VDRL) test**
   Baseline serology for syphilis should be obtained. The risk of acquiring syphilis from a sexual assault is estimated to be as high as 3%. Serology should be repeated in 3 to 4 weeks.
6. **Serology for human immunodeficiency virus**
   The risk of acquiring human immunodeficiency virus (HIV) from sexual assault is unknown. Baseline serology should be obtained and repeated in 3 to 6 months.
7. **Serology for herpes simplex virus**
   Baseline serology should be considered, and serology should be repeated in 3 to 4 weeks.
8. **Serology for hepatitis B**

Baseline serology should be considered, and serology should be repeated in 3 to 4 weeks.
9. **Serology for cytomegalovirus**
    Baseline serology should be considered, and serology should be repeated in 3 to 4 weeks.

■ MANAGEMENT

When managing a victim of sexual assault, the physician's responsibility is threefold: (1) medical evaluation and treatment, (2) documentation of injuries and collection of evidence for medical–legal reasons, and (3) emotional support.

1. **Medical evaluation and treatment**
    a. **Examine thoroughly for injuries and treat injuries**
    b. **Screen for and treat sexually transmitted infections**
        These sexually transmitted infections may not be detectable immediately. Nevertheless, baseline cultures and serology should be obtained initially and repeated in 3 to 4 weeks. Serology for HIV should be repeated in 3 to 6 months. Human papillomavirus (HPV) infection can be detected by the finding of genital warts or condylomata acuminata, by DNA hybridization testing, and by cytological smear of the cervix, which can show cellular changes suggestive of HPV infection.
    b. **Prophylactic antiobiotics**
        An antibiotic regimen that covers the prevention of gonorrhea, chlamydia, and syphilis should be used.
        (1) **Ceftriaxone 250 mg IM plus doxycycline 100 mg PO two times per day for 7 days** or
        (2) **Spectinomycin 2 g IM plus doxycycline 100 mg PO two times per day for 7 days**
        In pregnant patients, doxycycline should be substituted with **erythromycin 500 mg PO four times per day for 7 days.**
    c. **Prevention of pregnancy**
        If it is possible that pregnancy will result from the sexual assault, pregnancy prevention should be offered with the "morning after" prophylaxis. A pregnancy test should be performed before treatment, to determine if the victim is already pregnant.
        (1) **50-μg or "medium-dose" combination birth control pill: 2 pills initially and repeated in 12 hours** or
        (2) **35-μg or "low-dose" combination birth control pill: 4 pills initially and repeated in 12 hours** or
        (3) **5 mg ethinyl estradiol PO every day for 5 days** or
        (4) **20 to 30 mg conjugated estrogen PO every day for 5 days**

2. Documentation of injuries and collection of evidence for medical–legal reasons
   a. Obtain and record a detailed history.
   b. Document and describe in detail all injuries.

   The terms "sexual assault" and "rape" are legal terms and should therefore not be used in the physician's diagnosis. Instead, the phase **"consistent with the use of force"** should be used. Drawings of injuries often provide additional information to the written description.

   c. Collect the patient's clothing if she did not change her clothing.
   d. Collect fingernail scrapings.
   e. Collect hair samples by combing the pubic hair.
   f. Collect vaginal, rectal, and pharyngeal secretions for analysis for sperm or acid phosphatase.

   After ejaculation, motile sperm may be found in the vagina for up to 8 hours and in cervical mucus for up to 2 to 3 days. Nonmotile sperm may be detected in the vagina for up to 24 hours and in cervical mucus for up to 17 days. Acid phosphatase from seminal fluid can be detected in the vagina and in cervical mucus for up to 48 hours. Acid phosphatase should always be measured, because the assailant may have had a vasectomy.

3. Emotional support
   a. The physician should educate the patient concerning not only what to expect from a medical standpoint, but also what to expect in psychological and emotional recovery.

   She should be reassured that she will recover from her physical injuries and that it is unlikely that reproductive function has been jeopardized by the assault.

   b. The patient should be allowed to express her anxieties and to ask questions concerning her injuries and her recovery.
   c. Misconceptions should be corrected.

   Specifically, it should be emphasized that the patient is not to blame and that she did not deserve to be sexually assaulted.

   d. Experts who are trained specifically to work with victims of rape should be consulted to facilitate counseling and ongoing support.
   e. A follow-up evaluation should be planned to reevaluate her emotional state.

   Follow-up should be planned even if the patient initially appears to be calm and well controlled. This initial appearance is often just a defense mechanism and should not be interpreted as a sign that the patient does not need any emotional support.

32

SPONTANEOUS ABORTION

■ BACKGROUND AND DEFINITIONS

Spontaneous abortion: The spontaneous loss of a pregnancy before 20 weeks of gestation, also referred to as **"miscarriage"** in lay terminology. This condition can be more accurately defined by the following terms, which describe the clinical findings:

Threatened abortion: Vaginal bleeding alone

Inevitable abortion: Vaginal bleeding plus cervical dilatation

Incomplete abortion: Spontaneous passage of some but not all fetal tissue

Completed abortion: Spontaneous passage of all fetal tissue

Blighted ovum: Ultrasonographic absence of a fetus within a normal gestational sac after 6 weeks of gestation

Missed abortion: Ultrasonographic absence of fetal cardiac activity after 7 weeks of gestation, without bleeding or passage of tissue

Septic abortion: Any clinical presentation of spontaneous abortion associated with clinical signs of infection

Habitual or recurrent abortion: History of three or more spontaneous abortions

Approximately 15% of diagnosed pregnancies will undergo spontaneous abortion. Older women have higher incidences of spontaneous abortion than younger women. In approximately 50 to 60% of first trimester and 15% of second trimester spontaneous abortions, a fetal chromosomal abnormality is found. The distribution of chromosomal abnormalities found in aborted fetal tissue is as follows: 50% autosomal trisomy, 25% triploidy, 20% monosomy X (Turner's syndrome), and 5% translocation.

■ CLINICAL PRESENTATION

Vaginal bleeding
Uterine cramping
Passage of tissue through the vagina

■ PHONE CALL

Questions

1. **How heavy is the patient's vaginal bleeding?**
2. **What are the patient's vital signs?**
     Women undergoing spontaneous abortion can have bleeding significant enough to result in hypotension, tachycardia, and even shock. A fever is suggestive of a septic abortion.
3. **Has the patient passed any tissue from the vagina that she has saved?**

Orders

1. Perform a urine pregnancy test to confirm the diagnosis of pregnancy
2. Obtain a complete blood count (CBC)
3. Test for blood type and Rh factor
4. Start an IV if the patient is having heavy bleeding or if vital signs suggest significant blood loss
5. Crossmatch blood if the bleeding is severe or if the patient is unstable
6. If the patient passes tissue from the vagina, it should be collected and sent in a specimen bottle with formaldehyde solution for pathological evaluation.

Degree of Urgency

Spontaneous abortion is usually not life threatening. However, a patient who is bleeding heavily, complaining of severe pelvic pain, or exhibiting signs or symptoms of shock should be seen immediately.

■ ELEVATOR THOUGHTS

What are other causes of vaginal bleeding in early pregnancy?
- Ectopic pregnancy
- Cervical polyps and other cervical lesions
- Friable cervix
- Incompetent cervix
- Vaginal lesion
- Molar pregnancy

■ MAJOR THREAT TO LIFE

- Hypovolemic shock
    Patients with spontaneous abortion and molar pregnancy

can have vaginal bleeding significant enough to result in hypovolemic shock. In patients who exhibit signs and symptoms of shock without heavy vaginal bleeding, the diagnosis of tubal pregnancy with intraperitoneal bleeding should be considered.

■ BEDSIDE

Quick Look Test

Does the patient appear to be in shock?

Is the patient in significant pain?

The presence of crampy, midline pain is consistent with uterine cramping associated with a spontaneous abortion. Unilateral pain would be suggestive of a tubal pregnancy.

Vital Signs

Patients may be mildly hypertensive and tachycardic because of pelvic pain from uterine cramping. Patients who have had significant vaginal bleeding will usually be hypotensive and tachycardic. Postural hypotension might be revealed by the finding of changes in blood pressure and pulse when the patient is assisted in sitting or standing from a supine position. A fall in systolic or diastolic blood pressure (BP) of >15 mm Hg or a rise in pulse of >15 beats/min is evidence of hypovolemia.

Selective History and Chart Review

1. Has the patient had a positive pregnancy test?
2. When was the patient's last menstrual period, and what is the gestational age of the fetus?
3. Has the patient had a prior pelvic ultrasound examination confirming an intrauterine pregnancy, and what is the current gestational age of the fetus based on those fetal measurements?
4. How long has the patient been bleeding, and how severe has the vaginal bleeding been?
5. Has the patient passed any tissue through the vagina?
6. Does the patient have any risk factors for tubal pregnancy?
7. Does the patient have an intrauterine device (IUD)?

In patients who are pregnant and bleeding and have an IUD, the diagnosis of tubal pregnancy should be suspected, because the IUD is more effective in preventing intrauterine pregnancies than ectopic pregnancies.

Selective Physical Examination

Abdominal	Mildly tender and soft; the uterus is usually not palpable on abdominal examination in a pregnancy of less than 12 weeks' gestation. At 16 weeks, the uterus is usually halfway between the pubic symphysis and umbilicus, and at 20 weeks, it is usually palpable at the level of the umbilicus.
Pelvic	
External genitalia and vagina	Blood-stained with or without tissue in the vagina
Cervix	Threatened abortion: bleeding without cervical dilatation
	Inevitable abortion: bleeding with cervical dilatation
	Incomplete abortion: bleeding with cervical dilatation and tissue present at the cervical os
	Missed abortion: normal cervix without bleeding
	Completed abortion: small amount of bleeding with closed cervical os
Uterus	Tender and enlarged
Adnexae	Adnexal mass and tenderness suggests a tubal pregnancy.

■ DIAGNOSTIC TESTING

1. **Rapid qualitative urine or serum pregnancy test**
   A rapid urine pregnancy test should be performed in all patients suspected of having a spontaneous abortion. Enzyme-linked immunosorbent assay pregnancy tests such as Icon, Quest, and Confidot are simple and quick tests that can be performed on both urine and blood. These tests can detect levels of beta subunit of human chorionic gonadotropin (hCG) as low as 20 mIU/ml. In a normal intrauterine pregnancy, serum hCG is approximately 100 mIU/ml at a gestational age of 4 weeks. Therefore, with these tests, a pregnancy can be diagnosed even before a menstrual period is missed. The test can remain positive for up to a month after spontaneous abortion. A negative test rules out an ongoing pregnancy or a recent spontaneous abortion.
2. **Pelvic ultrasound examination**
   Ultrasonographic findings in spontaneous abortion can include any of the following:
   a. **Fetus with absence of fetal cardiac activity**
   b. **Collapsed gestational sac with or without a fetus**
   c. **Empty gestational sac**

Table 32–1 □ **ULTRASONOGRAPHIC MILESTONES IN NORMAL FIRST TRIMESTER PREGNANCY**

| Ultrasonographic Finding | Gestational Age at Detection (weeks) | |
	Transabdominal Examination	Transvaginal Examination
Gestational sac	6	5
Yolk sac	6	5
Fetus	7	6
Fetal cardiac activity	7	6

The absence of a fetus in a gestational sac with a diameter of ≥3.0 cm is evidence of a spontaneous abortion.

d. **Absent gestational sac**

An "endometrial stripe" is a bright longitudinal line found on ultrasound examination of the uterine cavity. The stripe is the result of the approximation of the anterior and the posterior endometrial surfaces and is ultrasonographic evidence of an empty uterine cavity.

Ultrasonographic milestones have been established for normal first trimester pregnancies (Table 32–1). By transabdominal ultrasound examination, the gestational sac and yolk sac should be identified by a gestational age of 6 weeks. The fetus and fetal cardiac activity should be identified by a gestational age of 7 weeks. The vaginal transducer used for transvaginal ultrasound examinations can be placed closer to the uterus than the transabdominal transducer and therefore can detect these same structures 1 week earlier.

Because the gestational age of the fetus is sometimes unknown, ultrasonographic milestones have been established that correlate with serum hCG levels. In normal pregnancies, a gestational sac should be seen by transabdominal ultrasound examination when the serum hCG level is >6500 mIU/ml (International Reference Preparation). On transvaginal ultrasound examination, the gestational sac should be seen when the serum hCG is >2000 mIU/ml. These two serum hCG levels define what is commonly referred to as the "discriminatory hCG zones."

Whenever these ultrasonographic milestones cannot be identified at the corresponding gestational age or serum hCG levels, an abnormal pregnancy should be suspected. This abnormal pregnancy can be either an abnormal intrauterine pregnancy that has undergone or is about to undergo spontaneous abortion or an ectopic pregnancy. The differentiation between an abnormal intrauterine pregnancy and an ectopic pregnancy depends on the physical examination, serial serum hCG determination, and ultrasound examination. Evidence of an intrauterine pregnancy on ultrasound examination makes the likelihood of ectopic pregnancy extremely rare. The incidence of concurrent intrauterine pregnancy and tubal pregnancy is nearly 1 in 3000. When neither physical examination nor ultrasound examination is conclusive, serial serum hCG testing can be used to help distinguish between a spontaneous abortion and ectopic pregnancy.

3. **Serial serum human chorionic gonadotropin testing**

   Human chorionic gonadotropin is produced by the syncytiotrophoblast in the placenta, and serum levels rise exponentially in the first trimester (Fig. 32–1). A peak level of approximately 100,000 mIU/ml is reached at 9 weeks of gestation, and hCG levels then fall to a plateau of 10,000 to 20,000 mIU/ml, where they remain for the duration of the pregnancy. Even with normal pregnancies, there is a wide range of serum hCG levels at any given gestational age, and therefore it may be difficult to confirm the diagnosis of spontaneous abortion with only a single serum hCG level (Table 32–2).

   When serum hCG levels are measured serially several days apart, an abnormally rising serum hCG is diagnostic of a abnormal pregnancy, either an ectopic pregnancy or a spontaneous abortion. In early pregnancy, with levels of serum hCG

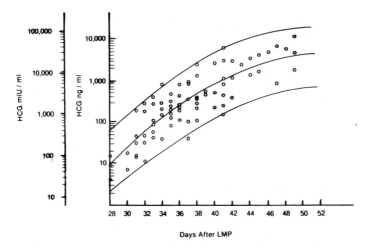

Figure 32–1 □ Rise in serum hCG in normal intrauterine pregnancies. (Modified from Pittaway DE, Reish RL, Wentz AC: Doubling times of human chorionic gonadotropin increase in early viable intrauterine pregnancies. Am J Obstet Gynecol 1985;152:299.)

Table 32–2 □ HUMAN CHORIONIC GONADOTROPIN LEVELS IN
NORMAL PREGNANCIES

Gestational Age (weeks)	Serum hCG (mIU/ml)
4	100
6	1000–10,000
7	10,000–50,000
9	50,000–100,000
20	10,000–20,000

hCG = human chorionic gonadotropin.

at <1200 mIU/ml, serum hCG normally doubles in 2 days. If there is not at least a 66% rise in serum hCG in 2 days, an abnormal pregnancy is diagnosed. At serum hCG levels of 1200 to 6000 mIU/ml, the normal hCG doubling time is almost 3 days, and at levels of >6000 mIU/ml, the doubling time is approximately 4 days. A falling hCG in early pregnancy is also indicative of an abnormal pregnancy. A rapidly declining serum hCG is more suggestive of a completed or ongoing spontaneous abortion than an ectopic pregnancy. The half-life of hCG is approximately 32 to 37 hours.

4. **Serum progesterone**

Women with normal intrauterine pregnancies almost always have a serum progesterone level of >25 ng/ml. Approximately 85 to 90% of women with spontaneous abortions or ectopic pregnancies have a serum progesterone of <10 ng/ml. Therefore, a serum progesterone level of <5 ng/ml is a strong indication of an abnormal pregnancy, although the level cannot differentiate between ectopic pregnancy and an abnormal intrauterine pregnancy.

5. **Complete blood count**

Bleeding from either a spontaneous abortion or an ectopic pregnancy can be significant enough to result in anemia. An elevated white blood cell count is suggestive of septic abortion.

6. **Blood Rh factor and antibody screen**

■ ADDITIONAL DIAGNOSTIC TESTING FOR SEPTIC ABORTION

In addition to the diagnostic tests listed above, the following tests may be helpful in diagnosing and managing a patient who is suspected of having a septic abortion:

1. **Serum chemistry including electrolytes**
2. **Urinalysis**
3. **Intrauterine culture and Gram stain**

4. Blood cultures
5. Coagulation studies
6. Chest x-ray

■ MANAGEMENT

1. Threatened abortion
   a. Conservative management
   b. Instruct patient to avoid strenuous physical activity and intercourse
   c. Instruct patient to return if bleeding, pelvic pain, or cramping increases

   Bleeding occurs in approximately 20 to 30% of women during the first 20 weeks of gestation. Spontaneous abortion will occur in about 50% of these women. Although women with threatened abortions are often warned to avoid strenuous activity and intercourse and are sometimes even placed on bedrest, there is no evidence that these measures decrease the risk of pregnancy loss. Furthermore, although hormonal therapy with progestins and estrogens such as diethylstilbestrol (DES) have been attempted in the past, there is no medical therapy that decreases the likelihood of pregnancy loss in normal patients.

2. Inevitable abortion
   a. Conservative management allowing spontaneous evacuation of the uterus or
   b. Surgical evacuation of the uterus or
   c. Induction of uterine contractions with prostaglandin E_2 vaginal suppositories or intravenous oxytocin

   Women with inevitable abortions can be given the option of either waiting for the passage of fetal tissue to occur spontaneously or undergoing surgical evacuation immediately. Patients who decide to wait should be warned to return to the hospital if they develop either severe or unremitting bleeding or pelvic pain. They should also be warned that suction curettage may still be necessary if not all of the fetal tissue is passed spontaneously. Suction curettage can be performed in an office or an emergency room and can be performed with either paracervical block or the use of intravenous drugs for sedation and analgesia. Some patients may elect to have the procedure performed in an operating room under general anesthesia. Suction curettage should be performed with a sterile suction cannula with a diameter in millimeters that corresponds to the number of weeks of gestation based on uterine size. For example, a 7- or 8-mm cannula should be used if the uterus is palpated to be 8-week size, and an 11- or 12-mm cannula should be used if the uterus is palpated to be 12-week size. All tissue obtained by surgical evacuation should be submitted for pathological evaluation to confirm the diagnosis of spontaneous abortion.

In women with inevitable abortions in the second trimester of pregnancy, rupture of membranes is usually found along with vaginal bleeding and cervical dilatation. Surgical evacuation in these patients can be accomplished by dilatation and evacuation, which is usually performed in an operating room, or by the use of either vaginal prostaglandin E_2 suppositories or an intravenous infusion of high doses of oxytocin to induce uterine contractions and delivery of the fetus and placenta. Prostin E_2 vaginal suppositories (Upjohn) containing 20 mg of prostaglandin E_2 can be placed high in the vagina every 3 to 5 hours until the abortion has been completed. As an alternative, an intravenous solution of oxytocin can be made by adding 10 ampules of oxytocin, each containing 10 IU of oxytocin, to 1000 ml of lactated Ringer's solution. This solution (with an oxytocin concentration of 100 mIU/ml) is infused starting at a rate of 0.5 ml or 50 mIU/min. The rate of infusion can be increased every 30 minutes to a maximum rate of 2 ml or 200 mIU/min. Because oxytocin has an antidiuretic effect, water restriction and administration of a more concentrated solution of oxytocin should be considered if the oxytocin induction is prolonged.

3. **Incomplete spontaneous abortion**
   a. **Surgical evacuation of the uterus** or
   b. **Induction of uterine contractions with prostaglandin E_2 vaginal suppositories or intravenous oxytocin**

   Women with incomplete spontaneous abortion usually have significant vaginal bleeding, which precludes conservative management. In some patients, speculum examination reveals fetal tissue protruding through the cervical os, and the abortion can be completed merely by grasping and removing the tissue. In the remaining patients, surgical evacuation by suction curettage is recommended for first trimester pregnancies. For second trimester pregnancies, dilatation and evacuation or medical induction of uterine contractions with either prostaglandin E_2 or intravenous oxytocin can be performed as described for the management of inevitable abortion.

4. **Completed spontaneous abortion**
   a. **Serum hCG in several days** or
   b. **Rapid pregnancy test in several weeks**

   Women with completed spontaneous abortion have passed all fetal and placental tissue. The cervical os is usually closed, and bleeding is minimal. Therefore, no surgical intervention is necessary. If tissue is not available for pathological evaluation or if evaluation does not reveal evidence of fetal tissue, a quantitative serum hCG level should be obtained in a few days or, as an alternative, a rapid qualitative urine or serum pregnancy test could be performed in several weeks to confirm that the abortion has been completed.

5. **Blighted ovum and missed abortion**
   a. **Surgical evacuation of the uterus by suction dilatation and curettage**

   Patients with either a blighted ovum or a missed abortion are usually asymptomatic. The cervical os is usually closed, and therefore, cervical dilatation followed by suction curettage is recommended. Women with a missed abortion who have retained nonviable fetal tissue for long periods of time are at risk for developing a coagulopathy, which is probably a result of thromboplastin released from the fetal tissue. This complication is rare and usually occurs only in pregnancies beyond the first trimester.

6. **Septic abortion**
   a. **Intravenous antibiotic therapy**
   b. **Surgical evacuation of the uterus**

   Septic abortion is a serious complication of spontaneous abortion resulting in a fatality rate of approximately 0.5 per 100,000 women with spontaneous abortions. Organisms causing septic abortion include anaerobic bacteria (*Bacteroides* species, *Clostridium perfringens, Peptostreptococcus* species) and aerobic species (beta-hemolytic streptococcus, *Enterococcus faecalis, Escherichia coli, Pseudomonas* species). Broad-spectrum antibiotics that provide adequate coverage for these organisms should be administered intravenously immediately. No one specific antibiotic regimen has been shown to be superior to others in all patients. A popular regimen is the following combination of gentamicin and clindamycin: **gentamicin 2.0 mg/kg IV loading dose followed by a maintenance dose of 1.5 mg/kg every 8 hours if renal function is normal, and clindamycin 900 mg IV every 8 hours.**

   Peak serum levels of antibiotics are usually attained 1 to 2 hours after administration, and the patient should then undergo surgical evacuation of the uterus. Postoperative care should include close monitoring of vital signs and urine output to detect septic shock.

7. **Rh-negative women**

   All Rh-negative women who have had spontaneous abortions should receive Rh immune globulin if (1) they are nonimmunized, as documented by a negative antibody screen and (2) the Rh factor of the father is either positive or unknown.

   In pregnancies with a gestational age of 12 weeks or less, the following should be given: **Rh immune globulin (MICRhoGAM) 50 μg IM within 72 hours of the spontaneous abortion.** After 12 weeks, a full dose of Rh immune globulin should be given as follows: **Rh immune globulin (RhoGAM) 300 μg within 72 hours of the spontaneous abortion.**

8. All women with spontaneous abortion

Almost all women who suffer pregnancy losses, even at an early gestational age, will undergo a grieving process. Both parents should be treated with sympathy and compassion. Furthermore, they should be educated concerning the common occurrence of spontaneous abortions, and it should be emphasized that in almost all cases, neither the patient nor her health care provider should be blamed for the loss. Information concerning support groups should be provided to both parents.

33

TOXIC SHOCK SYNDROME

■ BACKGROUND AND DEFINITION

Toxic shock syndrome (TSS): An acute, potentially fatal, multisystem illness caused by strains of *Staphylococcus aureus* that produce a toxin referred to as pyrogenic extoxin or enterotoxin F. The incubation period for TSS is 1 to 4 days. Ninety to 95% of cases of TSS occur in women, and >95% of these cases occur in menstruating women. White women younger than 30 years of age are at greatest risk. The incidence of TSS in menstruating women is 6 to 7 per 100,000 per year. TSS that is not associated with menstruation can occur in women of any age. The fatality rate of TSS is 3 to 6%. In patients who survive, there is a 30% recurrence rate.

The following two conditions must be present for TSS to develop:

1. The patient must be colonized with a strain of *Staphylococcus aureus* that produces the toxin.
2. There must be a portal of entry into the systemic circulation.

Toxins may enter into the systemic circulation through microulcerations that develop in the vagina secondary to trauma from tampons or tampon inserters. Nearly 99% of cases of TSS associated with menstruation occur in women who use tampons. Women who use tampons during menstruation are 18 times more likely to develop TSS than women who do not use them. Women who used the Rely brand of tampons were almost 8 times more likely to develop TSS than women who use other brands of tampons. The use of high-absorbency synthetic materials in newer tampon products may predispose a patient to TSS because of an effect on the colonization rate of *Staphylococcus aureus* or increased trauma to the vaginal wall. Patients who used the Rely brand of tampons were shown to have a 43% colonization rate for *Staphylococcus aureus* compared with a colonization rate of 8% in users of other brands of tampons.

■ CLINICAL PRESENTATION

The following signs and symptoms are found in >90% of patients with TSS:
Fever of >102°F
Hypotension

Shock
"Sunburn-like" skin rash with desquamation
Myalgias
Vomiting
Diarrhea

Other signs and symptoms that occur less frequently include the following:
Headache
Abdominal tenderness
Sore throat
Hyperemia of the pharynx and tongue
Conjunctivitis
Photophobia
Altered sensorium
Hyperemia of the vagina
Vaginal discharge
Arthralgia
Adnexal tenderness

■ PHONE CALL

Questions

1. **How ill does the patient appear?**
2. **What are the vital signs?**

Orders

1. Start IV
2. Insert urethral catheter to monitor urine output
3. Record intake and output
4. Administer oxygen via face mask or nasal cannula
5. Obtain a complete blood count (CBC) with differential
6. Obtain a chemistry panel
7. Perform coagulation studies: prothrombin time (PT), partial thromboplastin time (PTT), platelet count, fibrinogen, fibrin split products
8. Perform urinalysis

Degree of Urgency

TSS is a potentially fatal disease, so patients should be seen immediately.

■ ELEVATOR THOUGHTS

What is the differential diagnosis of TSS?

- Streptococcal scarlet fever

    This infection is rare after the age of 10 years and is usually preceded by an upper respiratory infection. Serum antibodies to streptococcus such as antistreptolysin O are positive.

- Mucocutaneous lymph node syndrome (Kawasaki's disease)

    This syndrome is usually encountered in pediatric patients of <5 years of age. Furthermore, hypotension, shock, and adult respiratory distress syndrome (ARDS) are rarely present in this syndrome.

- Rubeola (measles)
- Rubella (German measles)
- Rocky Mountain spotted fever (*Ricksettsia rickettsii*)

    This infection is caused by a gram-negative bacterium for which small rodents and occasionally larger mammals are the reservoir. Transmission to humans is by bites from multiple tick species.

- Leptospirosis

    This infection is caused by *Leptospira interrogans*, a spirochete found in domestic livestock, dogs, rodents, skunks, and foxes. Transmission is by contact with infected tissue, body fluids, or contaminated water. Those who work with animals such as dairy or slaughterhouse workers are at highest risk, although nearly 50% of cases are contracted during recreation in water contaminated by drainage from nearby farmland.

■ MAJOR THREATS TO LIFE

- ARDS
- Hypotensive shock
- Hemorrhage secondary to disseminated intravascular coagulation

■ BEDSIDE

Quick Look Test

Does the patient appear to be severely ill and in shock?

    A patient in shock will usually appear distressed, ill, and apprehensive. She will appear pale and have cold and clammy skin.

Vital Signs

    A patient with TSS will be in hypotensive shock with a systolic blood pressure of ≤90 mm Hg and tachycardia. Furthermore, the patient might have postural hypotension. Changes in blood pressure (BP) and pulse should be measured when the patient is assisted in sitting or standing from a supine position. A fall in systolic or diastolic BP of >15 mm Hg or a rise in pulse of >15 beats/min is evidence of orthostatic hypotension.

Selective History and Chart Review

1. Has the patient menstruated recently?
2. Does the patient use tampons?
3. Has the patient had a history of TSS?
4. Has the patient suffered any type of trauma or surgical procedure that might provide a portal of entry for bacteria?
5. Has the patient had any recent exposure to livestock or engaged in any outdoor activities such as hiking and camping, which would place her at risk for Rocky Mountain spotted fever or leptospirosis?

Selective Physical Examination

Dermatological	Sunburn-like macular rash
	Desquamation of the palms or soles
Head and neck	"Strawberry" tongue
	Hyperemia of the pharynx
	Conjunctivitis
Abdominal	Tender to palpation
Pelvic	
External genitalia and vagina	Hyperemia of the vagina
	Vaginal discharge
	Tampon or diaphragm may be found in the vagina
Cervix	Hyperemia of the cervix
Uterus and adnexae	Adnexal tenderness

■ DIAGNOSTIC TESTING

There are no specific laboratory tests that are pathognomonic for TSS. Instead, the diagnosis is based on a constellation of physical findings and laboratory tests. The case definition proposed in 1982 by the Centers for Disease Control and Prevention for TSS is as follows:

1. **Fever (≥38.9°C or ≥102°F)**
2. **Diffuse macular rash**
3. **Desquamation occurring 1 to 2 weeks after the onset of illness**
4. **Hypotension or orthostatic syncope**

5. **Involvement of three or more of the following organ systems:**
   a. Gastrointestinal system (vomiting or diarrhea at onset of illness)
   b. Muscular system (myalgia, creatine phosphokinase level $2\times$ normal)
   c. Mucous membranes (vaginal, oropharyngeal, or conjunctival hyperemia)
   d. Renal system (blood urea nitrogen [BUN] or creatinine level $\geq 2\times$ normal or urinalysis with ≥ 5 white blood cells per high-power field in the absence of urinary tract infection)
   e. Hepatic system (total bilirubin, serum glutamic-oxoloacetic transaminase [SGOT], or serum glutamic-pyruvic transaminase [SGPT] $2\times$ normal level)
   f. Hematological system (platelets $\leq 100,000/mm^3$)
   g. Central nervous system (disorientation or alterations in consciousness without focal neurological signs in the absence of fever and hypotension)
6. **Negative throat and cerebrospinal fluid cultures**
7. **Negative serological tests for Rocky Mountain spotted fever, leptospirosis, and rubeola**

   Tests that are often abnormal and therefore helpful in confirming the diagnosis of TSS are listed below along with the frequency with which abnormal findings are encountered.

1. **CBC with differential**
   a. Anemia (60%)
   b. Leukocytosis (60%)
2. **Coagulation studies**
   a. Thrombocytopenia (55%)
   b. Prolonged PT (55%)
   c. Prolonged PTT (50%)
3. **Blood chemistries**
   a. Hypoproteinemia (80%)
   b. Hypokalemia (80%)
   c. Elevated SGOT (75%)
   d. Hypocalcemia (70%)
   e. Elevated serum creatinine (65%)
   f. Hypophosphatemia (60%)
   g. Elevated lactate dehydrogenase (60%)
   h. Elevated creatine phosphokinase (CPK) (55%)
   i. Elevated BUN (55%)
   j. Hyponatremia (50%)
   k. Elevated SGPT (50%)
4. **Urinalysis**
   a. Sterile pyuria (80%)
   b. Proteinuria (60%)
   c. Hematuria (60%)
5. **Serological studies**

Acute and convalescent serological testing can rule out the following infections, which can present in a fashion similar to TSS:

a. Rocky Mountain spotted fever
b. Leptospirosis
c. Rubeola

6. **Cultures for *Staphylococcus aureus***

If physical examination does not reveal an obvious site of entry, cultures should be obtained from the vagina, rectum, conjunctivae, oropharynx, and nares. Blood, urine, and cerebrospinal fluid can also be cultured.

7. **Arterial blood gas**

a. Metabolic acidemia (80%)
b. Hypoxemia

8. **Chest x-ray**

a. Diffuse infiltrations consistent with ARDS
b. Pulmonary edema

■ MANAGEMENT

1. **Fluid resuscitation**

Aggressive fluid resuscitation is the initial step in the management of patients with TSS. Patients can require >8 L of fluid/day.

2. **Hemodynamic monitoring**

A pulmonary artery catheter (Swan-Ganz catheter) and arterial line will provide intensive hemodynamic monitoring that is necessary for the maintenance of cardiac output and blood pressure. Normal pulmonary artery catheter measurements are listed in Table 33–1.

4. **Vasopressor therapy**

Dopamine, a vasoactive amine, has a positive inotropic effect resulting in increased myocardial contractility and heart rate. Furthermore, dopamine increases organ perfusion through vasodilation of the renal, mesenteric, coronary, and cerebral vasculatures. Dosage is as follows: **dopamine 5 μg/kg/min by IV infusion with dose increased by 5 μg/kg/min increments to a maximum of 50 μg/mg/min.**

The dose is monitored by Swan-Ganz catheter measurements of pulmonary artery and wedge pressure.

5. **Respiratory support**

Oxygen should be administered by face mask or nasal cannula at a flow rate of 8 to 10 L/min. Arterial blood gas determination should be used to monitor the patient. Intubation may be necessary in the acutely ill patient.

6. **Beta-lactamase–resistant antistaphylococcal antibiotics**

a. **Nafcillin sodium 500 to 1000 mg IV every 4 hours**

Table 33–1 □ **NORMAL CENTRAL HEMODYNAMIC MEASUREMENTS IN NONPREGNANT AND PREGNANT PATIENTS**

	Nonpregnant	Pregnant
Cardiac output (L/min)	4.3 ± 0.9	6.2 ± 1.0
Heart rate (beats/min)	71 ± 10.0	83 ± 10.0
Systemic vascular resistance (dyne $\times$ cm $\times$ sec^{-5})	1530 ± 520	1210 ± 266
Pulmonary vascular resistance (dyne $\times$ cm $\times$ sec^{-5})	119 ± 47.0	78 ± 22
Colloid oncotic pressure (mm Hg)	20.8 ± 1.0	18.0 ± 1.5
Colloid oncotic pressure–pulmonary capillary wedge pressure (mm Hg)	14.5 ± 2.5	10.5 ± 2.7
Mean arterial pressure (mm Hg)	86.4 ± 7.5	90.3 ± 5.8
Pulmonary capillary wedge pressure (mm Hg)	6.3 ± 2.1	7.5 ± 1.8
Central venous pressure (mm Hg)	3.7 ± 2.6	3.6 ± 2.5
Left ventricular stroke work index (g $\times$ m $\times$ m^{-2})	41 ± 8	48 ± 6

From Clark SL, Cotton DB, Lee W, et al: Central hemodynamic assessment of normal term pregnancy. Am J Obstet Gynecol 1989; 161:1439.

 b. In patients who are allergic to penicillin, vancomycin should be administered: **vancomycin hydrochloride 500 mg IV every 4 hours**

7. **Treatment of coagulopathy**

 a. **Platelets**

  Platelets should be transfused for a platelet count of <20,000/mm^3. Each unit of platelets should increase the platelet count by 5000 to 10,000/mm^3.

 b. **Fresh frozen plasma**

  Fresh frozen plasma (FFP) is transfused for coagulopathy due to clotting factor deficiency, manifested by a PT or PTT that is >1.5 times normal. Each unit of FFP will increase any clotting factor by 2 to 3%. The usual initial dose is 2 units, and each unit has a volume of 200 to 250 ml.

 c. **Cryoprecipitate**

  Cryoprecipitate is transfused for coagulopathy due to deficiency of factor VIII, von Willebrand factor, factor XIII, fibrinogen, or fibronectin. Cryoprecipitate is concentrated from FFP, and each bag has a volume of 10 to 15 ml. Each bag contains at least 150 mg of fibrinogen.

34

VULVAR LESIONS AND ULCERS

■ BACKGROUND AND DEFINITIONS

Vulvar lesions and ulcers can be placed into one of the following four categories:

Infectious lesions: Many are caused by sexually transmitted diseases

Vulvar dystrophies: Nonneoplastic epithelial disorders of the vulvar skin and mucosa

Vulvar malignancies: Most often encountered in postmenopausal women; the most common vulvar malignancy is squamous cell carcinoma

Vulvar trauma: Can be a result of sexual assault, vaginal delivery, or saddle-injury falls

■ CLINICAL PRESENTATION

Vulvar pain
Vulvar bleeding
Itching or burning
Inguinal lymphadenopathy
Vulvar rash, papule, or nodule
Vulvar vesicles or ulcer, with or without pain

■ PHONE CALL

Questions

1. **What is the patient's age?**
   Vulvar lesions and ulcers caused by sexually transmitted diseases are more common in younger patients who are sexually active, especially with multiple partners. Vulvar dystrophy and malignancy are encountered more commonly in older patients.
2. **What are the patient's symptoms, and how severe are those symptoms?**
   Severe vulvar pain is usually associated with genital herpes, chancroid, and granuloma inguinale. Vulvar itching is usually associated with yeast vulvovaginitis, scabies, pediculosis pubis, vulvar dystrophy, and vulvar malignancy.

3. Has the patient suffered any trauma?

Trauma from falls can result in vulvar trauma such as "saddle injuries." Vulvar trauma can also be caused by sexual assault.

Orders

1. Prepare the patient for a pelvic examination and have materials available for vaginal smears, vulvar biopsy, dark-field smear, herpes culture, chlamydia culture, and bacterial culture
2. Obtain a Venereal Disease Research Laboratory (VDRL) test if the patient has a painless vulvar ulcer
3. Obtain a complete blood count (CBC) if the patient had suffered trauma or assault

Degree of Urgency

Vulvar lesions and ulcers may be extremely uncomfortable but are rarely life threatening. Therefore, patients do not usually need to be seen immediately.

■ ELEVATOR THOUGHTS

What are causes of vulvar lesions and ulcers?

1. Infection
   a. Genital herpes simplex virus (HSV)

   Genital herpes is a sexually transmitted disease caused by HSV. HSV type 2 (HSV-2) causes approximately 85% of primary genital herpes, and HSV type 1 (HSV-1) is responsible for 15%. Genital herpes is endemic in the United States. The incidence of symptomatic disease is 1 to 2%, and 50 to 80% of adults have antibodies to HSV. Genital herpes is a recurrent disease, and HSV-2 has a frequency of recurrence that is three to four times higher than that of HSV-1. Nearly 25% of recurrences are asymptomatic and manifested only by viral shedding. Primary infections are characterized by severe local pain with multiple lesions that progress from the vesicular to the ulcerative stages. Clinically, patients may experience prodromal symptoms consisting of mild paresthesia and burning. Inguinal lymphadenopathy is common, and the patient may have systemic symptoms such as fever, malaise, headaches, and myalgia. The incubation period is 3 to 7 days. Patients with primary infections can have lesions for 2 to 6 weeks. Patients with recurrent infection have milder local symptoms and rarely have systemic symptoms. The duration of recurrent infections is also shorter, usually 3 to 5 days. There is currently no cure for HSV infection.

b. **Human papillomavirus (HPV)**

There have been over 60 subtypes of HPVs described, and 21 have been implicated in genital disease. HPV infection is a sexually transmitted disease that results not only in lesions of the lower genital tract, but also in premalignant or dysplastic changes. Condylomata acuminata, also referred to as venereal or genital warts, and low-grade dysplasia of the lower genital tract are usually associated with HPV subtypes 6, 11, 41, 42, 43, and 44. High-grade dysplasia and carcinoma are associated with HPV subtypes 16, 18, 31, 33, 35, 39, 45, 51, 52, and 56.

There are three levels of HPV infection: clinical infection, subclinical infection, and latent infection.

(1) **Clinical infection**

This is manifested by the appearance of genital warts in the lower genital tract. Approximately one-third of patients with clinical infection have vulvar or external involvement alone, another one-third have both external as well as cervical and vaginal or internal involvement, and the remaining one-third have internal involvement alone.

(2) **Subclinical infection**

This is manifested by lesions that are visible only under the magnification of a colposcope or by cytological changes that are detectable by Pap smear.

(3) **Latent infection**

This is detected only by DNA hybridization testing, and no lesions are visible even under magnification.

HPV is highly contagious, with a transmission rate of 25 to 60%. The average incubation period is 3 months. HPV infection undergoes continuous remissions and recurrences. Although the visible lesions can be eradicated, there is no permanent cure for HPV.

c. **Syphilis**

Syphilis is a chronic sexually transmitted infection caused by an anaerobic spirochete, *Treponema pallidum.* It is moderately contagious, with a transmission rate of nearly 10%. The incubation period is 10 to 90 days, with an average of approximately 3 weeks. The clinical course of syphilis is divided into primary, secondary, and tertiary phases.

(1) **Primary syphilis**

The manifestation of primary syphilis is the appearance of a hard, painless chancre. If untreated, the chancre resolves in 3 to 6 weeks, and hematogenous dissemination of the spirochete results in the secondary stage.

(2) Secondary syphilis

Secondary syphilis is a systemic disease that lasts 2 to 6 weeks and is characterized by lymphadenopathy, skin rash, and vulvar condylomata lata. If the patient is untreated, the secondary phase resolves, and the patient enters a latent phase in which there are usually no clinical manifestations. Latent syphilis lasts 2 to 20 years.

(3) Tertiary syphilis

Without treatment, approximately one-third of patients will develop tertiary syphilis, which consists of progressive damage to the central nervous system, cardiovascular system, and musculoskeletal system. Clinical manifestations of tertiary syphilis include tabes dorsalis, generalized paresis, aortic aneurysm, and gummata of soft tissues and bones.

d. Chancroid

Chancroid, also referred to as "soft chancre," is a highly contagious sexually transmitted disease caused by *Haemophilus ducreyi*, a gram-negative nonmotile bacillus. The incubation period is 3 to 5 days. The initial presentation includes vulvar pain and a papule that progresses in 2 to 3 days to a painful, tender ulcer. In 50% of women, a bubo characterized by acute and tender inguinal lymphadenopathy develops 7 to 10 days after the initial lesion. The bubo is unilateral in two-thirds of patients, and if untreated, rupture and the formation of a large ulcer occur.

e. Granuloma inguinale

Granuloma inguinale, also referred to as donovanosis, is caused by *Calymmatobacterium granulomatis*, a nonmotile gram-negative bacillus. It is not highly contagious, and repeated sexual contact or close nonsexual contact is necessary for transmission. The incubation period is 1 to 12 weeks. The initial manifestation is a painless papule or nodule that ulcerates and forms into enlarging, beefy red granulation tissue. There is usually little lymphadenopathy. If untreated, lesions can coalesce and result in vulvar scarring and fibrosis.

f. Lymphogranuloma venereum (LGV)

LGV is a sexually transmitted infection caused by *Chlamydia trachomatis* serotypes L1, L2, and L3. The incubation period is 4 to 21 days. The clinical course of LGV can be divided into three phases, primary, secondary, and tertiary.

(1) Primary LGV

This is manifested by the appearance of a painless papular or vesicular lesion that may progress to an ulcer but heals within a few days.

(2) Secondary LGV

This develops 1 to 4 weeks after the primary lesion

and is characterized by painful inguinal lymphadenopathy that is usually unilateral. Approximately 50% of patients will have systemic symptoms such as fever, myalgias, and malaise. If untreated, the inguinal nodes become enlarged and progressively more tender. The nodes can become matted to each other and become adherent to the subcutaneous tissue and skin. If the femoral lymph nodes also become infected, the inguinal ligament forms a groove between the two groups of nodes. This "groove sign" is found in 10 to 20% of patients.

(3) **Tertiary LGV**

This is characterized by tissue destruction, scarring, and multiple draining sinuses arising from the lymph nodes.

g. **Molluscum contagiosum**

Molluscum contagiosum is caused by a pox virus and is transmitted both sexually and nonsexually by close physical contact. The incubation period is 2 to 7 weeks. The disease is only mildly contagious. The infection is usually asymptomatic, although some patients will complain of pruritus. The characteristic lesion is a smooth papule, 2 to 5 mm in diameter, with an umbilicated center. The lesions are multiple and may number up to 20. The lesions are usually present for 6 to 9 months but can persist for several years.

h. **Scabies**

Scabies is caused by the mite *Sarcoptes scabiei* and is transmitted both sexually and nonsexually by close physical contact. The infection can be widespread throughout the entire body. The mite moves rapidly across the skin at a speed of 2.5 cm/min. The adult female mite digs burrows in the skin and deposits her eggs, which hatch in 3 to 4 days. The entire life span of the mite is 1 month. Clinical manifestations appear 4 to 6 weeks after infection. The primary presentation of scabies is a papular or vesicular rash and gradual onset of severe and intermittent itching, which is usually worse at night.

i. **Pediculosis pubis or crab lice**

Pediculosis pubis is transmitted both sexually and nonsexually by close contact or by fomites. It is caused by *Pthirus pubis,* the crab or pubic louse. The incubation period is 30 days. It is highly contagious, with a transmission rate of 95% after a single sexual encounter. The primary presentation of pubic louse is constant irritation and pruritus due to allergic sensitization to bites.

2. **Vulvar dystrophy**

a. **Squamous cell hyperplasia**

Squamous cell hyperplasia was formerly referred to as

"hyperplastic dystrophy." This lesion is associated with epithelial thickening and hyperkeratosis. However, the clinical appearance of the lesion is highly variable. The primary symptom is itching.

  b. Lichen sclerosus

    The lesion of lichen sclerosus is characterized by epithelial thinning resulting in an atrophic appearance to the vulva and perineum. The primary symptoms are itching and dyspareunia.

  c. Mixed dystrophy

3. Vulvar malignancy

  a. Squamous cell carcinoma

    Squamous cell carcinoma of the vulva accounts for 90% of all vulvar malignancies. It is primarily a disease of older, postmenopausal women. The most common presentation is pruritus.

  b. Melanoma

    Melanoma is the second most common vulvar malignancy, accounting for 5 to 10% of all vulvar malignancies. The most common presenting symptom is a vulvar mass.

4. Vulvar trauma

■ MAJOR THREAT TO LIFE

- Vulvar malignancy

■ BEDSIDE

Quick Look Test

Patients with vulvar lesions will usually not appear to be ill but may appear distressed by the amount of vulvar pain and discomfort.

Vital Signs

Vital signs are usually normal.

Selective History and Chart Review

1. What type of local symptoms, if any, does the patient have?
2. Does the patient have any systemic symptoms such as fever, malaise, or myalgias?
3. Is the patient sexually active?
4. If the patient is sexually active, does the patient's partner have similar symptoms?

5. Does the patient have a history of sexually transmitted diseases?

Patients with prior sexually transmitted diseases are at greater risk of having recurrent disease. This is especially true of genital herpes and human papillomavirus infection.

6. Does the patient have a history of abnormal Pap smears?

Changes on Pap smear such as koilocytotic atypia and multinucleated giant cell can be detected in the presence of cervical HPV and HSV infections, respectively.

7. Has the patient had a previous vulvar biopsy?

A prior vulvar biopsy will often help in confirming the diagnosis of vulvar dystrophy.

8. Is the patient pregnant?

Pregnancy limits the options of antibiotic treatment in patients with vulvar lesions secondary to infection.

Selective Physical Examination (Table 34–1)

Dermatological	Secondary syphilis: maculopapular rash, especially on the palms and soles
Inguinal region	Inguinal lymphadenopathy in: genital herpes simplex, syphilis, and chancroid
	Groove sign in lymphogranuloma venereum
Pelvic	
External genitalia and vagina	Genital herpes: Multiple small vesicles progressing to ulcers
	HPV: genital warts or condylomata acuminata appearing as flesh-colored to gray excrescences that can be broad based or on pedicles, varying in size from a pinpoint to a large cauliflower-like lesion
	Primary syphilis: chancre that is a painless, round or oval ulcer with a sharp border and a firm, button-like base that is initially glistening and later covered with a gray film

Table 34–1 □ DIFFERENTIAL DIAGNOSIS OF GENITAL ULCERS

Characteristic	HSV	Syphilis	Chancroid	Granuloma Inguinale	LGV
Lesion	Multiple vesicles	Single ulcer	Single or multiple ulcers	Single or multiple ulcers	Single ulcer
Depth	Shallow	Shallow	Deep	Elevated	Shallow
Induration	Absent	Hard	Soft	Hard	Absent
Adenopathy	Present	Present	Present	Absent	Present
Pain	Present	Absent	Present	Absent	Variable
Incubation	3–7 days	3 weeks	3–5 days	1–12 weeks	4–21 days

HSV = herpes simplex virus; LGV = lymphogranuloma venereum.

Secondary syphilis: condylomata lata that are raised, white lesions similar to genital warts

Chancroid: tender papule that ulcerates and forms a painful soft ulcer with sharp borders and a base that is covered with a yellow or gray exudate

Granuloma inguinale: painless papule or nodule that progresses to an enlarging, painless ulcer with beefy red granulation tissue

LGV: in early LGV, painless papular or vesicular lesions that progress to ulcers with local edema; in late LGV, ulcerations become invasive and destructive, resulting in severe distortion of the normal anatomy, vaginal stenosis, and fistula formation

Molluscum contagiosum: smooth, firm, spherical papule with a diameter of 2 to 5 mm and a umbilicated center; lesions usually number 1 to 20 but can be more numerous and are found not only on the external genitalia, but also the lower abdominal wall and inner thighs

Scabies: papular erythematous rash often associated with burrows 5 to 10 mm long that have the appearance of wavy lines of dirt

Crab lice: erythema and excoriation secondary to scratching; "blue spots" may appear secondary to the crab louse bite

Squamous cell hyperplasia: gross appearance highly variable and may be affected by chronic scratching; classic lesions are well demarcated and raised with a dusky red or white color

Lichen sclerosus: skin of the vulva and perianal region with a crinkled, pale, parchment-like appearance; labia minora may be absent and vaginal introitus may be stenotic secondary to atrophy; fissure may be present in the natural folds of the skin

Squamous cell cancer: gross appearance variable; initial lesion may be a small itchy nodule that ulcerates; alternatively, lesion may appear as a cauliflower-like growth similar to genital warts

Melanoma: gross appearance similar to melanoma elsewhere on the body; lesions usually pigmented, raised, and may be ulcerated with bleeding; most lesions appear on the labia minora and clitoris

Trauma: highly variable appearance that is dependent on the type of trauma; falls often associated with obvious lacerations and hematomas; trauma from sexual assault may

	appear more subtle with abrasions and erythema
Cervix	Genital herpes: friable and erythematous with multiple ulcers
	HPV: flat or raised coarse white lesions
	Primary syphilis: chancre similar to that found on the vulva
	Chancroid: ulcer similar to that found on the vulva
	Granuloma inguinale: ulcer similar to that found on the vulva
	LGV: papule and ulcer is most commonly found on the posterior lip of the cervix

■ DIAGNOSTIC TESTING

1. Genital herpes simplex

a. Herpes culture

Viral isolation by tissue culture is the most sensitive and specific diagnostic test for genital herpes. Culture usually becomes positive in 1 to 4 days.

b. Serology for herpes simplex virus

Anti-HSV-1 and anti-HSV-2 antibodies can be detected and measured in the acute and convalescent phases.

c. Cytology smear

The finding on Pap smear of multinucleated giant cells is suggestive of genital HSV.

2. Human papillomavirus

HPV infection can usually be diagnosed by the appearance of classic condylomata acuminata. Laboratory testing is necessary only to confirm the diagnosis when the clinical presentation is unclear.

a. Tissue biopsy

Tissue biopsy is the most sensitive and specific diagnostic test for HPV.

b. DNA hybridization testing

DNA hybridization testing can be performed for HPV subtypes 6, 11, 16, and 18. However, up to 30% of women will test positive even in the absence of any lesions.

c. Cytology smear

The cytological finding of koilocytotic atypia is highly suggestive of HPV infection.

3. Syphilis

a. Dark-field microscopy

Dark-field examination is the most specific diagnostic test for syphilis. It is the test of choice in the presence of a chancre, because nonspecific serology such as the VDRL may be nonreactive at this early stage. This test can be performed on lesions of primary and secondary syphilis.

To obtain an adequate specimen, the following steps should be taken:

(1) Cleanse the lesion with normal saline.
(2) Abrade the lesion with a scalpel blade or sterile gauze until bleeding appears.
(3) Express serum from the lesion, and place it on a microscope slide.
(4) Place coverslip over the specimen, and seal the edges with petroleum jelly.

b. Nonspecific serology
(1) VDRL (Venereal Disease Research Laboratory) test: slide flocculation test
(2) RPR (rapid plasma reagin) test: agglutination test

Both of these tests are nonspecific antibody tests for cardiolipin antibodies that are used for the screening of syphilis. Unfortunately, these tests have a high false-positive rate. In patients with syphilis, these tests turn positive 1 to 2 weeks after the appearance of a chancre. Approximately two-thirds of patients who have primary syphilis will have a positive nonspecific serology test, and 99% of patients who have secondary syphilis will be positive. In addition to the qualitative VDRL, quantitative VDRL is sometimes helpful in making the diagnosis of syphilis and is especially useful in monitoring the therapeutic response. Most patients with a false-positive VDRL will have a titer of <1:8, whereas most patients with secondary syphilis will have a titer of at least 1:16. A fourfold rise in the titer is highly suggestive of acute syphilis.

4. Chancroid
a. Gram stain smear
A Gram stain smear of the exudates reveals gram-negative rods in the form of chains that appear as a "school of fish."

b. Culture

5. Granuloma inguinale
a. Tissue smear stained with Giemsa's, Leishman's, or Wright's stain
No culture exists for granuloma inguinale. The diagnosis is best made by crushing a tissue specimen between two microscope slides and staining with an appropriate stain. The diagnosis is made by the demonstration of Donovan bodies, encapsulated bipolar reddish bacteria within a monocyte.

6. Lymphogranuloma venereum
a. LGV complement fixation test
A titer of 1:64 or above is considered to be positive.

b. Microimmunofluorescence test

This test is more specific than the complement fixation test. A titer of 1:512 or above is consistent with LGV.

7. **Molluscum contagiosum**
   a. **Cytological smear**
   b. **Tissue biopsy**
      The diagnosis is confirmed by the demonstration of intracytoplasmic inclusion bodies on biopsy or Pap smear of scrapings of the lesion stained with Giemsa's, Gram, or Wright's stain.

8. **Scabies**
   a. **Microscopic examination of skin scrapings**
      To obtain adequate skin scrapings, a fresh burrow is chosen. Mineral oil is placed on the burrow, and the top of the burrow is scraped with a sterile scalpel. The scrapings are placed on a glass slide and examined for the mite, eggs, or fecal pellets.
   b. **Burrow ink test**
      This test is painless, but there may be false-negative results. To perform the test, a fountain pen is used to cover the papule with ink. An alcohol pad is then used to wipe off the ink, and an examination is performed for a burrow with ink tracking down it forming a dark, wavy line.

9. **Pediculosis pubis or crab lice**
   Visualization with magnifying glass or microscope of the lice, larvae, or eggs.

10. **Vulvar dystrophy or malignancy**
    a. **Vulvar biopsy**

■ MANAGEMENT

1. **Genital herpes simplex**
   a. **Primary infection**
      (1) Acyclovir (Zovirax)
         (a) **400 mg PO three times per day for 7 to 10 days or until clinical resolution is attained** or
         (b) **200 mg PO five times per day for 7 to 10 days or until clinical resolution is attained**
   b. **Recurrent infection**
      (1) Acyclovir (Zovirax)
         (a) **400 mg PO three times per day for 5 days** or
         (b) **800 mg PO two times per day for 5 days**
   c. **Severe, hospitalized patients**
      (1) Acyclovir (Zovirax)
         (a) **5 mg/kg IV every 8 hours for 5 to 7 days**
   d. **Prophylaxis for recurrent infection (≥4 infections per year)**
      (1) Acyclovir (Zovirax)

(a) **400 mg PO two times per day** or
(b) **200 mg PO 2 to 5 times per day**

2. Human papillomavirus

a. 80 to 90% topical trichloroacetic or bichloroacetic acid

The acid is applied in small amounts with a cotton-tipped applicator and can be repeated weekly. Petroleum jelly can be used on adjacent normal skin to prevent spreading or running of the acid. These acids work best on mucosal warts such as those on the cervix and on the vaginal side walls but can also be used for external cutaneous warts. Most important, these acids can be used during pregnancy.

b. Podofilox (Condylox) 0.5% solution or podophyllin resin 10 to 25% solution in benzoin

The recommended use of podofilox is to apply the solution twice daily, morning and evening, for 3 consecutive days followed by a hiatus of 4 days. This weekly regimen can be repeated up to four times or until no visible warts are seen.

Podophyllin is applied to the lesions and allowed to dry. It is washed off after 3 to 4 hours, although subsequent applications can be washed off after 24 hours. Applications can be repeated once or twice weekly until the lesions have disappeared.

Because of the potential complications of myelotoxicity and neurotoxicity, these agents cannot be used in pregnancy and furthermore cannot be used in the vagina or on the cervix.

c. Local sharp excision

Excision with a scalpel is most appropriate for large pedunculated lesions.

d. Carbon dioxide laser vaporization

Laser vaporization can be performed with colposcopic guidance to magnify small and subtle lesions. Laser vaporization is the treatment of choice for extensive disease. It can be used for internal lesions on the cervix and vaginal wall and external lesions of the vulva.

e. Electrocauterization

f. Cryocautery

Cryocautery is most appropriate for small lesions.

3. Syphilis

a. Primary, secondary, or early latent syphilis

(1) **Benzathine penicillin G 2.4 million units IM once** or
(2) **Doxycycline 100 mg PO two times per day for 2 weeks** or
(3) **Tetracycline 500 mg PO four times per day for 2 weeks** or

        (4) **Erythromycin 500 mg PO four times per day for 2 weeks**

    b. **Late latent syphilis of undertermined duration**

        (1) **Benzathine penicillin G 2.4 million units IM weekly for 3 weeks** or

        (2) **Doxycycline 100 mg PO two times per day for 4 weeks** or

        (3) **Tetracycline 500 mg PO four times per day for 4 weeks** or

        (4) **Erythromycin 500 mg PO four times per day for 4 weeks**

4. **Chancroid**

    a. **Azithromycin 1 PO once** or

    b. **Ceftriaxone 250 mg IM once** or

    c. **Erythromycin 500 mg PO four times per day for 7 days** or

    d. **Ciprofloxacin 500 mg PO two times per day for 3 days**

5. **Granuloma inguinale**

    a. **Tetracycline 500 mg PO four times per day for 21 days** or

    b. **Erythromycin 500 mg PO four times per day for 21 days**

6. **Lymphogranuloma venereum**

    a. **Doxycycline 100 mg PO two times per day for 21 days** or

    b. **Erythromycin 500 mg PO four times per day for 21 days** or

    c. **Sulfisoxazole 500 mg PO four times per day for 21 days**

7. **Molluscum contagiosum**

    a. **Sharp scraping of the lesion followed by electrocautery or application of silver nitrate, trichloroacetic acid, or carbonic acid** or

    b. **Cryocautery of the lesions**

8. **Scabies**

    Any of the following three drugs can be used. Clothing and linen should be cleaned in hot water or should be dry-cleaned.

    a. **Crotamiton (Eurax) 10% cream or lotion** applied as follows:

        (1) Take routine shower or bath

        (2) Apply cream or lotion from neck down to toes

        (3) Repeat application 24 hours later

        (4) Take a cleansing bath 48 hours after last application

        Crotamiton can be used in pregnant and lactating women.

    b. **Lindane (Kwell) 1% cream or lotion** applied from neck down, left on for 8 to 12 hours, then washed off.

        Because this drug does not kill the eggs, treatment should be repeated in 1 week. Lindane is not recommended for pregnant or lactating women.

    c. **Permethrin (Elimite) 5% cream** applied once on the skin from head to toes and washed off with shower or bath in 8 to 14 hours.

Permethrin can be used in pregnant and lactating women.

9. **Pediculosis pubis**
    a. **Lindane (Kwell) 1% cream or lotion** applied to affected area for 8 to 12 hours, then washed off.

    As an alternative, **Lindane (Kwell) 1% shampoo** applied for 4 minutes, then washed off. Lindane is not recommended for pregnant or lactating women.
    b. **Pyrethrins (A-200 Pediculicide shampoo and gel)** applied to dry hair or other affected areas for 10 minutes, then washed off.

    With either drug, repeat treatment may be necessary in 1 week if lice or eggs are still seen. Clothing and bed linen used by the patient within the past 2 days should be washed in hot water or should be dry-cleaned.

10. **Squamous cell hyperplasia**
    a. **Fluocinolone acetonide 0.025% or 0.01% cream or lotion applied two or three times per day** or
    b. **Triamcinolone acetonide 0.01% cream or lotion applied two or three times per day**

11. **Lichen sclerosus**
    a. **Testosterone propionate 2% in petroleum jelly applied locally two or three times per day** for at least 3 to 6 months or until pruritus is relieved.

    The frequency of application can then be reduced to a maintenance dose of once or twice per week.
    b. **Mixture of 1% or 2.5% hydrocortisone and testosterone propionate 2% in petroleum jelly applied locally two or three times per day** can be used in patients with severe pruritus.
    c. **Triamcinolone (10 mg/ml) diluted 2:1 in saline injected intradermally in an amount of 0.1 ml at 1-cm intervals over the affected area** can be used if the above measures do not result in relief of pruritus.

    After the injection, the tissue should be massaged gently.

35

VULVOVAGINAL INFECTIONS

■ BACKGROUND AND DEFINITION

Vulvovaginal infections: Infections involving the vulva and vagina resulting in symptoms of vaginal discharge, itching, burning, dyspareunia, or foul odor

Vulvovaginal infection is one of the most common gynecological problems in adult women. The symptoms of vaginal discharge and itching are often the primary complaints of women presenting to an urgent care facility or even an emergency room. Furthermore, acute vulvovaginal infection can affect women admitted to any inpatient service. Most patients with vulvovaginitis have one of the following three common infections (Table 35–1): (1) yeast or *Candida* vulvovaginitis caused by *Candida albicans* and other *Candida* species, (2) bacterial vaginosis caused by *Gardnerella vaginalis* and other anaerobic vaginal bacteria, or (3) *Trichomonas* vulvovaginitis caused by the protozoan *Trichomonas vaginalis*. The evaluation of a patient with a vulvovaginal infection can be accomplished in the matter of minutes, and the treatment is often simple and effective.

■ CLINICAL PRESENTATION

Vaginal itching or burning
Vaginal discharge
Malodorous discharge
Dyspareunia
Vulvar or vaginal erythema

■ PHONE CALL

Questions

1. **What symptoms is the patient complaining of?**
2. **Does the patient have pelvic pain or a fever?**
   These symptoms would be suggestive of pelvic inflammatory disease (PID).

Orders

1. Prepare the patient for a pelvic examination, and have available materials necessary for the preparation of wet smears

Table 35-1 □ COMPARISON OF THE THREE MOST COMMON VULVOVAGINAL INFECTIONS

	Yeast Vulvovaginitis	Bacterial Vaginosis	Trichomonas Vulvovaginitis
Cause	*Candida* species	*Gardnerella vaginalis*, mixed anaerobes	*Trichomonas vaginalis*
Major symptoms	Itching, burning	Malodorous, watery discharge	Itching, burning, variable
Discharge	White, cottage cheese	White, skim milk	Frothy, variable
Odor	Absent	Present	Variable
Vulvovaginal inflammation	Present	Absent	Variable
Vaginal wet smear	Hyphae, spores	"Clue cells"	Trichomonads
"Whiff test"	Negative	Positive	Negative
Vaginal pH	Normal, 3–4	Basic, 5–6	Basic, 6–7
Treatment	Antifungal drugs	Metronidazole	Metronidazole

of the vaginal discharge with both normal saline and 10% potassium hydroxide solutions
2. Obtain a complete blood count (CBC) with differential if the patient has signs and symptoms of PID
3. Obtain cervical cultures for *Chlamydia trachomatis* and *Neisseria gonorrhoeae* if PID is suspected.

Degree of Urgency

Vulvovaginal infection is rarely serious or life-threatening and the patient does not need to be seen immediately.

■ ELEVATOR THOUGHTS

What is the differential diagnosis of vulvovaginal infection?
- Cervicitis
- PID
- Normal physiological cervical discharge

■ BEDSIDE

Quick Look Test

Patients with vulvovaginal infection will not usually appear ill or distressed. If the patient appears ill and is febrile, PID should be suspected.

Vital Signs

Patients with vulvovaginal infections will usually have normal vital signs. The finding of fever is suggestive of PID.

Selective History and Chart Review

1. Is the patient pregnant?
    Certain antibiotics are contraindicated in pregnancy. Furthermore, pregnancy increases the risk of yeast vulvovaginitis.
2. How long has the patient had symptoms of a vulvovaginal infection?
3. Does the patient have a history of recurrent vulvovaginal infections?
4. Does the patient have a history of any sexually transmitted diseases?
5. Is the patient on antibiotics?

Chronic use of antibiotics can predispose to vulvovaginitis.

6. Is the patient using oral contraceptive pills?

The use of birth control pills increases the risk of vulvovaginal infection.

Selective Physical Examination

Abdominal	Soft and nontender; a tender abdomen, especially with guarding and rebound tenderness, is suggestive of PID
Pelvic	
External genitalia and vagina	Yeast vulvovaginitis: erythematous with a white "cottage cheese"–like discharge
	Bacterial vaginosis: nonerythematous with white, watery, skim milk–like malodorous discharge
	Trichomonas vulvovaginitis: erythematous with frothy, foul-smelling discharge
	PID and cervicitis: normal
Cervix	*Trichomonas* vulvovaginitis: erythematous "flea-bitten" or "strawberry" cervix, often friable and bleeding
	PID and cervicitis: usually with mucopurulent discharge with cervical motion tenderness
Uterus and adnexae	PID: usually tender to palpation

In any case of vulvovaginitis, the pelvic examination can be normal with the absence of discharge, and therefore, confirmation of the diagnosis should depend on laboratory testing and not just pelvic examination. The clinical manifestations of *Trichomonas* vulvovaginitis are especially variable, with an estimated 10 to 50% of infected women being asymptomatic.

■ DIAGNOSTIC TESTING (see Table 35–1)

1. **Yeast vulvovaginitis**
   a. **Vaginal wet smear with 10% potassium hydroxide**
      Hyphae and spores are noted.
   b. **Vaginal fungal culture**
      Vaginal cultures are rarely necessary to make the diagnosis of vulvovaginitis. Fungal cultures are indicated only in patients with symptoms of yeast vulvovaginitis with negative vaginal wet smears.
2. **Bacteria vaginosis**
   a. **Vaginal wet smear with normal saline shows "clue cells"**
      In patients with bacterial vaginosis, clue cells are vaginal epithelial cells with a stippled cell wall because of the ad-

herence of the causative bacteria onto the cell wall. The presence of clue cells signifies a high concentration of bacteria and is a more sensitive indicator of clinical infection than cultures.

   b. **Positive "whiff test" or amine test**

   A positive whiff test or amine test is the detection of a fishy or nitrogen odor when vaginal secretions are mixed with 10% potassium hydroxide.

   c. **pH of vaginal secretions is basic with a pH value of 5 to 6**

   The pH of normal vaginal secretions is acidic with a pH value of 3 to 4. Patients with bacterial vaginosis have a more basic vaginal secretion with a pH of 5 to 6.

3. *Trichomonas* **vulvovaginitis**

   a. **Normal saline shows motile trichomonads and abundant white blood cells**

   The diagnosis of this vulvovaginal infection is most easily made because of the finding of the motile trichomonas protozoa on vaginal wet smear. The organism has an ovoid body and a posterior flagellum and is usually found moving in circles in a jerky fashion.

   b. **Trichomonads can occasionally be detected on routine cervical Pap smear**

   c. **pH of vaginal secretions is very basic with a pH of 6 to 7**

■ MANAGEMENT

1. **Yeast vulvovaginitis**
   a. **Acute infection**
      (1) Antifungal medication (Table 35–2)
   b. **Recurrent infection**
      (1) **Clotrimazole 500 mg vaginal suppository weekly** or
      (2) **Fluconazole 150 mg tablet PO once a month** or
      (3) **Ketoconazole 200 mg tablet PO daily** or
      (4) **Ketoconazole 400 mg tablet PO daily for 5 days each month starting with menses**
      (5) Eliminate predisposing causes

Yeast or candidal infection is usually caused by *Candida albicans*, although approximately 10% of cases are caused by *Candida glabrata*. One or more species of *Candida* can be recovered in approximately 30% of pregnant and 15% of nonpregnant asymptomatic women. These asymptomatic patients do not require treatment. In symptomatic patients, yeast vaginitis can usually be easily and effectively treated with any of several antifungal imidazole and triazole derivatives, many of which are now available over the counter. These medications are available in the form of a vaginal cream or vaginal suppository

Table 35–2 □ **ANTIFUNGAL MEDICATIONS FOR ACUTE YEAST VULVOVAGINITIS**

Medication	Formulation	Dose
Butoconazole		
Femstat	2% vaginal cream	5 g every night for 3 nights
Clotrimazole		
Gyne-Lotrimin	100-mg vaginal tablet	1 tablet every night for 7 nights
	1% vaginal cream	5 g every night for 7 nights
Mycelex-G	500-mg vaginal tablet	1 tablet once
Mycelex-7	100-mg vaginal insert	1 insert every night for 7 nights
	1% vaginal cream	5 g every night for 7 nights
Fluconazole		
Diflucan	150-mg oral tablet	1 tablet orally once
Miconazole		
Monistat 3	200-mg suppository	1 every night for 3 nights
Monistat 7	2% cream	5 g every night for 7 nights
	100-mg suppository	1 every night for 7 nights
Terconazole		
Terazol 3	80-mg suppository	1 every night for 3 nights
	0.8% vaginal cream	5 g every night for 3 nights
Terazol 7	0.4% vaginal cream	5 g every night for 7 nights
Tioconazole		
Vagistat-1	6.5% ointment	4.6 g once

or an oral pill. All of these antifungal agents have comparable efficacy, with cure rates greater than 90%.

Despite this high cure rate, some patients continue to have recurrent yeast infections, and this is often frustrating to both the patients and their physicians. A patient is considered to have recurrent yeast vulvovaginitis if she has four or more episodes of yeast vulvovaginitis in a year. Possible causes of recurrent yeast infections are listed in Table 35–3. Unfortunately in many patients, no specific cause is found. Nevertheless, the management of patients with recurrent yeast infection begins with the elimination of these causes where possible. Oral antifungal medication has been recommended to decrease the amount of yeast in the gastrointestinal tract. Both oral ketoconazole and fluconazole have been shown to be effective in treating patients with recurrent infections. The weekly use of a 500-mg clotrimazole vaginal suppository has also been shown to be effective.

2. Bacterial vaginosis
   a. **Metronidazole (Flagyl) 500 mg PO two times per day for 7 days** or

Table 35–3 ▫ CAUSES OF RECURRENT YEAST VULVOVAGINITIS

Diabetes mellitus
Immunosuppressed state
    Steroid treatment
    Chemotherapy administration
    AIDS
Antibiotic therapy
Oral contraceptive pills
Pregnancy
Increased yeast colonization of the gastrointestinal tract
Infection with *Candida* species resistant to current antifungal drugs

---

    b. **Metronidazole 0.75% vaginal gel (MetroGel-Vaginal) 5 g (1 applicator full) intravaginally two times per day for 5 days** or

    c. **Cleocin 2% vaginal cream 5 g (1 applicator full) intravaginally every night for 7 days** or

    d. **Ampicillin 500 mg PO four times per day for 7 days** for patients allergic to metronidazole or in the first trimester of pregnancy or

    e. **Cephradine 500 mg PO four times per day for 7 days** for patients allergic to penicillin and in whom metronidazole is contraindicated

    Bacterial vaginosis has implications beyond that of a vulvovaginal infection. A positive correlation has been found between bacterial vaginosis and premature labor as well as PID. Metronidazole has a cure rate of 90 to 95%. Broad-spectrum antibiotics such as ampicillin, erythromycin, and doxycycline are somewhat less effective, with cure rates of 40 to 50%. Sulfonamide-containing vaginal creams are also only minimally effective. Based on the Food and Drug Administration classification of drugs with regard to possible adverse fetal effects, metronidazole is a category B drug because of findings of carcinogenic effects on rodents. Although human studies have not shown any increase in congenital anomalies in infants born to women who used metronidazole in pregnancy, it is recommended that the drug be avoided in the first trimester of pregnancy. Patients being treated with metronidazole should be warned to avoid ingestion of alcohol.

3. *Trichomonas* **vulvovaginitis**

    a. **Metronidazole (Flagyl) 250 mg PO three times per day for 7 days** or

    b. **Metronidazole (Flagyl) 2.0 g PO once** or

    c. **Clotrimazole (Gyne-Lotrimin or Mycelex-7) 100-mg vaginal tablet every night for 7 nights or 1% vaginal cream 5**

g every night for 7 nights for patients in the first trimester of pregnancy

Trichomonas vulvovaginitis is a sexually transmitted disease, and therefore, patients should be advised to have their partners evaluated and treated if necessary. Approximately 40 to 60% of male partners of infected women will harbor the organism. The 7-day regimen of metronidazole has been shown to be slightly superior to the one-time dose. However, if poor patient compliance is suspected, the one-time dose should be prescribed. As discussed above, metronidazole should not be prescribed for women in the first trimester of pregnancy. Intravaginal clotrimazole should be used in these patients, although the cure rate is significantly lower than that of metronidazole. Patients taking metronidazole should not ingest alcohol.

APPENDIX A

GUIDELINES, ILLUSTRATIONS, AND TABLES FOR OBSTETRICS

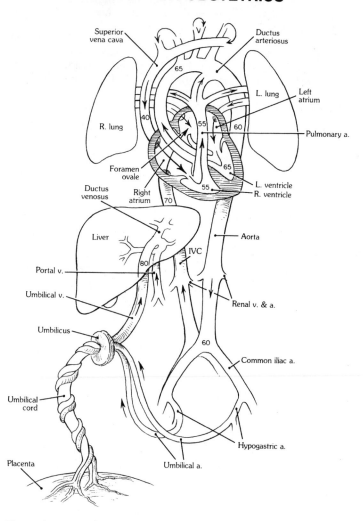

Figure A–1 □ Normal fetal circulation. (From Parer JJ: Fetal circulation. In Sciarra JJ, ed: Obstetrics and Gynecology, Vol 3, Maternal and Fetal Medicine. Hagerstown, MD, Harper & Row, 1984, p 2.)

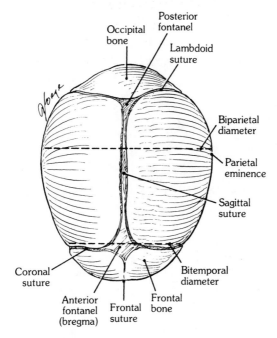

Figure A–2 □ Superior view of fetal skull and diameters. (From Hacker NF, Moore JG: Essentials of Obstetrics and Gynecology, 2nd ed. Philadelphia, WB Saunders Co, 1992, p 110.)

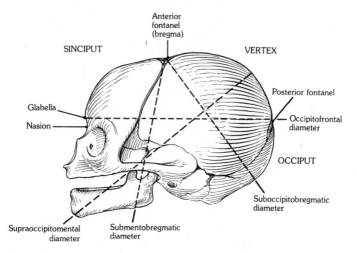

Figure A–3 □ Lateral view of fetal skull and diameters. (From Hacker NF, Moore JG: Essentials of Obstetrics and Gynecology, 2nd ed. Philadelphia, WB Saunders Co, 1992, p 111.)

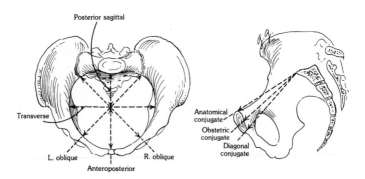

Figure A–4 □ Pelvic inlet. (From Hacker NF, Moore JG: Essentials of Obstetrics and Gynecology, 2nd ed. Philadelphia, WB Saunders Co, 1992, p 113.)

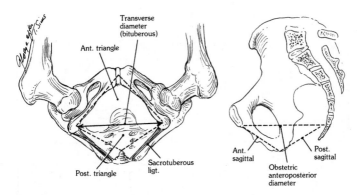

Figure A–5 □ Pelvic outlet. (From Hacker NF, Moore JG: Essentials of Obstetrics and Gynecology, 2nd ed. Philadelphia, WB Saunders Co, 1992, p 114.)

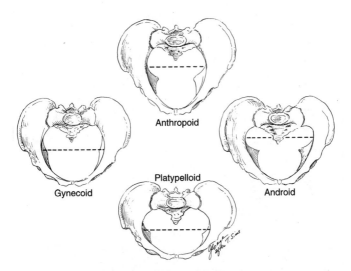

Figure A–6 □ Pelvic types. (From Hacker NF, Moore JG: Essentials of Obstetrics and Gynecology, 2nd ed. Philadelphia, WB Saunders Co, 1992, p 115.)

1. Head floating, before engagement

5. Complete extension

2. Engagement; descent, flexion

6. Restitution (external rotation)

3. Further descent, internal rotation

7. Delivery of anterior shoulder

4. Complete rotation, beginning extension

8. Delivery of posterior shoulder

Figure A–7 □ Movements in the mechanism of labor and delivery, left occiput anterior position. (From Cunningham FG, MacDonald PC, Gant NF, et al: Williams Obstetrics, 19th ed. Norwalk, Connecticut, Appleton & Lange, 1993, p 364.)

Figure A–8 ▫ Oxygen dissociation curves of fetal and maternal blood at pH 7.4 and 37°C. (From Hellegers AE, Schruefer JJ: Nomograms and empirical equations relating oxygen tension, percentage saturation, and pH in maternal and fetal blood. Am J Obstet Gynecol 1961;81:377.)

Figure A–9 ▫ Technique for measuring amniotic fluid index. The uterus is divided into quadrants. The transducer is held perpendicular to the floor, and the largest vertical pocket of amniotic fluid without loops of umbilical cord is measured in each quadrant and summed. (From Creasy RK, Resnik R: Maternal-Fetal Medicine: Principles and Practice, 3rd ed. Philadelphia, WB Saunders Co, 1994, p 621.)

Figure A–10 □ Mean and percentiles for amniotic fluid index. (Redrawn from Moore TR, Cayle JE: Amniotic fluid index in normal human pregnancy. Am J Obstet Gynecol 1990;162:1168.)

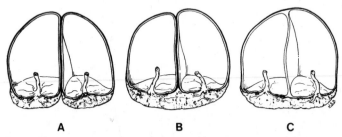

Figure A–11 □ Placenta and membranes in twin gestations. *A,* Two placentas, diamniotic, dichorionic (from either dizygotic or monozygotic twins). *B,* Single placenta, diamniotic, dichorionic (from either dizygotic or monozygotic twins). *C,* Single placenta, diamniotic, monochorionic (from monozygotic twins). (From Cunningham FG, MacDonald PC, Gant NF, et al: Williams Obstetrics, 19th ed. Norwalk, Connecticut, Appleton & Lange, 1993, p 892.)

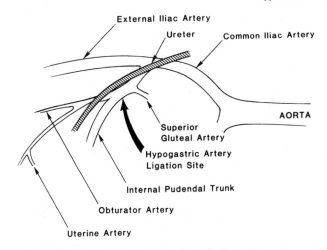

Figure A–12 □ Site of hypogastric artery ligation. (From Creasy RK, Resnik R: Maternal-Fetal Medicine: Principles and Practice, 3rd ed. Philadelphia, WB Saunders Co, 1994, p 882.)

Figure A–13 □ Amniotic fluid phospholipid levels and gestational age. L/S = lecithin/sphingomyelin ratio; PG = phosphatidylglycerol; PI = phosphatidylinositol. (Data from Gluck L, et al: Am J Obstet Gynecol 1974;120:142, and Hallman M, et al: Am J Obstet Gynecol 1976;125:613, as shown in Jobe A: The developmental biology of the lung. In Fanaroff AA, Martin RJ, eds: Neonatal-Perinatal Medicine. St. Louis, Mosby-Year Book, 1992, p 792. From Creasy RK, Resnik R: Maternal-Fetal Medicine: Principles and Practice, 3rd ed. Philadelphia, WB Saunders Co, 1994, p 435.)

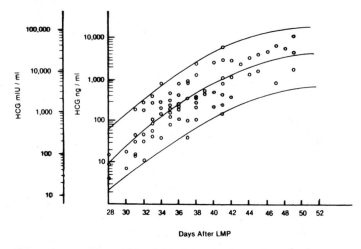

Figure A–14 □ Rise in serum hCG in normal intrauterine pregnancies. LMP = last menstrual period. (From Pittaway DE, Reish RL, Wentz AC: Doubling times of human chorionic gonadotropin increase in early viable intrauterine pregnancies. Am J Obstet Gynecol 1985;152:299.)

Table A–1 □ **COMPONENTS OF THE FETAL CIRCULATION**

Fetal Structure	From/To	Adult Remnant
Umbilical vein	Umbilicus/ductus venosus	Ligamentum teres hepatis
Ductus venosus	Umbilical vein/inferior vena cava (bypasses liver)	Ligamentum venosum
Foramen ovale	Right atrium/left atrium	Closed atrial wall
Ductus arteriosus	Pulmonary artery/descending aorta	Ligamentum arteriosum
Umbilical artery	Common iliac artery/ umbilicus	Superior vesical arteries Lateral vesicoumbilical ligaments

Adapted from Main DM, Main EK: Obstetrics and Gynecology, A Pocket Reference. Chicago, Year Book, 1984, p 34.

Table A–2 □ COMMON LABORATORY VALUES IN PREGNANCY

Test	Normal Range (Nonpregnant)	Change in Pregnancy	Timing
Serum Chemistries			
Albumin	3.5–4.8 g/dl	→ 1 g/dl	Most by 20 wk, then gradual
Calcium (total)	9–10.3 mg/dl	→ 10%	Gradual fall
Chloride	95–105 mEq/L	No significant change	Gradual rise
Creatinine	0.6–1.1 mg/dl	→ 0.3 mg/dl	Most by 20 wk
Fibrinogen	1.5–3.6 g/L	↑ 1–2 g/L	Progressive
Glucose, fasting (plasma)	65–105 mg/dl	→ 10%	Gradual fall
Potassium (plasma)	3.5–4.5 mEq/L	→ 0.2–0.3 mEq/L	By 20 wk
Protein (total)	6.5–8.5 g/dl	→ 1 g/dl	By 20 wk, then stable
Sodium	135–145 mEq/L	→ 2–4 mEq/L	By 20 wk, then stable
Urea nitrogen	12–30 mg/dl	→ 50%	First trimester
Uric acid	3.5–8 mg/dl	→ 33%	First trimester, rise at term
Urinary Chemistries			
Creatinine	15–25 mg/kg/day (1–1.4 g/day)	No significant change	
Protein	Up to 150 mg/day	Up to 250–300 mg/day	By 20 wk
Creatinine clearance	90–130 ml/min per 1.73 m²	↑ 40–50%	By 16 wk

Table continued on following page

Table A–2 □ COMMON LABORATORY VALUES IN PREGNANCY *Continued*

Test	Normal Range (Nonpregnant)	Change in Pregnancy	Timing
Serum Enzymatic Activities			
Amylase	23–84 IU/L	↑ 50–100%	Controversial
Transaminase			
Glutamic pyruvic (SGPT)	5–35 mU/ml	No significant change	
Glutamic oxaloacetic (SGOT)	5–40 mU/ml	No significant change	
Hematocrit	36–46%	↓ 4–7%	Bottoms at 30–34 wk
Hemoglobin	12–16 g/dl	↓ 1.5–2 g/dl	Bottoms at 30–34 wk
Leukocyte count	$4.8–10.8 \times 10^3/mm^3$	↑ $3.5 \times 10^3/mm^3$	Gradual
Platelet count	$150–400 \times 10^3/mm^3$	Slight decrease	
Serum Hormone Values			
Cortisol (plasma)	8–21 μg/dl	↑ 20 μg/dl	Gradual, peaks at term
Prolactin	25 ng/ml	↑ 50–400 ng/ml	Early sustained
Thyroxine, total (T_4)	5–11 μg/dl	↑ 5 μg/dl	Early sustained
Triiodothyronine, total (T_3)	125–245 ng/dl	↑ 50%	

Adapted from Main DM, Main EK: Obstetrics and Gynecology. A Pocket Reference. Chicago, Year Book, 1984, p 7.

Table A–3 □ WEIGHT GAIN IN PREGNANCY

Tissues and Fluids	Increase in Weight (g) Up to			
	10 Weeks	*20 Weeks*	*30 Weeks*	*40 Weeks*
Fetus	5	300	1500	3400
Placenta	20	170	430	650
Amniotic fluid	30	350	750	800
Uterus	140	320	600	970
Mammary gland	45	180	360	405
Blood	100	600	1300	1250
Interstitial fluid (no edema or leg edema)	0	30	80	1680
Maternal stores	310	2050	3480	3345
Total weight gained	650	4000	8500	12,500

Adapted from Hyten F, Chamberlain G, eds: Clinical Physiology in Obstetrics. Oxford, Blackwell Scientific, 1980, p 221.

Table A–4 □ NORMAL CENTRAL HEMODYNAMIC MEASUREMENTS IN NONPREGNANT AND PREGNANT PATIENTS

	Nonpregnant	Pregnant
Cardiac output (L/min)	4.3 ± 0.9	6.2 ± 1.0
Heart rate (beats/min)	71 ± 10.0	83 ± 10.0
Systemic vascular resistance (dyne $\times$ cm $\times$ sec^{-5})	1530 ± 520	1210 ± 266
Pulmonary vascular resistance (dyne $\times$ cm $\times$ sec^{-5})	119 ± 47.0	78 ± 22
Colloid oncotic pressure (mm Hg)	20.8 ± 1.0	18.0 ± 1.5
Colloid oncotic pressure–pulmonary capillary wedge pressure (mm Hg)	14.5 ± 2.5	10.5 ± 2.7
Mean arterial pressure (mm Hg)	86.4 ± 7.5	90.3 ± 5.8
Pulmonary capillary wedge pressure (mm Hg)	6.3 ± 2.1	7.5 ± 1.8
Central venous pressure (mm Hg)	3.7 ± 2.6	3.6 ± 2.5
Left ventricular stroke work index (g $\times$ m $\times$ m^{-2})	41 ± 8	48 ± 6

From Clark SL, Cotton DB, Lee W, et al: Central hemodynamic assessments in normal term pregnancy. Am J Obstet Gynecol 1989;161:1439.

Table A–5 □ NORMAL DURATION OF THE STAGES OF LABOR

Stages of Labor	Nullipara	Multipara
First stage		
Latent phase	≤20 hr	≤14 hr
Active phase	5–8 hr	2–5 hr
Rate of dilatation	≥1.2 cm/hr	≥1.5 cm/hr
Second stage	≤2 hr	≤1 hr
Third stage	≤30 min	≤30 min

Table A–6 □ LENGTH OF PELVIC DIAMETERS

Pelvic Plane	Diameter	Average Length (cm)
Inlet	True conjugate	11.5
	Obstetric conjugate	11
	Transverse	13.5
	Oblique	12.5
	Posterior sagittal	4.5
Greatest diameter	Anteroposterior	12.75
	Transverse	12.5
Midplane	Anteroposterior	12
	Bispinous	10.5
	Posterior sagittal	4.5–5
Outlet	Anatomical anteroposterior	9.5
	Obstetric anteroposterior	11.5
	Bituberous	11
	Posterior sagittal	7.5

From Hacker NF, Moore JG: Essentials of Obstetrics and Gynecology, 2nd ed. Philadelphia, WB Saunders Co, 1992, p 113.

Table A–7 ▫ **BIOPHYSICAL PROFILE SCORING: TECHNIQUE AND INTERPRETATION***

Biophysical Variable	Normal Score	Abnormal (Score = 0)
Fetal breathing movements	At least 1 episode of FBM of at least 30 sec duration in 30 min observation	Absent FBM or no episode of ≥30 sec in 30 min
Gross body movement	At least 3 discrete body/limb movements in 30 min (episodes of active continuous movement considered as single movement)	2 or fewer episodes of body/limb movements in 30 min
Fetal tone	At least 1 episode of active extension with return to flexion of fetal limb(s) or trunk. Opening and closing of hand considered normal tone	Either slow extension with return to partial flexion or movement of limb in full extension or absent fetal movement with fetal hand held in complete or partial deflection
Reactive FHR	At least two episodes of FHR acceleration of ≥15 beat/min and of at least 15 sec duration associated with fetal movement in 30 min	Less than 2 episodes of acceleration of FHR or acceleration of <15 beats/min in 30 min
Qualitative AFV†	At least 1 pocket of AF that measures at least 2 cm in 2 perpendicular planes	Either no AF pockets or a pocket <2 cm in 2 perpendicular planes

*FBM = fetal breathing movement; FHR = fetal heart rate; AFV = amniotic fluid volume; AF = amniotic fluid.

†Modification of the criteria for reduced amniotic fluid from <1 cm to <2 cm would seem reasonable.

From Creasy RK, Resnik R: Maternal-Fetal Medicine: Principles and Practice. Philadelphia, WB Saunders Co, 1994, p 345.

Table A–8 □ BIOPHYSICAL PROFILE SCORING: MANAGEMENT

Score	Interpretation	Recommended Management
10	Normal infant, low risk for chronic asphyxia	Repeat testing at weekly intervals; repeat twice weekly in diabetic patients and patients ≥42 wk gestation
8	Normal infant, low risk for chronic asphyxia	Repeat testing at weekly intervals; repeat twice weekly in diabetic patients and patients ≥42 wk; oligohydramnios indication for delivery
6	Suspected chronic asphyxia	Repeat testing in 4–6 hr; deliver if oligohydramnios present
4	Suspected chronic asphyxia	If ≥36 wk and favorable, then deliver; if ≥36 wk and L/S <2.0, repeat test in 24 hr; if repeat score <4, deliver
0–2	Strong suspicion of chronic asphyxia	Extend testing time to 120 min; if persistent score <4, deliver, provided gestational age is sufficiently advanced to permit possible neonatal survival

L/S = amniotic fluid lecithin/sphingomyelin ratio.
From Creasy RK, Resnik R: Maternal-Fetal Medicine: Principles and Practice. Philadelphia, WB Saunders Co, 1994, p 346.

Table A–9 □ APGAR SCORING SYSTEM

	Score		
Sign	*0*	*1*	*2*
Heart rate	Absent	<100 beats/min	>100 beats/min
Respiratory effort	Absent	Slow, irregular	Good, crying
Muscle tone	Limp	Some flexion of extremities	Active motion
Reflex irritability	Absent	Grimace	Vigorous cry
Color	Pale, blue	Body pink, extremities blue	Completely pink

Table A–10 □ STEPS FOR PERFORMING AMNIOTIC FLUID "SHAKE TEST"

Materials needed:	Amniotic fluid recently collected
	95% ethanol (19 parts of absolute alcohol mixed with 1 part of distilled water), 0.9% saline
	Two 13 × 100-mm glass tubes with Teflon-lined plastic screw cap
Steps of test:	1. Mix 1 ml of amniotic fluid and 1 ml of ethanol in one tube.
	2. Mix 0.5 ml of amniotic fluid, 0.5 ml of saline, and 1 ml of ethanol in the second tube.
	3. Shake both tubes for 15 seconds and place tubes upright.
	4. Wait for 15 minutes and look for a ring of bubble or foam at the air–liquid interface.
Results:	Positive test: ring of bubble observed in both tubes
	Equivocal test: ring of bubble observed only in first tube
	Negative test: rings of bubble not observed in either tube

Table A–11 □ INTERPRETATION OF RESULTS OF DIAGNOSTIC PERITONEAL LAVAGE* FOLLOWING BLUNT TRAUMA

Positive†
  Grossly bloody lavage fluid
  RBC count >100,000/mm^3
  WBC count >175/mm^3
  Amylase >175/dl
  Lavage fluid identified in Foley catheter
Indeterminate‡
  RBC count >50,000 but <100,000/mm^3
  WBC count >100 but <500/mm^3
  Amylase >75 but <175/dl
Negative
  RBC count <50,000/mm^3
  WBC count <100/mm^3
  Amylase <75/dl

*Peritoneal lavage performed with 1 L of Ringer's lactated solution.
†Positive lavage (any one criterion) suggests need for surgical exploration.
‡Recommendations are to repeat lavage.
Modified from Rothenberger DA, Quattlesbaum FW, Zabel J, et al: Diagnostic peritoneal lavage for blunt trauma in pregnant women. Am J Obstet Gynecol 1977;129:479.

Table A–12 □ ESTIMATED OVARIAN RADIATION EXPOSURE FROM COMMON RADIOLOGIC PROCEDURES*

Procedure	Estimated Ovarian Dose (millirad)	Average Number of Films per Examination
Chest examination		
Radiography	8	1.4
Fluoroscopy	71	
Upper GI series		
Total	558	4.4
Radiography	360	
Fluoroscopy	198	
Barium enema		
Total	805	3.5
Radiography	439	
Fluoroscopy	366	
Intravenous or retrograde pyelography	407	5.0
Abdominal x-rays	289	1.7
Lumbar spine x-rays	275	2.5
Pelvic x-rays	41	1.5

*Ovarian dose approximates fetal exposure.
Adapted from Penfil RL, Brown ML: Genetically significant dose to the United States population from diagnostic medical roentgenology. Radiology 1968;90:209.

Table A–13 □ SONOGRAPHIC FINDINGS IN NORMAL FIRST-TRIMESTER PREGNANCIES

Sonographic Finding	Gestational Age at Detection (weeks)	
	Transabdominal Examination	*Transvaginal Examination*
Gestational sac	6	5
Yolk sac	6	5
Fetus	7	6
Fetal cardiac activity	7	6

APPENDIX B

GUIDELINES, ILLUSTRATIONS, AND TABLES FOR GYNECOLOGY

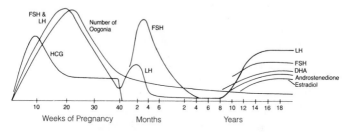

Figure B–1 □ Changes in gonadotropins and oocytes from fetal life to puberty. DHA = dehydroepiandrosterone; FSH = follicle-stimulating hormone; HCG = human chorionic gonadotropin; LH = luteinizing hormone. (From Speroff L, Glass RH, Kase NG: Neuroendocrinology. In Clinical Gynecologic Endocrinology and Infertility. Baltimore, Williams & Wilkins, 1989, p 83.)

Figure B–2 □ Tanner stages of breast development. Stage 1: Preadolescent—elevation of the papilla only. Stage 2: Breast bud stage—elevation of the breast and papilla with enlargement of the areolar region. Stage 3: Further enlargement of the breast and areola without separation of their contours. Stage 4: Projection of the areola and papilla to form a secondary mound above the level of the breast. Stage 5: Mature stage—projection of the papilla only, resulting from recession of the areola to the general contour of the breast. (From Tanner M, Eveleth PB: Variability between populations in growth and development at puberty. In Bereberg SR, ed: Puberty, Biologic and Physiological Correlations. Leiden, The Netherlands, HF Stenfert Kroese, 1976, p 256.)

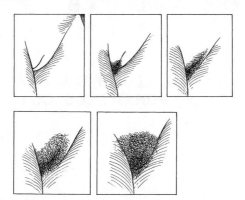

Figure B–3 □ Tanner stages of female pubic hair development. Stage 1: Preadolescent—absence of pubic hair. Stage 2: Sparse hair along the labia. Stage 3: Hair sparsely over the junction of the pubes. Hair is darker and coarser. Stage 4: Adult-type hair without spread to the medial surface of the thighs. Stage 5: Adult-type hair with spread to the medial thighs. (From Hacker NF, Moore JG: Essentials of Obstetrics and Gynecology, 2nd ed. Philadelphia, WB Saunders Co, 1992, p 516.)

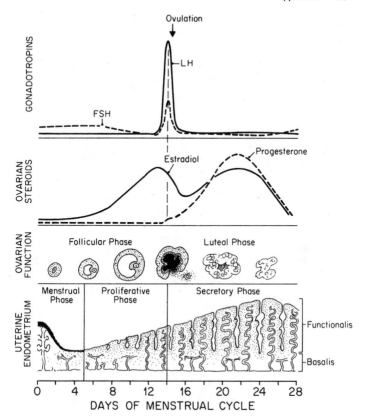

Figure B–4 □ Events of the normal menstrual cycle. FSH = follicle-stimulating hormone; LH = luteinizing hormone. (From Hacker NF, Moore JG: Essentials of Obstetrics and Gynecology, 2nd ed. Philadelphia, WB Saunders, 1992, p 39.)

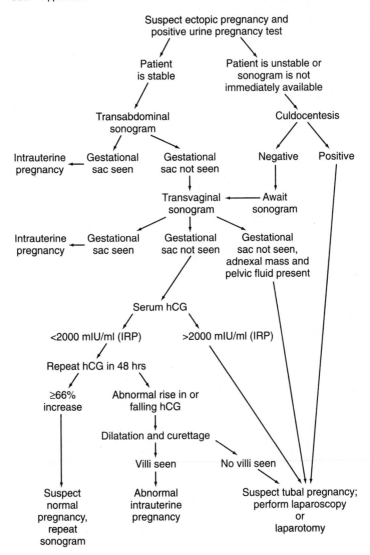

Figure B–5 □ Diagnostic scheme for ectopic pregnancy. IRP = International Reference Preparation.

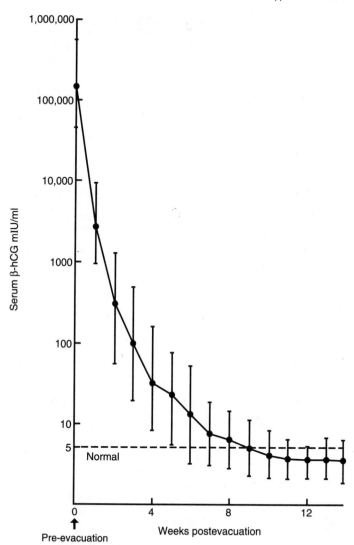

Figure B–6 □ Normal regression curve of hCG following surgical evacuation of hydatidiform mole. (From Morrow CP, Kletzky OA, DiSaia PJ, et al: Clinical and laboratory correlates of molar pregnancy and trophoblastic disease. Am J Obstet Gynecol 1977;128:424.)

Table B–1 □ STAGES OF PUBERTAL DEVELOPMENT

Stage	Mean Age (yr)	Age Range (yr)
Thelarche (breast budding)	9.8	8–13
Adrenarche (pubic or axillary hair)	11	8–14
Peak height velocity (maximal growth)	11.5	10–14
Menarche	13	9–16
Mature pubic hair	14	12–18
Mature breasts	14.5	12–18

Table B–2 □ GONADOTROPIN AND STEROID LEVELS

	Follicular Phase	Midcycle	Luteal Phase	Postmenopausal
Serum FSH (mIU/ml)	5–20	10–40	5–20	>40
Serum LH (mIU/ml)	5–20	15–60	5–20	>40
Serum estradiol (pg/ml)	25–75	200–600	100–300	5–25
Serum progesterone (ng/ml)	<1	<1	5–20	<1
Serum testosterone (ng/dl)	20–80	20–80	20–80	10–40

Table B–3 □ DIFFERENTIAL DIAGNOSIS OF THE PELVIC MASS

	Sonographic Characteristic	
Source	Cystic	Solid or Complex

Ovaries	Functional cyst
	Endometrioma
	Neoplasm
	  Benign
	  Malignant
		Neoplasm
		  Benign
		  Malignant

Fallopian tubes	Hydrosalpinx Tubo-ovarian abscess Pyosalpinx Paratubal cyst	Neoplasm Tubo-ovarian abscess Tubal pregnancy
Uterus		Intrauterine pregnancy Uterine anomaly Leiomyoma Adenomyosis Sarcoma
Bowel	Ileus	Appendiceal abscess Diverticular abscess Neoplasm Stool
Bladder and kidneys	Distended bladder	Pelvic kidney

Table B–4 □ DIFFERENTIAL DIAGNOSIS OF GENITAL ULCERS

	HSV	Syphilis	Chancroid	Granuloma Inguinale	LGV
Lesion	Multiple vesicles	Single ulcer	Single or multiple ulcers	Single or multiple ulcers	Single ulcer
Depth	Shallow	Shallow	Deep	Elevated	Shallow
Induration	Absent	Hard	Soft	Hard	Absent
Adenopathy	Present	Present	Present	Absent	Present
Pain	Present	Absent	Present	Absent	Variable
Incubation	3–7 days	3 weeks	3–5 days	1–12 weeks	4–21 days

HSV = herpes simplex virus; LGV = lymphogranuloma venereum.

Table B–5 □ COMPARISON OF THE THREE MOST COMMON VULVOVAGINAL INFECTIONS

	Yeast Vulvovaginitis	Bacterial Vaginosis	Trichomonas Vulvovaginitis
Cause	*Candida* species	*Gardnerella vaginalis*, mixed anaerobes	*Trichomonas vaginalis*
Major symptoms	Itching, burning	Malodorous, watery discharge	Itching, burning, variable
Discharge	White, cottage cheese	White, skim milk	Frothy, variable
Odor	Absent	Present	Variable
Vulvovaginal inflammation	Present	Absent	Variable
Vaginal wet smear	Hyphae, spores	"Clue cells"	Trichomonads
"Whiff test"	Negative	Positive	Negative
Vaginal pH	Normal, 3–4	Basic, 5–6	Basic, 6–7
Treatment	Antifungal drugs	Metronidazole	Metronidazole

APPENDIX C

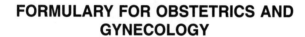

FORMULARY FOR OBSTETRICS AND GYNECOLOGY

FOOD AND DRUG ADMINISTRATION'S USE-IN-PREGNANCY RATINGS

Category	Interpretation
A	**Controlled studies show no risk.** Adequate, well-controlled studies in pregnant women have failed to demonstrate risk to the fetus.
B	**No evidence of risk in humans.** Either animal findings show risk but human findings do not, or, if no adequate human studies have been done, animal findings are negative.
C	**Risk cannot be ruled out.** Human studies are lacking, and animal studies are either positive for fetal risk or also lacking. However, potential benefits may justify the potential risk.
D	**Positive evidence of risk.** Investigational or postmarketing data show risk to the fetus. Nevertheless, potential benefits may outweigh the potential risk.
X	**Contraindicated in pregnancy.** Studies in animals or humans, or investigational or postmarketing reports, have shown fetal risk that clearly outweighs any possible benefit to the patient.

ACETAMINOPHEN WITH CODEINE   *Class: Analgesic*
(Tylenol with codeine)

Category:	C
Indications:	Mild to moderate pain
Actions:	Acetaminophen: peripherally acting analgesic; codeine: centrally acting analgesic
Side effects:	Nausea, vomiting, lightheadedness, dizziness, shortness of breath
Dose:	Acetaminophen 300 mg with codeine 15 mg (No. 2), 30 mg (No. 3), or 60 mg (No. 4). Give the number of tablets that provides 15 to 60 mg codeine PO every 4 hours.

ACYCLOVIR (Zovirax)   *Class: Antiviral*

Category: C
Indications: Treatment and prophylaxis for herpes simplex, herpes zoster, and chicken pox
Actions: Synthetic purine nucleoside analogue inhibiting viral DNA replication
Side effects: Nausea, vomiting, headaches
Dose: 400 mg PO 3 times per day or 200 mg PO 5 times per day for 7 to 10 days or until clinical resolution is attained for primary infection
                400 mg PO 3 times per day for 5 days or 800 mg PO 2 times per day for 5 days for recurrent infection
                400 mg PO 2 times per day or 200 mg PO 2 to 5 times per day for prophylaxis against recurrent infection
                5% ointment applied to cover all lesions every 3 hours, 6 times per day, for 7 days

ALBUTEROL (Airet, Proventil, Ventolin)   *Class: Bronchodilator*

Category: C
Indications: Treatment of bronchospasm
Actions: Beta-sympathomimetic
Side effects: Tremors, dizziness, nervousness, nausea, hypertension
Dose: Bronchodilator aerosol: 2 inhalations every 4 to 6 hours
                Syrup: 1 to 2 teaspoons PO 3 to 4 times per day
                Tablets: 2 to 4 mg PO 3 to 4 times per day

ALPRAZOLAM (Xanax)   *Class: Benzodiazepine*

Category: D
Indications: Anxiety disorder
Actions: Binding specific receptors within the central nervous system
Side effects: Drowsiness, lightheadedness
Dose: 0.25 to 0.5 mg PO 3 times per day, maximum dose of 4 mg per day

AMINOPHYLLINE   *Class: Bronchodilator*

Category: C
Indications: Bronchospasm
Actions: Relaxation of smooth muscles of the bronchi
Side effects: Nausea, vomiting, irritability, tachycardia, arrhythmias, seizures
Dose: Loading dose of 6 mg/kg IV followed by maintenance dose of 0.4 to 0.9 mg/kg/hr IV
                24 mg/kg PO per day in 4 divided doses

AMITRIPTYLINE (Elavil)   *Class: Tricyclic antidepressant*

Category: D
Indications: Depression
Actions: Unknown
Side effects: Cardiovascular: myocardial infarction, stroke, nonspecific electrocardiographic changes

Central nervous system and neuromuscular: coma, seizure, hallucinations, delusions, confusion

Anticholinergic: paralytic ileus, hyperpyrexia, urinary retention, constipation

Hematological: bone marrow depression, leukopenia, thrombocytopenia

Gastrointestinal: hepatitis

Withdrawal symptoms

Dose: 75 to 300 mg/day PO in divided doses

AMOXICILLIN (Amoxil, Augmentin, Moxilin)   *Class: Antibiotic*

Category: B
Indications: Treatment of infection with gram-negative organisms *(Haemophilus influenzae, Escherichia coli, Proteus mirabilis,* or *Neisseria gonorrhoeae)* and gram-positive organisms (streptococci, non–penicillinase-producing staphylococci)
Actions: Inhibition of cell wall synthesis
Side effects: Nausea, vomiting, diarrhea, urticaria, erythematous maculopapular rashes
Dose: 250 to 500 mg PO 3 times per day for 10 days

AMPHOTERICIN B (Fungizone)   *Class: Antifungal agent*

Category: B
Indications: Systemic fungal infection
Actions: Interferes with cell membrane by inhibition of ergosterol
Side effects: Fever, hypotension, tachypnea, gastrointestinal symptoms, anemia, generalized pain, elevated liver enzymes, decreased renal function tests
Dose: Test dose of 1 mg administered IV over 20 to 30 minutes followed by a gradual increase of 5 to 10 mg per day to a final daily maintenance dose of 0.5 to 0.7 mg/kg IV

AMPICILLIN (Omnipen, Ampicillin)   *Class: Antibiotic*

Category: B
Indications: Treatment of infection with gram-negative organisms *(Haemophilus influenzae, Escherichia coli, Neisseria gonorrhoeae, N. meningitidis, Proteus mirabilis, Salmonella,* or *Shigella)* and gram-positive organisms (streptococci, non–penicillinase-producing staphylococci, *Bacillus anthracis, Clostridium, Corynebacterium,* or enterococci)
Actions: Inhibition of cell wall synthesis
Side effects: Gastrointestinal: nausea, vomiting, diarrhea, glossitis, stomatitis, enterocolitis, pseudomembranous colitis
Dose: 0.5 to 2.0 g IV every 6 hours
                   250 to 500 mg PO 4 times per day

AMPICILLIN AND SULBACTAM (Unasyn)   *Class: Antibiotic*

Category: B
Indications: Treatment of gynecological infection due to beta-lacta-

mase–producing strains of *Escherichia coli* and *Bacteroides*

Actions:	Inhibition of cell wall synthesis, beta-lactamase inhibitor
Side effects:	Gastritis, stomatitis, enterocolitis
Dose:	1.5 g (1.0 g ampicillin and 0.5 g sulbactam) to 3.0 g (2.0 g ampicillin and 1.0 g sulbactam) IV every 6 hours

ASTEMIZOLE (Hismanal)   *Class: Antihistamine*

Category:	C
Indications:	Allergic rhinitis, chronic idiopathic urticaria
Actions:	Histamine H_1-receptor antagonist
Side effects:	Drowsiness, headache, fatigue, appetite increase, weight increase, nausea, nervousness, dizziness
Dose:	10 mg PO once daily

AZITHROMYCIN (Zithromax)   *Class: Antibiotic*

Category:	C
Indications:	Treatment of sexually transmitted diseases due to *Chlamydia trachomatis, Staphylococcus aureus, Streptococcus, Haemophilus influenzae,* or *Moraxella catarrhalis*
Actions:	Macrolide antibiotic
Side effects:	Nausea, diarrhea, vomiting, abdominal pain
Dose:	1 g PO once for chlamydia
	500 mg PO on first day followed by 250 mg PO every day for a total of 5 days of therapy for other indications

AZTREONAM (Azactam)   *Class: Antibiotic*

Category:	B
Indications:	Treatment of endometritis and pelvic infections caused by *Escherichia coli, Klebsiella pneumoniae, Enterobacter,* or *Proteus mirabilis*
Actions:	Inhibition of cell wall synthesis
Side effects:	Diarrhea, nausea, vomiting, rash
Dose:	1.0 to 2.0 g IV every 8 hours

BROMOCRIPTINE (Parlodel)   *Class: Dopamine receptor agonist*

Category:	C
Indications:	Hyperprolactinemia
Actions:	Dopamine receptor agonist
Side effects:	Nausea, headache, dizziness, fatigue, lightheadedness, vomiting, abdominal cramps, constipation, diarrhea, drowsiness, nasal congestion
Dose:	2.5 to 15 mg PO per day

BUTOCONAZOLE (Femstat)   *Class: Antifungal agent*

Category:	C
Indications:	Vulvovaginal candidal infection
Actions:	Imidazole derivative, interferes with cell membrane by inhibition of ergosterol
Side effects:	Vulvovaginal itching and burning
Dose:	2% vaginal cream: 5 g every night before bed for 3 nights

CALCIUM GLUCONATE *Class: Calcium supplement*

Category:	B
Indications:	Cardiac or respiratory arrest due to magnesium toxicity
Actions:	Calcium replacement, increases myocardial contractility and ventricular automaticity
Side effects:	Electrocardiographic changes, arrhythmias, sensitivity to digoxin
Dose:	10% solution: administer 10 ml (1 g) IV over 3 minutes

CARBAMAZEPINE (Tegretol, Atretol) *Class: Anticonvulsant*

Category:	C
Indications:	Seizures, trigeminal neuralgia
Actions:	Reduction of polysynaptic responses and blockage of posttetanic potentiation
Side effects:	Aplastic anemia, agranulocytosis, dizziness, nausea, vomiting
Dose:	800 to 1200 mg PO per day

CEFIXIME (Suprax) *Class: Antibiotic*

Category:	B
Indications:	Uncomplicated urinary tract infection caused by *Escherichia coli* or *Proteus mirabilis*
	Uncomplicated gonorrhea
Actions:	Inhibition of cell wall synthesis
Side effects:	Diarrhea, dyspepsia, nausea, vomiting, abdominal pain
Dose:	400 mg PO once for uncomplicated gonorrhea
	200 mg 2 times per day or 400 mg every day for urinary tract infection

CEFOPERAZONE (Cefobid) *Class: Antibiotic*

Category:	B
Indications:	Pelvic inflammatory disease caused by *Neisseria gonorrhoeae, Escherichia coli, Clostridium, Bacteroides,* or group B beta-hemolytic streptococci
Actions:	Inhibition of cell wall synthesis
Side effects:	Hypersensitivity reaction, neutropenia, hepatitis, diarrhea
Dose:	0.5 to 1.0 g IV every 6 hours

CEFOTAXIME (Claforan) *Class: Antibiotic*

Category:	B
Indications:	Pelvic inflammatory disease (PID) due to *Staphylococcus, Streptococcus, Enterobacter,* enterococci, *Klebsiella, Escherichia coli, Proteus mirabilis, Bacteroides, Clostridium, Peptococcus,* or *Peptostreptococcus*
	Gonococcal bacteremia and arthritis
Actions:	Inhibition of cell wall synthesis
Side effects:	Local inflammation at IM injection site or IV site
Dose:	1 to 2 g IM or IV every 8 hours for PID
	1 g IV every 8 hours for 2 to 3 days for gonococcal bacteremia and arthritis

CEFOTETAN (Cefotan)   *Class: Antibiotic*

Category: B
Indications: Pelvic inflammatory disease due to *Staphylococcus, Streptococcus, Neisseria gonorrhoeae, Proteus mirabilis, Bacteroides, Peptococcus,* or *Peptostreptococcus*
Actions: Inhibition of cell wall synthesis
Side effects: Nausea, diarrhea, pseudomembranous colitis, prolonged prothrombin time
Dose: 1.0 to 2.0 g IV every 12 hours

CEFOXITIN (Mefoxin)   *Class: Antibiotic*

Category: B
Indications: Pelvic inflammatory disease due to group B streptococci, *Escherichia coli, Neisseria gonorrhoeae, Bacteroides, Clostridium, Peptococcus,* or *Peptostreptococcus*
Actions: Inhibition of cell wall synthesis
Side effects: Local inflammation at IM injection site or IV site, diarrhea
Dose: 1.0 to 2.0 g IV every 6 hours

CEFTIZOXIME (Cefizox)   *Class: Antibiotic*

Category: B
Indications: Pelvic inflammatory disease due to *Streptococcus agalactiae, Escherichia coli,* or *Neisseria gonorrhoeae*
                 Gonococcal bacteremia and arthritis
Actions: Inhibition of cell wall synthesis
Side effects: Hypersensitivity reaction, elevation of liver enzymes, eosinophilia, thrombocytosis, local inflammation
Dose: 1 g IV every 8 hours

CEFTRIAXONE (Rocephin)   *Class: Antibiotic*

Category: B
Indications: Infection caused by *Neisseria gonorrhoeae*
Actions: Inhibition of cell wall synthesis
Side effects: Hypersensitivity reaction, elevation of liver enzymes, eosinophilia, thrombocytosis, leukopenia, elevation of blood urea nitrogen, diarrhea, and local inflammation
Dose: 250 mg IM once for uncomplicated gonorrhea
                 1 g IV daily for 7 to 10 days for gonococcal bacteremia and arthritis

CEPHRADINE (Velosef)   *Class: Antibiotic*

Category: B
Indications: Bacterial vaginosis in patients allergic to penicillin
Actions: Inhibition of cell wall synthesis
Side effects: Nausea, vomiting, diarrhea
Dose: 500 mg PO 4 times per day for 7 days

CHLORAMPHENICOL (Chloromycetin)   *Class: Antibiotic*

Category: C
Indications: Serious infection caused by *Salmonella, Haemophilus in-*

fluenzae, Rickettsia, or other gram-negative aerobic and anaerobic bacteria
Gonococcal meningitis

Actions:	Bacteriostatic effect due to interference with protein synthesis
Side effects:	Bone marrow depression
	"Gray syndrome," a potentially fatal toxic reaction encountered in neonates
Dose:	50 to 100 mg/kg/day in divided doses at 6-hour intervals
	4 to 6 g IV daily for at least 10 days for gonococcal meningitis

CHLORPROMAZINE (Thorazine) *Class: Antipsychotic*

Category:	C
Indications:	Psychosis, nausea, vomiting, intractable hiccups, restlessness
Actions:	Unknown, antiadrenergic and anticholinergic activity
Side effects:	Drowsiness, jaundice, hematological disorders, agranulocytosis, extrapyramidal reactions, hypotension
Dose:	10 to 25 mg PO 2 to 3 times per day
	25 mg IM, repeated in 1 hour if necessary

CIMETIDINE (Tagamet) *Class: Histamine antagonist*

Category:	B
Indications:	Peptic ulcer disease, gastrointestinal reflux
Actions:	Inhibition of gastric acid secretion induced by histamine
Side effects:	Diarrhea, headache, gynecomastia, leukopenia, thrombocytopenia, elevation of liver enzymes
Dose:	400 to 800 mg PO every night before bed
	300 mg IM or IV every 6 to 8 hours

CIPROFLOXACIN (Cipro) *Class: Antibiotic*

Category:	C
Indications:	Uncomplicated gonorrhea
	Urinary tract infection and other infections caused by gram-positive or gram-negative aerobic bacteria
Actions:	Interference with enzyme DNA gyrase, which is necessary for DNA synthesis
Side effects:	Nausea, diarrhea, vomiting, abdominal discomfort, headache, restlessnesss, rash
Dose:	250 to 750 mg PO every 12 hours
	500 mg PO once for uncomplicated gonorrhea
	200 to 400 mg IV every 12 hours

CLINDAMYCIN (Cleocin) *Class: Antibiotic*

Category:	B
Indications:	Gynecological infections caused by anaerobic bacteria
	Infections caused by susceptible strains of streptococci, pneumococci, and staphylococci
	Bacterial vaginosis

Actions:	Interference with protein synthesis
Side effects:	Pseudomembranous colitis caused by *Clostridium difficile*
Dose:	300 to 600 mg IV every 6 hours or
	900 mg IV every 8 hours
	150 to 450 mg PO every 6 hours
	2% vaginal cream: 5 g (1 applicator full) intravaginally every night before bed for 7 nights

CLOMIPHENE CITRATE
(Clomid, Serophene)   *Class: Ovulation stimulant*

Category:	X
Indications:	Oligo-ovulation resulting in infertility
Actions:	Increases gonadotropins
Side effects:	Hyperstimulation of the ovaries
Dose:	50 to 100 mg PO every day for 5 days at the beginning of the menstrual cycle

CLOTRIMAZOLE (Mycelex, Gyne-Lotrimin)   *Class: Antifungal agent*

Category:	C
Indications:	Candida vulvovaginitis, dermatitis
Actions:	Imidazole derivative, interferes with cell membrane by inhibition of ergosterol
Side effects:	Vaginal administration: vaginal itching, irritation, cramping, headaches
	Topical administration: erythema, blistering, peeling, edema, pruritus

Dose:		
	100-mg vaginal tablet:	1 tablet every night before bed for 7 nights
	1% vaginal cream:	5 g every night before bed for 7 nights
	500-mg vaginal tablet:	1 tablet once
	1% lotion or cream:	Apply 2 times per day

CROTAMITON (Eurax)   *Class: Antiparasitic*

Category:	C
Indications:	Infection with scabies *(Sarcoptes scabiei)*
Actions:	Scabicidal and antipruritic actions
Side effects:	Allergic sensitivity and primary irritation
Dose:	10% cream or lotion applied to the skin from chin to toes. A second application is recommended 24 hours later. Bed linens and clothing should be changed the next day. A cleansing bath should be taken 48 hours after the last application.

DIAZEPAM (Valium)   *Class: Benzodiazepine*

Category:	D
Indications:	Treatment of anxiety disorder, seizure disorder, and muscle spasms
Actions:	Acts on parts of the limbic system, the thalamus, and the hypothalamus

Side effects:	Drowsiness, fatigue, ataxia, phlebitis at injection site
Dose:	2 to 10 mg PO 3 to 4 times per day
	2 to 20 mg IM or IV

DICLOXACILLIN (Pathocil, Dicloxacillin)   *Class: Antibiotic*

Category:	B
Indications:	Infection due to penicillinase-producing staphylococci
Actions:	Inhibition of cell wall synthesis
Side effects:	Nausea, vomiting, epigastric discomfort, diarrhea, hypersensitivity reaction
Dose:	125 to 250 mg PO 4 times per day for 10 days

DIGOXIN (Lanoxicaps, Lanoxin)   *Class: Inotropic agent*

Category:	C
Indications:	Heart failure, atrial fibrillation, atrial flutter, paroxysmal atrial tachycardia
Actions:	Increases myocardial contractility, slows atrioventricular (AV) conduction
Side effects:	Premature ventricular contractions, ventricular tachycardia, AV dissociation, atrial tachycardia, accelerated junctional rhythm
Dose:	Oral: 0.5 to 0.75 mg PO, then 0.125 to 0.375 mg PO every 6 to 8 hours until clinical effect is achieved, then maintenance dose of 0.125 to 0.25 mg PO every day
	IV: 0.4 to 0.6 mg IV, then 0.1 to 0.3 mg IV every 4 to 8 hours until clinical effect is achieved, then maintenance dose of 0.125 to 0.25 mg IV every day

DIPHENHYDRAMINE (Benadryl)   *Class: Antihistamine*

Category:	B
Indications:	Allergic reaction, motion sickness, parkinsonism
Actions:	Antihistamine, anticholinergic, and sedative effects
Side effects:	Drowsiness, dizziness, epigastric distress, thickening of bronchial secretions
Dose:	25 to 50 mg PO 3 to 4 times per day, 50 mg PO every night before bed
	10 to 50 mg IV or IM

DIPHENOXYLATE WITH ATROPINE (Lomotil)   *Class: Antidiarrheal*

Category:	C
Indications:	Diarrhea
Actions:	Direct effect on circular smooth muscle of the bowel resulting in prolonged transit time
Side effects:	Numbness of the extremities, depression, euphoria, confusion, sedation, dizziness, toxic megacolon, paralytic ileus, nausea, vomiting, abdominal discomfort
Dose:	2 tablets PO 4 times per day
	10 ml PO 4 times per day

DOPAMINE (Intropin, Dopastat) *Class: Cardiovascular agent*

Category:	C
Indications:	Treatment of hemodynamic imbalances caused by shock, myocardial infarction, septicemia, and trauma
Actions:	Vasoactive amine with positive inotropic effects
	Increases cardiac heart rate and contractility
	Vasodilatation
Side effects:	Hypotension, ectopic heart beats, nausea, vomiting, tachycardia, anginal pain, palpitation, dyspnea, and headache
Dose:	2 to 5 μg/kg/min IV infusion with dose increased by 5 μg/kg/min increments to a maximum of 50 μg/mg/min

DOXYCYCLINE *Class: Antibiotic*
(Doryx, Vibramycin, Doxycycline, Monodox)

Category:	D
Indications:	Infection caused by *Chlamydia trachomatis, Neisseria gonorrhoeae, Treponema pallidum, Mycoplasma pneumoniae, Haemophilus ducreyi,* or *Bacteroides*
Actions:	Interference with protein synthesis
Side effects:	Nausea, vomiting, diarrhea, rash, rise in blood urea nitrogen, hypersensitivity reaction
Dose:	100 mg PO 2 times per day for 7 days
	100 mg IV every 12 hours

EPHEDRINE SULFATE *Class: Cardiovascular agent*

Category:	C
Indications:	Hypotension from conduction anesthesia, acute bronchospasm
Actions:	Sympathomimetic
Side effects:	Tremulousness, excitation, nervousness, palpitations, tachycardia
Dose:	25 to 50 mg IM or IV

ERYTHROMYCIN *Class: Antibiotic*
(Erythrocin, E-Mycin, ERYC, Ery-Tab, Ilosone)

Category:	B
Indications:	Treatment of infection with *Chlamydia trachomatis, Neisseria gonorrhoeae, Treponema pallidum,* group A beta-hemolytic streptococci, *Streptococcus pneumoniae,* or *Staphylococcus aureus*
Actions:	Interference with protein synthesis
Side effects:	Nausea, vomiting, abdominal pain, diarrhea
Dose:	250 to 500 mg PO 4 times per day for 7 days
	500 to 1000 mg IV 4 times per day

ESTRADIOL (Estrace) *Class: Hormone*

Category:	X
Indications:	Hypoestrogenic symptoms from menopause, perimenopause, and premenopausal castration

Actions:	Estrogen replacement
Side effects:	Nausea, breast tenderness, irregular bleeding, fluid retention, enlargement of fibroid tumors of the uterus, endometrial hyperplasia, endometrial adenocarcinoma
Dose:	1 to 2 mg PO every day either continuously or cyclically

0.01% vaginal cream: 2 to 4 g intravaginally every day for 1 to 2 weeks, then reduced gradually to a maintenance dose of 1 g 1 to 3 times per week

Progestin should be administered to those patients who have not undergone hysterectomy, to prevent endometrial hyperplasia or adenocarcinoma

ESTRADIOL TRANSDERMAL SYSTEM   *Class: Hormone*
(Estraderm, Climara, Vivelle)

Category:	X
Indications:	Hypoestrogenic symptoms from menopause, perimenopause, and premenopausal castration
Actions:	Estrogen replacement
Side effects:	Nausea, breast tenderness, irregular bleeding, fluid retention, enlargement of fibroid tumors of the uterus, endometrial hyperplasia, endometrial adenocarcinoma
Dose:	0.0375-, 0.05-, 0.075-, or 0.1-mg transdermal patch applied twice weekly

Progestin should be administered to those patients who have not undergone hysterectomy, to prevent endometrial hyperplasia or adenocarcinoma

ESTROGEN, CONJUGATED (Premarin)   *Class: Hormone*

Category:	X
Indications:	Hypoestrogenic symptoms from menopause, perimenopause, and premenopausal castration
Actions:	Estrogen replacement
Side effects:	Nausea, breast tenderness, irregular bleeding, fluid retention, enlargement of fibroid tumors of the uterus, endometrial hyperplasia, endometrial adenocarcinoma
Dose:	0.3, 0.625, 0.9, or 1.25 mg PO every day either continuously or cyclically

2 to 4 g intravaginal cream every day for short-term use, tapered or discontinued every 3 to 6 months

25 mg IV every 6 to 12 hours for severe dysfunctional uterine bleeding

Progestin should be administered to those patients who are using estrogen chronically and who have not undergone hysterectomy, to prevent endometrial hyperplasia or adenocarcinoma

ESTROGEN, CONJUGATED WITH   *Class: Hormone*
METHYLTESTOSTERONE (Premarin
with methyltestosterone)

Category:	X
Indications:	Hypoestrogenic symptoms from menopause, perimenopause, and premenopausal castration with hypoandrogenic symptoms such as decreased libido

Actions: Estrogen and androgen replacement

Side effects: Nausea, breast tenderness, irregular bleeding, fluid retention, enlargement of fibroid tumors of the uterus, endometrial hyperplasia, endometrial adenocarcinoma, hirsutism, acne

Dose: 0.625 mg estrogen with 5 mg methyltestosterone or 1.25 mg estrogen with 10 mg methyltestosterone PO every day either continuously or cyclically

Progestin should be administered to those patients who have not undergone hysterectomy, to prevent endometrial hyperplasia or adenocarcinoma

ESTROGEN, ESTERIFIED (Estratab, Menest) *Class: Hormone*

Category: X

Indications: Hypoestrogenic symptoms from menopause, perimenopause, and premenopausal castration

Actions: Estrogen replacement

Side effects: Nausea, breast tenderness, irregular bleeding, fluid retention, enlargement of fibroid tumors of the uterus, endometrial hyperplasia, endometrial adenocarcinoma

Dose: 0.3, 0.625, 0.9, or 1.25 mg PO every day either continuously or cyclically

Progestin should be administered to those patients who have not undergone hysterectomy, to prevent endometrial hyperplasia or adenocarcinoma

ESTROGEN, ESTERIFIED WITH METHYLTESTOSTERONE (Estratest) *Class: Hormone*

Category: X

Indications: Hypoestrogenic symptoms from menopause, perimenopause, and premenopausal castration with hypoandrogenic symptoms such as decreased libido

Actions: Estrogen and androgen replacement

Side effects: Nausea, breast tenderness, irregular bleeding, fluid retention, enlargement of fibroid tumors of the uterus, endometrial hyperplasia, endometrial adenocarcinoma, hirsutism, acne

Dose: 0.625 mg estrogen with 1.25 mg methyltestosterone or 1.25 mg estrogen with 2.5 mg methyltestosterone PO every day either continuously or cyclically

Progestin should be administered to those patients who have not undergone hysterectomy, to prevent endometrial hyperplasia or adenocarcinoma

ESTROPIPATE (Ogen) *Class: Hormone*

Category: X

Indications: Hypoestrogenic symptoms from menopause, perimenopause, and premenopausal castration

Actions: Estrogen replacement

Side effects: Nausea, breast tenderness, irregular bleeding, fluid retention, enlargement of fibroid tumors of the uterus, endometrial hyperplasia, endometrial adenocarcinoma

Dose:	0.625, 1.25, or 2.5 mg; 1 to 2 tablets PO either continuously or cyclically
	Progestin should be administered to those patients who have not undergone hysterectomy, to prevent endometrial hyperplasia or adenocarcinoma

FLUCONAZOLE (Diflucan) *Class: Antifungal agent*

Category:	C
Indications:	Candida vulvovaginitis, candidal systemic infection
Actions:	Imidazole derivative, interferes with cell membrane by inhibition of ergosterol
Side effects:	Hepatotoxicity, nausea, vomiting, headache, skin rash, abdominal pain, diarrhea
Dose:	Systemic infection: 400 mg IV on the first day, followed by 200 mg IV every day for a minimum of 3 weeks
	Vulvovaginitis: 150 mg PO once
	Recurrent vulvovaginitis: 150 mg PO once each month

FLUOCINOLONE ACETONIDE (Synalar) *Class: Dermatological*

Category:	C
Indications:	Squamous cell hyperplasia of the vulva, inflammatory and pruritic dermatoses
Actions:	Topical corticosteroid
Side effects:	Local adverse reaction
Dose:	0.025% to 0.2% cream or lotion applied 2 or 3 times per day

FLUOXETINE (Prozac) *Class: Antidepressant*

Category:	B
Indications:	Depression
Actions:	Inhibition of central nervous system neuronal uptake of serotonin
Side effects:	Anxiety, nervousness, insomnia, drowsiness, fatigue, gastrointestinal symptoms
Dose:	20 to 60 mg/day PO

FLURAZEPAM (Dalmane) *Class: Hypnotic*

Category:	D
Indications:	Insomnia
Actions:	Benzodiazepine
Side effects:	Dizziness, drowsiness, lightheadedness, ataxia
Dose:	15 to 30 mg PO every night before bed

FUROSEMIDE (Lasix) *Class: Diuretic*

Category:	C
Indications:	Edema, hypertension
Actions:	Diuretic effect on distal tubule inhibiting reabsorption of sodium and chloride
Side effects:	Electrolyte depletion, hypotension, pancreatitis, jaundice
Dose:	20 to 80 mg PO or IV initial dose followed by a repeat dose or increased dose 6 to 8 hours later

GENTAMICIN (Garamycin)   *Class: Antibiotic*

Category:	C
Indications:	Treatment of infections due to *Pseudomonas aeruginosa, Proteus, Escherichia coli, Enterobacter, Klebsiella, Serratia,* or *Staphylococcus*
Actions:	Interference with protein synthesis
Side effects:	Renal toxicity, ototoxicity, neurotoxicity
Dose:	1.0 to 1.5 mg/kg IV every 8 hours

HALOPERIDOL (Haldol)   *Class: Antipsychotic*

Category:	C
Indications:	Treatment of psychosis
Actions:	Unknown
Side effects:	Tardive dyskinesia, extrapyramidal symptoms
Dose:	0.5 to 5.0 mg PO 2 to 3 times per day
	2 to 5 mg IM initially for acute psychosis

HEPARIN   *Class: Anticoagulant*

Category:	C
Indications:	Treatment or prevention of venous thrombosis, pulmonary embolism
Actions:	Synergistic activity with antithrombin III to produce antithrombin effect
Side effects:	Bleeding, thrombocytopenia
Dose:	Prophylaxis: 5000 units SC every 8 to 12 hours
	Treatment: 5000 to 10,000 units IV bolus followed by 1000 to 2000 units IV per hour with dose adjusted to prolong partial thromboplastin time to 1.5 times control

HYDRALAZINE (Apresoline)   *Class: Antihypertensive*

Category:	C
Indications:	Hypertension
Actions:	Vasodilator
Side effects:	Headache, anorexia, nausea, vomiting, diarrhea, palpitations, tachycardia, angina
Dose:	1 mg IV over 1 minute as a test dose to detect idiosyncratic hypotension, then 5 to 25 mg IV over 2 to 4 minutes. After 20 minutes, if a diastolic blood pressure of 90 to 100 mm Hg is not attained, a repeat dose or lower dose can be given.
	10 to 40 mg IM as needed
	10 mg PO 4 times per day for first 2 to 4 days, then if necessary, increase to 25 mg PO 4 times per day for rest of the week. Then, if necessary, increase to 50 mg PO 4 times per day.

HYDROCHLOROTHIAZIDE (Esidrix, HydroDIURIL)   *Class: Diuretic*

Category:	B
Indications:	Congestive heart failure, edema, hypertension
Actions:	Diuretic effect on distal tubule inhibiting reabsorption of sodium and chloride

| Side effects: | Electrolyte depletion, hypotension, pancreatitis, jaundice |
| Dose: | 25 to 100 mg PO every day in single or divided doses |

IBUPROFEN (Motrin, Nuprin, Advil)   *Class: Nonsteroidal anti-inflammatory agent*

Category:	B
Indications:	Treatment of dysmenorrhea, mild to moderate pain
Actions:	Nonsteroidal anti-inflammatory agent
Side effects:	Gastrointestinal complaints
Dose:	600 to 800 mg 3 to 4 times per day with a maximum dosage of 3200 mg/day

IMIPRAMINE (Tofranil)   *Class: Tricyclic antidepressant*

Category:	B
Indications:	Depression
Actions:	Unknown, may block norepinephrine uptake
Side effects:	Hypotension, tachycardia, palpitations, confusion, numbness, tingling, anticholinergic effects (dry mouth, disturbances of pupillary accommodation, mydriasis, constipation, blurred vision), bone marrow suppression, nausea, vomiting
Dose:	100 to 300 mg/day IM or PO in divided doses 75 to 150 mg/day initially with a maintenance dose of 50 to 150 mg/day in divided doses

INDOMETHACIN (Indocin)   *Class: Nonsteroidal anti-inflammatory agent*

Category:	B
Indications:	Arthritis Preterm labor
Actions:	Nonsteroidal anti-inflammatory agent
Side effects:	Gastrointestinal complaints, headache, dizziness, vertigo, somnolence, depression, tinnitus
Dose:	100-mg rectal suppository as a loading dose followed by 25 mg PO every 6 hours for premature labor 25 to 50 mg PO 3 times per day for arthritis

ISONIAZID (INH)   *Class: Antituberculosis drug*

Category:	C
Indications:	Active tuberculosis, prophylaxis against tuberculosis
Actions:	Bactericidal
Side effects:	Peripheral neuropathy, hepatitis, nausea, vomiting
Dose:	5 mg/kg to 300 mg PO every day in a single dose Prophylactic dose: 300 mg PO every day for 6 to 12 months

ISOPROTERENOL (Isuprel)   *Class: Cardiovascular drug*

Category:	C
Indications:	Heart block, cardiac arrest, bronchospasm, hypovolemic and septic shock
Actions:	Beta-sympathomimetic
Side effects:	Nervousness, headache, dizziness, tachycardia, angina, palpitations

Dose: Shock: 0.5 to 5.0 μg/min IV
                      Bronchospasm: 0.01 to 0.02 mg IV
                      Heart block and cardiac arrest: 5 μg/min IV

KETOCONAZOLE (Nizoral)   *Class: Antifungal agent*

Category: C
Indications: Systemic fungal infection
                      Fungal dermatitis
                      Recurrent candida vulvovaginitis
Actions: Inhibition of cell wall synthesis
Side effects: Reversible idiosyncratic hepatitis
Dose: 200- to 400-mg tablet PO daily
                      400-mg tablet PO for 5 days each month starting with
                        menses may also be given for recurrent candida vulvo-
                        vaginitis
                      2% cream applied once daily

LABETALOL (Normodyne, Trandate)   *Class: Antihypertensive*

Category: C
Indications: Hypertension
Actions: Beta-adrenergic blocker
Side effects: Dizziness, nausea, vomiting, fatigue, dyspepsia, pares-
                        thesias
Dose: 20-mg IV bolus dose, followed by 10 to 50 mg IV every
                        10 minutes
                      100 to 400 mg PO 2 times per day

LEUPROLIDE ACETATE (Lupron)   *Class: Hormone*

Category: X
Indications: Endometriosis, uterine leiomyomata
Actions: Gonadotropin-releasing hormone agonist with antago-
                        nist effect
Side effects: Vasomotor symptoms, genitourinary atrophy, osteoporo-
                        sis
Dose: Lupron: 1 mg SC every day
                      Lupron Depot: 3.75 to 7.5 mg SC once monthly

LEVOTHYROXINE (Levothyroid,   *Class: Thyroid supplement*
Levoxine, Synthroid)

Category: A
Indications: Hypothyroidism
Actions: Synthetic T_4
Side effects: Hyperthyroidism
Dose: Initial dose: 50 μg PO every day, with daily dose in-
                        creased in increments of ≤25 μg every 2 to 3 weeks
                        as needed
                      Usual maintenance dose: 100 to 200 μg PO every day

LINDANE (Kwell)   *Class: Antiparasitic*

Category: B
Indications: Infection with scabies *(Sarcoptes scabiei)*, crab lice *(Pedicu-
                        losis pubis)*

Actions:	Scabicidal and antipruritic actions
Side effects:	Allergic sensitivity and primary irritation
Dose:	Lindane (Kwell) 1% cream or lotion applied to affected area for 8 to 12 hours, then washed off
	Lindane (Kwell) 1% shampoo applied for 4 minutes, then washed off

LITHIUM (Eskalith, Lithobid, Lithonate, Lithotab)   *Class: Antipsychotic*

Category:	D
Indications:	Manic episodes of manic-depressive illness
Actions:	Alteration of sodium transport in nerve and muscle cells and change in the metabolism of catecholamines
Side effects:	Diarrhea, vomiting, drowsiness, muscular weakness, ataxia, blurred vision, tinnitus
Dose:	Acute mania: 600 mg PO 3 times per day
	Maintenance dose: 300 mg PO 3 to 4 times per day

LOPERAMIDE (Imodium)   *Class: Antidiarrheal*

Category:	B
Indications:	Diarrhea
Actions:	Slowing of intestinal motility, change in water and electrolyte movement through the bowel, inhibition of peristaltic activity of the bowel
Side effects:	Hypersensitivity reactions, abdominal pain, constipation, fatigue, drowsiness
Dose:	Initial dose: 4 mg PO followed by 2 mg PO after each loose stool
	Dose not to exceed 16 mg/day

MAGNESIUM GLUCONATE or MAGNESIUM OXIDE (Magonate, Mag-Ox, Uro-Mag, Beelith)   *Class: Magnesium salt*

Category:	B
Indications:	Magnesium supplementation
	Preterm labor
Actions:	Decreases myometrial contractility
Side effects:	None
Dose:	0.5 to 2.0 g PO every 2 to 4 hours

MAGNESIUM SULFATE   *Class: Anticonvulsant, uterine tocolytic*

Category:	B
Indications:	Preeclampsia, eclampsia, preterm labor, uterine hypertonus
Actions:	Decreases myometrial contractility, inhibition of neuromuscular transmission and the cardiac conducting system, depression of central nervous system irritability
Side effects:	Flushing, nausea, vomiting, hypocalcemia, magnesium toxicity (somnolence, respiratory and cardiac depression)
Dose:	2.0 to 6.0 g IV over 20 minutes as a loading dose
	1.0 to 3.0 g/hr IV as the maintenance dose
	5.0 IM every 4 hours can also be used as a maintenance dose for preeclampsia.

MECLIZINE (Antivert, Bonine)   *Class: Antihistamine*

Category:	B
Indications:	Vertigo, motion sickness
Actions:	Blockage of H_1-histamine receptor
Side effects:	Drowsiness, dry mouth, blurred vision
Dose:	Vertigo: 25 to 100 mg PO every day in divided doses
	Motion sickness: 25 to 50 mg PO 1 hour before trip; dose can be repeated every 24 hours

MEDROXYPROGESTERONE (Provera,   *Class: Hormone*
Depo-Provera, Amen, Cycrin)

Category:	D
Indications:	Hormone replacement, anovulatory bleeding, endometrial hyperplasia
	Contraception
Actions:	Progestin supplementation
Side effects:	Irregular bleeding, breast tenderness, amenorrhea, thromboembolic disease
Dose:	2.5 to 10 mg PO daily for 10 to 14 days each month for anovulatory bleeding or treatment of endometrial hyperplasia
	2.5 mg PO daily or 5.0 mg PO for 12 days each month for postmenopausal hormone replacement if a patient is taking estrogen replacement and has not had a hysterectomy
	Depo-Provera: 150 mg IM every 3 months for contraception

MEPERIDINE HYDROCHLORIDE (Demerol)   *Class: Narcotic analgesic*

Category:	B
Indications:	Sedation, relief of moderate to severe pain
Actions:	Agonist interacting with receptors in the brain and spinal cord
Side effects:	Respiratory depression, nausea, vomiting, hypotension, constipation, agitation, skin rash
Dose:	50 to 100 mg IM or SC every 4 hours for analgesia in labor

METAPROTERENOL (Alupent, Metaprel)   *Class: Bronchodilator*

Category:	C
Indications:	Bronchial asthma, bronchospasm, emphysema
Actions:	Beta-sympathomimetic
Side effects:	Nervousness, headache, dizziness, palpitations, gastrointestinal distress, nausea, vomiting, tremor
Dose:	Inhalation aerosol: 2 to 3 inhalations, repeated not more than every 3 to 4 hours
	Tablet: 20 mg PO 3 to 4 times per day

METHADONE (Dolophine)   *Class: Analgesic*

Category:	B
Indications:	Severe pain, treatment of narcotic addiction
Actions:	Agonist interacting with receptors in the brain and spinal cord

Side effects:	Lightheadedness, dizziness, sedation, nausea, vomiting, respiratory depression and arrest, cardiac arrest, shock
Dose:	Analgesic effect: 2.5 to 10 mg IM or SC every 3 to 4 hours
	Detoxification: Initial dose of 15 to 20 mg PO every day for 2 to 3 days for stabilization, then dose is decreased every 1 to 2 days

METHIMAZOLE (Tapazole)   *Class: Thyroid suppressant*

Category:	D
Indications:	Hyperthyroidism
Actions:	Inhibits organification of iodine and therefore inhibits production of T_3 and T_4
Side effects:	Bone marrow suppression, hepatitis, dermatitis
Dose:	20 to 30 mg PO every 12 hours

METHOTREXATE   *Class: Antimetabolite*

Category:	X
Indications:	Treatment of tubal pregnancy, gestational trophoblastic disease
Actions:	Inhibition of folic acid synthesis
Side effects:	Bone marrow suppression, stomatitis, nausea, abdominal distress
Dose:	50 mg/m^2 IM for tubal pregnancy; dose is repeated depending on the response in serum hCG levels

METHYLERGONOVINE (Methergine)   *Class: Oxytocic*

Category:	C
Indications:	Postpartum atony and hemorrhaging, subinvolution of the uterus
Actions:	Ergot alkaloid that acts directly on smooth muscle of the uterus resulting in increased tone, frequency, and amplitude of uterine contractions
Side effects:	Hypertension, nausea, vomiting
Dose:	0.2 mg PO 3 to 4 times per day for maximum of 1 week
	0.2 mg IM or IV, repeated every 2 to 4 hours

METRONIDAZOLE (Flagyl, Protostat, MetroGel)   *Class: Antibiotic*

Category:	B
Indications:	Trichomoniasis, bacterial vaginosis, amebiasis, pseudomembranous colitis caused by *Clostridium difficile* infection, anaerobic infection
Actions:	Interference with DNA synthesis
Side effects:	Gastrointestinal symptoms, peripheral neuropathy
Dose:	250 mg PO 3 times per day for 7 days or 500 mg PO 2 times per day for 7 days for trichomoniasis or bacterial vaginosis
	2 g PO once for trichomoniasis
	500 mg PO 3 times per day for 7 to 10 days for *C. difficile*
	Metronidazole vaginal gel 5 g (1 applicator full) intravaginally 2 times per day for 5 days

MICONAZOLE (Monistat)   *Class: Antifungal agent*

Category:	C
Indications:	Candida vulvovaginitis, dermatitis, or systemic infection
Actions:	Imidazole derivative, interferes with cell membrane by inhibition of ergosterol
Side effects:	IV administration: phlebitis, pruritus, rash, nausea, vomiting, diarrhea, anorexia, flushes
	Vaginal administration: vaginal itching, irritation, cramping, headaches
Dose:	Systemic infection: 200 to 1200 mg IV 3 times per day
	Vulvovaginitis: 200-mg suppository every night before bed for 3 nights; 100-mg suppository every night before bed for 7 nights
	2% cream 5 g every night before bed for 7 nights

MIDAZOLAM (Versed)   *Class: Benzodiazepine*

Category:	C
Indications:	Conscious sedation or premedication for short diagnostic or surgical procedure
Actions:	Short-acting central nervous system depressant
Side effects:	Respiratory depression, headache, fluctuation of vital signs, hiccups, nausea, vomiting, drowsiness
Dose:	0.07 to 0.08 mg/kg IM 1 hour before procedure
	0.02 to 0.05 mg/kg IV before procedure

MORPHINE SULFATE (Morphine sulfate, MS Contin, MSIR, Rescudose, Roxanol, MS/L, OMS Concentrate)   *Class: Narcotic analgesic*

Category:	C
Indications:	Sedation, relief of moderate to severe pain
Actions:	Agonist interacting with receptors in the brain and spinal cord
Side effects:	Respiratory depression, nausea, vomiting, hypotension, dizziness, sweating, constipation, agitation, flushing, skin rash
Dose:	10 to 30 mg PO every 4 hours
	5 to 20 mg IM every 4 hours
	2.5 to 15 mg IV every 4 hours

NAFARELIN ACETATE (Synarel)   *Class: Hormone*

Category:	X
Indications:	Pelvic pain and dysmenorrhea secondary to endometriosis
Actions:	Gonadotropin-releasing hormone agonist with antagonist effect
Side effects:	Vasomotor symptoms, genitourinary atrophy, osteoporosis
Dose:	200 µg intranasal spray 2 times per day (patients who do not achieve amenorrhea can be placed on 400 µg 2 times per day)

NAFCILLIN (Unipen)   *Class: Antibiotic*

Category:	B
Indications:	Treatment of infection due to penicillinase-producing staphylococci
Actions:	Inhibition of cell wall synthesis
Side effects:	Hypersensitivity reaction, transient leukopenia, thrombocytopenia, skin rash
Dose:	250 to 500 mg PO every 4 to 6 hours
	500 to 1000 mg IV every 4 hours

NALOXONE (Narcan)   *Class: Narcotic antagonist*

Category:	B
Indications:	Reversal of narcotic effects
Actions:	Competitive antagonism of narcotics
Side effects:	Nausea, vomiting, tachycardia, hypertension, tremulousness, seizures
Dose:	0.4 to 2 mg SC, IM, or IV, repeated at 2- to 3-minute intervals until a maximum dose of 10 mg has been administered

NAPROXEN (Naprosyn,   *Class: Nonsteroidal anti-inflammatory agent*
Anaprox, Anaprox DS)

Category:	B
Indications:	Treatment of dysmenorrhea, mild to moderate pain
Actions:	Nonsteroidal anti-inflammatory agent
Side effects:	Gastrointestinal complaints
Dose:	Naprosyn: 250 to 500 mg PO every 6 to 8 hours with maximum dose of 1250 mg/day
	Anaprox: 275 to 550 mg PO every 6 to 8 hours with maximum dose of 1375 mg/day

NIFEDIPINE (Adalat,   *Class: Antihypertensive, uterine tocolytic*
Procardia)

Category:	C
Indications:	Hypertension
	Vasospastic and chronic stable angina
	Preterm labor
Actions:	Calcium channel blocker
Side effects:	Dizziness, lightheadedness, flushing, headache, weakness, nausea, muscle cramps, peripheral edema
Dose:	Hypertension: 10 to 30 mg PO 3 to 4 times per day
	Preterm labor: 10 mg PO or sublingual, repeat after 20 minutes if necessary; 10 to 20 mg every 4 to 6 hours, maintenance dose

NITROFURANTOIN (Macrodantin)   *Class: Antibiotic*

Category:	B
Indications:	Treatment of urinary tract infection
Actions:	Inactivation and alteration of bacterial ribosomal proteins and other macromolecules resulting in inhibition of protein synthesis, DNA and RNA synthesis, aerobic energy metabolism, and cell wall synthesis

Side effects:	Pulmonary hypersensitivity reactions, hepatitis, nausea, vomiting, peripheral neuropathy, dermatitis
Dose:	50 to 100 mg PO 4 times per day
	Suppressive therapy: 50 to 100 mg PO every night before bed

NYSTATIN (Mycostatin, Mytrex) *Class: Antifungal agent*

Category:	B
Indications:	Candida vulvovaginitis or dermatitis
Actions:	Polyene compound, binds to ergosterol causing cell membrane permeability
Side effects:	Topical application: skin irritation
	Oral administration: nausea
Dose:	Vaginal: 100,000 units every night before bed for 14 days
	Oral: 200,000 to 400,000 units 4 to 5 times per day for 14 days
	Topical: Apply 2 to 3 times every day

OFLOXACIN (Floxin) *Class: Antibiotic*

Category:	C
Indications:	Uncomplicated infection with *Neisseria gonorrhoeae* or *Chlamydia trachomatis*
	Lower respiratory infection due to *Haemophilus influenzae* or *Streptococcus pneumoniae*
	Urinary tract infection due to *Enterobacter aerogenes, Escherichia coli, Klebsiella pneumoniae, Proteus mirabilis,* or *Pseudomonas aeruginosa*
Actions:	Interference with enzyme DNA gyrase, which is necessary for DNA synthesis
Side effects:	Nausea, diarrhea, vomiting, insomnia, headache, dizziness, rash
Dose:	200 to 400 mg PO or IV 2 times per day
	Chlamydia: 300 mg PO 2 times per day for 7 days
	Gonorrhea: 400 mg PO once

OXYCODONE (Percodan, Percocet) *Class: Analgesic*

Category:	C
Indications:	Moderate to severe pain
Actions:	Agonist interacting with receptors in the brain and spinal cord
Side effects:	Lightheadedness, dizziness, sedation, nausea, vomiting
Dose:	1 tablet PO every 6 hours

OXYTOCIN (Pitocin, Syntocinon) *Class: Oxytocic*

Category:	C
Indications:	Induction or augmentation of labor
	Treatment of uterine atony
Actions:	Promotes contractility of uterine smooth muscle by increasing intracellular calcium
Side effects:	Hypertonus, antidiuretic effect with high doses given over a prolonged period of time
Dose:	Induction or augmentation of labor: A solution of 10 IU

of oxytocin in 1000 ml of 5% dextrose and lactated Ringer's solution or 5% dextrose and 0.5 normal saline is used. Infusion is started at a rate of 0.1 ml/min or 1 mIU/min and increased until regular uterine contractions are achieved. The infusion rate is increased by 1 mIU/min every 20 to 30 minutes up to a dose of 8 mIU/min. Above this dose, the rate can be increased in increments of 2 mIU/min every 20 to 30 minutes up to a dose of 20 mIU/min.

Treatment of uterine atony: A solution of 20 to 40 IU of oxytocin in 1000 ml of 5% dextrose and lactated Ringer's solution or 5% dextrose and 0.5 normal saline is infused at rates of 250 to 500 ml/hr

PENICILLIN G BENZATHINE SUSPENSION (Bicillin)   *Class: Antibiotic*

Category:	B
Indications:	Syphilis, upper respiratory infection due to streptococci, prophylactic therapy for rheumatic heart disease and acute glomerulonephritis
Actions:	Inhibition of cell wall synthesis
Side effects:	Hypersensitivity reactions
Dose:	Primary, secondary, and latent syphilis: 2.4 million units IM once
	Tertiary and neurosyphilis: 2.4 million units IM 1 time per week for 3 weeks

PENICILLIN G PROCAINE (Wycillin)   *Class: Antibiotic*

Category:	B
Indications:	Syphilis, infection caused by *Neisseria gonorrhoeae, Streptococcus,* or *Staphylococcus*
Actions:	Inhibition of cell wall synthesis
Side effects:	Hypersensitivity reactions
Dose:	Uncomplicated gonorrhea: 4.8 million units IM divided into two doses and given in two different sites with 1 g probenecid PO given just before injection
	Disseminated gonorrhea: 10 million units IV daily for at least 10 days
	Primary, secondary, and latent syphilis: 600,000 units IM daily for 8 days
	Tertiary, neurosyphilis, and latent syphilis with positive cerebrospinal fluid: 600,000 units IM daily for 10 to 15 days

PENICILLIN V POTASSIUM (Pen-Vee K)   *Class: Antibiotic*

Category:	B
Indications:	Mild to moderate infection due to gram-positive bacteria such as *Staphylococcus, Streptococcus, Clostridium,* or *Corynebacterium*
Actions:	Inhibition of cell wall synthesis
Side effects:	Nausea, vomiting, diarrhea, epigastric distress, hypersensitivity reactions
Dose:	250 to 500 mg PO 4 times per day

PENTOBARBITAL (Nembutal)   *Class: Anticonvulsant, hypnotic sedative*

Category:	D
Indications:	Insomnia, preanesthetic, sedation
	Seizure disorder
Actions:	Central nervous system depressant
Side effects:	Somnolence
Dose:	100- to 200-mg capsule PO for hypnosis and sedation in early labor
	150 to 200 mg IM
	100 to 500 mg IV by slow infusion not to exceed 50 mg/min

PERMETHRIN (Elimite)   *Class: Antiparasitic*

Category:	B
Indications:	Treatment of *Sarcoptes scabiei* (scabies)
Actions:	Disrupts sodium channel current by which polarization of the membrane is regulated, resulting in delayed re-polarization and paralysis of the organism
Side effects:	Burning, pruritus, erythema, numbness, tingling, rash
Dose:	5% cream: massage into skin from head to toes and wash off after 8 to 14 hours

PHENAZOPYRIDINE (Pyridium, Prodium)   *Class: Urinary tract agent*

Category:	B
Indications:	Urinary tract infection
Actions:	Topical analgesic effect on mucosa of urinary tract
Side effects:	Headache, rash, pruritus, gastrointestinal symptoms, orange discoloration of the urine
Dose:	200 mg PO 3 times per day

PHENOBARBITAL   *Class: Barbiturate*

Category:	D
Indications:	Sedation, anticonvulsant
Actions:	Central nervous system depressant
Side effects:	Respiratory depression, residual sedation
Dose:	Sedation: 30 to 120 mg PO or IM, doses repeated as needed with maximum of 400 mg in 24 hours
	Anticonvulsant effect: 60 to 200 mg PO or IM every day

PHENYTOIN (Dilantin)   *Class: Anticonvulsant*

Category:	D
Indications:	Treatment and prevention of seizures
Actions:	Inhibition of spread of seizure activity in the motor cortex, possibly by promoting the efflux of sodium from neurons
Side effects:	Nystagmus, ataxia, slurred speech, mental confusion, nausea, vomiting, atrial and ventricular conduction depression, ventricular fibrillation
Dose:	Sedation: 30 to 120 mg PO or IM every day
	Anticonvulsant effect: 100 mg PO 3 to 4 times per day
	Status epilepticus: Loading dose of 10 to 15 mg/kg by

slow IV infusion not to exceed 50 mg/min, followed by a maintenance dose of 100 mg PO or IV every 6 to 8 hours

PROCHLORPERAZINE (Compazine)   *Class: Antiemetic*

Category:	C
Indications:	Nausea, vomiting, nonpsychotic anxiety
Actions:	Phenothiazine effect
Side effects:	Drowsiness, dizziness, amenorrhea, blurred vision, hypotension, tardive dyskinesia, neuroleptic malignant syndrome (hyperpyrexia, muscle rigidity, altered mental status, autonomic instability)
Dose:	Nausea: 5 to 10 mg PO 3 to 4 times per day; 5 to 10 mg IM every 3 to 4 hours; 25-mg rectal suppository 2 times per day; or 2.5 to 10 mg by slow IV infusion, not to exceed 5 mg/min
	Nonpsychotic anxiety: 5 mg PO 3 to 4 times per day; or 10 to 20 mg IM, repeated if necessary every 2 to 4 hours

PROGESTERONE IN OIL   *Class: Hormone*

Category:	X
Indications:	Anovulatory or dysfunctional bleeding
Actions:	Progestin supplementation
Side effects:	Irregular bleeding, breast tenderness, amenorrhea, thromboembolic disease
Dose:	50 to 100 mg IM each month

PROMETHAZINE (Phenergan)   *Class: Antiemetic*

Category:	C
Indications:	Nausea, vomiting, motion sickness, sedation
Actions:	Phenothiazine derivative with antihistaminic, sedative, antimotion sickness, and anticholinergic effects
Side effects:	Drowsiness, tachycardia, bradycardia, constipation, dry mouth
Dose:	Nausea: 12.5 to 25 mg PO, IM, rectally, or IV every 4 to 6 hours
	Sedation: 25 to 50 mg PO, IM, rectally, or IV for preoperative or obstetrical sedation

PROPOXYPHENE   *Class: Analgesic*
(Darvon, Darvocet-N, Darvon-N, Darvon compound)

Category:	C
Indications:	Mild to moderate pain
Actions:	Narcotic analgesic with central nervous system effect
Side effects:	Dizziness, sedation, nausea, vomiting
Dose:	1 tablet PO every 4 hours

PROPRANOLOL (Inderal)   *Class: Beta blocker*

Category:	C
Indications:	Hypertension, cardiac arrhythmias, myocardial infarction, migraine headaches, tremors, hypertrophic subaortic stenosis, pheochromocytoma, thyrotoxicosis

Actions:	Beta-adrenergic receptor–blocking agent
Side effects:	Bradycardia, hypotension, congestive heart failure, light-headedness, mental depression, nausea, vomiting, bronchospasm, hallucinations, vivid dreams
Dose:	10 to 80 mg PO 2, 3, or 4 times per day

PROPYLTHIOURACIL (PTU)   *Class: Thyroid suppressant*

Category:	D
Indications:	Hyperthyroidism
Actions:	Inhibits organification of iodine and therefore inhibits production of T_3 and T_4, inhibits conversion of T_4 to T_3
Side effects:	Leukopenia, skin rash
Dose:	100 to 150 mg PO every 8 hours

PROSTAGLANDIN E₂ (Prostin E2, Prepidil Gel)   *Class: Prostaglandin*

Category:	C
Indications:	Termination of pregnancy from 12 to 20 weeks of gestation
	Management of missed abortion or intrauterine fetal demise up to 28 weeks of gestation
	Ripening of unfavorable cervix
Actions:	Stimulation of myometrium
	Induces biochemical changes in the cervix, resulting in collagen degradation
Side effects:	Vomiting, diarrhea, nausea, fever, headache, chills, backache, joint pain, flushing, dizziness, arthralgia, vaginal pain, chest pain, dyspnea
Dose:	Prostin E2: 20-mg vaginal suppositories inserted every 4 hours until the patient is in labor
	Prepidil Gel: 0.5 mg intracervically every 6 hours for 2 to 3 doses for cervical ripening

PROTAMINE SULFATE   *Class: Heparin antagonist*

Category:	C
Indications:	Heparin overdose
Actions:	Binds with heparin, neutralizing anticoagulant effect
Side effects:	Hypotension, bradycardia, flushing, dyspnea, nausea, vomiting
Dose:	Solution of 10 mg/ml given by slow IV infusion at a rate not to exceed 20 mg/min or 50 mg in a 10-minute period
	Each mg of protamine will neutralize 90 to 115 units of heparin

PYRETHRINS (A-200 Pediculicide shampoo and gel) *Class: Antiparasitic*

Category:	C
Indications:	Treatment of pediculosis pubis or crab lice
Actions:	Kills lice and eggs
Side effects:	Skin irritation
Dose:	Apply undiluted to dry hair. Wet entirely and leave on for 10 minutes, and then wash thoroughly. Repeat treatment in 7 to 10 days.

RANITIDINE (Zantac)   *Class: Histamine H$_2$-receptor antagonist*

Category:	B
Indications:	Duodenal ulcer, hypersecretory conditions, gastroesophageal reflux, esophagitis
Actions:	Inhibition of histamine-induced secretion of gastric acid by binding histamine H$_2$-receptor sites in gastric cells
Side effects:	Headache, malaise, dizziness, hepatitis, jaundice, leukopenia
Dose:	Oral: 150 mg PO 2 times per day or 300 mg PO every day
	Maintenance dose: 150 mg PO every night before bed
	Parenteral: 50 mg IM or IV every 6 to 8 hours

RIFAMPIN (Rifadin)   *Class: Antibiotic*

Category:	C
Indications:	Tuberculosis, *Neisseria meningitidis* carriers
Actions:	Inhibition of DNA-dependent RNA polymerase activity
Side effects:	Epigastric distress, nausea, vomiting, thrombocytopenia, headache, drowsiness, dizziness, hepatitis
Dose:	Tuberculosis: 600 mg PO or IV every day
	N. meningitidis: 600 mg PO or IV 2 times per day for 2 days

RITODRINE (Yutopar)   *Class: Tocolytic*

Category:	B
Indications:	Preterm labor, uterine hypertonus
Actions:	Beta-sympathomimetic
Side effects:	Nausea, emesis, restlessness, agitation, hypotension, pulmonary edema, cardiac insufficiency, cardiac arrhythmia, myocardial ischemia, hyperglycemia, hypokalemia
Dose:	0.050 to 0.350 mg/min IV or 5 to 10 mg IM every 2 to 4 hours or 20 mg PO every 2 to 4 hours

SECOBARBITAL (Seconal)   *Class: Sedative, hypnotic*

Category:	D
Indications:	Insomnia, sedation prior to administration of anesthesia
Actions:	Central nervous system depresssant
Side effects:	Somnolence, confusion, agitation, respiratory depression, bradycardia, hypotension, nausea, vomiting, headache
Dose:	100 mg PO every night before bed
	200 to 300 mg PO 1 to 2 hours before procedure

SERTRALINE (Zoloft)   *Class: Antidepressant*

Category:	B
Indications:	Depression
Actions:	Inhibition of central nervous system neuronal uptake of serotonin
Side effects:	Nausea, diarrhea, dyspepsia, tremor, dizziness, insomnia, dry mouth

Dose: Initial dose of 50 mg PO every day followed by maintenance dose of 50 to 200 mg PO every day

SPECTINOMYCIN (Trobicin)   *Class: Antibiotic*

Category: B
Indications: Uncomplicated gonorrhea
Actions: Inhibition of protein synthesis
Side effects: Nausea, chills, fever, urticaria, insomnia
Dose: 2 g IM

SULFASALAZINE (Azulfidine)   *Class: Antibiotic*

Category: B
Indications: Ulcerative colitis
Actions: Anti-inflammatory effect
Side effects: Anorexia, headache, nausea, vomiting, gastric distress
Dose: Initial dose of 3 to 4 g PO every day in divided doses, followed by maintenance dose of 2 g PO every day in divided doses

SULFISOXAZOLE (Gantrisin)   *Class: Antibiotic*

Category: C
Indications: Urinary tract infection due to *Escherichia coli, Klebsiella, Staphylococcus,* and *Proteus mirabilis*
Meningococcal meningitis
Acute otitis media
Infection due to *Chlamydia trachomatis*
Actions: Inhibition of synthesis of dihydrofolic acid
Side effects: Hypersensitivity reactions, gastrointestinal symptoms
Dose: 500 to 1000 mg PO 4 times per day
500 mg PO 4 times per day for 10 days for chlamydial infections

TAMOXIFEN (Nolvadex)   *Class: Antineoplastic*

Category: D
Indications: Breast cancer
Actions: Nonsteroidal agent with antiestrogenic properties
Side effects: Vasomotor symptoms, nausea, vomiting, irregular bleeding, vaginal discharge, endometrial hyperplasia, endometrial carcinoma
Dose: 10 to 20 mg PO 2 times per day

TERBUTALINE (Brethine, Bricanyl)   *Class: Bronchodilator, tocolytic*

Category: B
Indications: Bronchial asthma, bronchospasm
Preterm labor
Actions: Beta-sympathomimetic
Side effects: Nausea, vomiting, palpitations, tachycardia, tremors, nervousness, dizziness, headache, drowsiness, dyspnea, chest discomfort, weakness, flushing, sweating
Dose: 0.01 to 0.08 mg/min IV
0.25 to 0.50 mg IM or SC every 3 to 4 hours

2.5 to 5.0 mg PO every 2 to 4 hours

If decrease in uterine activity is not achieved in 15 to 30 minutes, a second dose can be administered

TERCONAZOLE (Terazol)   *Class: Antifungal agent*

Category:	C
Indications:	Candida vulvovaginitis
Actions:	Imidazole derivative, interferes with cell membrane by inhibition of ergosterol
Side effects:	Vaginal itching, irritation, dysmenorrhea, headaches
Dose:	Terazol 3: 80-mg suppository, 1 every night before bed for 3 nights
	0.8% vaginal cream, 5 g every night before bed for 3 nights
	Terazol 7: 0.4% vaginal cream, 5 g every night before bed for 7 nights

TETRACYCLINE (Achromycin)   *Class: Antibiotic*

Category:	D
Indications:	Infection caused by *Chlamydia trachomatis, Neisseria gonorrhoeae, Treponema pallidum, Mycoplasma pneumoniae, Haemophilus ducreyi,* or *Bacteroides*
Actions:	Interference with protein synthesis
Side effects:	Nausea, vomiting, diarrhea, rash, rise in blood urea nitrogen, hypersensitivity reaction
Dose:	250 to 500 mg PO 4 times per day for 10 to 14 days

THEOPHYLLINE (Aerolate, Asbron, Quibron, Respbid, Theo-Dur, Theolair, Theo-X, T-PHYL, Uniphyl)   *Class: Bronchodilator*

Category:	C
Indications:	Asthma, bronchospasm associated with bronchitis and emphysema
Actions:	Relaxation of smooth muscle of the bronchi
Side effects:	Nausea, vomiting, irritability, tachycardia, arrhythmias, seizures
Dose:	13 mg/kg PO per day in divided doses, not to exceed 900 mg/day

TICARCILLIN AND CLAVULANIC ACID (Timentin)   *Class: Antibiotic*

Category:	B
Indications:	Infection due to beta-lactamase–producing strains of *Escherichia coli, Klebsiella pneumoniae, Staphylococcus aureus,* or *Enterobacter*
Actions:	Inhibition of cell wall synthesis
Side effects:	Hypersensitivity reactions
Dose:	50 to 75 mg/kg IV every 6 hours

TIOCONAZOLE (Vagistat-1)   *Class: Antifungal agent*

Category:	C
Indications:	Vulvovaginal candidal infection
Actions:	Imidazole derivative, interferes with cell membrane by inhibition of ergosterol

Side effects: Vulvovaginal burning, itching
Dose: 6.5% ointment: 4.6 g inserted with prefilled applicator into the vagina once

TOBRAMYCIN (Nebcin)   *Class: Antibiotic*

Category: D
Indications: Treatment of infections due to *Pseudomonas aeruginosa, Proteus, Escherichia coli, Enterobacter, Klebsiella, Serratia, Staphylococcus aureus, Providencia,* or *Citrobacter* species
Actions: Inhibition of protein synthesis
Side effects: Ototoxicity, neurotoxicity, renal toxicity
Dose: 3 mg/kg/day IM or IV in 3 divided doses every 8 hours
5 mg/kg/day may be given for life-threatening infection

TRIAMCINOLONE ACETONIDE   *Class: Anti-inflammatory agent*
(Aristocort A)

Category: C
Indications: Treatment of inflammatory and pruritic manifestations of dermatoses
Treatment of squamous cell hyperplasia of the vulva
Actions: Topical corticosteroid
Side effects: Burning, itching, skin irritation, dryness
Dose: 0.01% cream or lotion applied 2 or 3 times per day

TRIMETHOBENZAMIDE (Tigan)   *Class: Antiemetic*

Category: C
Indications: Nausea and vomiting
Actions: Unclear, may act centrally on medulla oblongata
Side effects: Hypersensitivity reactions, Parkinson-like symptoms, hypotension
Dose: Oral: 250 mg PO 3 to 4 times per day
Rectal suppository: 200 mg rectally, 3 to 4 times per day
Intramuscular: 200 mg IM 3 to 4 times per day

TRIMETHOPRIM AND SULFAMETHOXAZOLE   *Class: Antibiotic*
(Bactrim, Septra)

Category: C
Indications: Urinary tract infection due to *Escherichia coli, Klebsiella, Enterobacter, Proteus mirabilis, Proteus vulgaris,* or *Morganella morganii*
Acute otitis media, chronic bronchitis, travelers' diarrhea, shigellosis, and *Pneumocystis carinii* pneumonia
Actions: Sulfamethoxazole: inhibition of synthesis of dihydrofolic acid
Trimethoprim: inhibition of synthesis of tetrahydrofolic acid from dihydrofolic acid
Side effects: Nausea, vomiting, anorexia, skin reaction, leukopenia, hepatitis
Dose: 2 tablets PO every 12 hours for 10 to 14 days
1 double-strength (DS) tablet PO every 12 hours for 10 to 14 days
4 teaspoons or 20 ml PO every 12 hours for 10 to 14 days

Shigellosis and travelers' diarrhea can be treated with one of the above regimens for a total of 5 days.

VANCOMYCIN (Vancocin, Vancoled)   *Class: Antibiotic*

Category:	C
Indications:	Parenteral administration: treatment of methicillin-resistant staphylococcus
	Oral administration: treatment of staphylococcal enterocolitis and pseudomembranous colitis caused by *Clostridium difficile*
Actions:	Interference with protein synthesis
Side effects:	Nephrotoxicity, ototoxicity, neutropenia
Dose:	250 to 500 mg PO 4 times per day for 10 days
	500 mg IV every 6 hours or 1000 mg IV every 12 hours

WARFARIN SODIUM (Coumadin)   *Class: Anticoagulant*

Category:	X
Indications:	Prophylaxis and treatment of deep vein thrombosis, pulmonary embolism, atrial fibrillation with embolization
Actions:	Inhibition of production of vitamin K–dependent clotting factors (II, VII, IX, and X)
Side effects:	Hemorrhaging, necrosis of the skin and other organs, nausea, alopecia
Dose:	Initial dose of 2 to 5 mg PO every day, followed by a maintenance dose of 2 to 10 mg PO every day with dose adjusted to prolong prothrombin time by 1.2 to 1.5 times control

INDEX

Note: Page numbers in *italics* refer to illustrations;
page numbers followed by t refer to tables